T0336424

Exploration and Analysis of DNA Microarray and Other High-Dimensional Data

WILEY SERIES IN PROBABILITY AND STATISTICS

Established by WALTER A. SHEWHART and SAMUEL S. WILKS

A complete list of the titles in this series appears at the end of this volume.

Exploration and Analysis of DNA Microarray and Other High-Dimensional Data

Second Edition

DHAMMIKA AMARATUNGA

Janssen Pharmaceutical Companies of Johnson and Johnson
USA

JAVIER CABRERA

Rutgers University
USA

ZIV SHKEDY

Hasselt University
Belgium

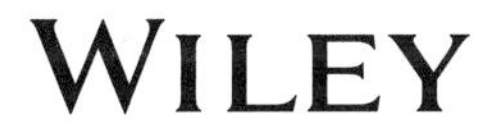

Published by John Wiley & Sons, Inc., Hoboken, New Jersey.
Published simultaneously in Canada.

Library of Congress Cataloging-in-Publication Data:

Amaratunga, Dhammika, 1956–
Exploration and analysis of DNA microarray and other high-dimensional data / Dhammika Amaratunga, Janssen Pharmaceutical Companies of Johnson and Johnson, USA, Javier Cabrera, Rutgers University, USA, Ziv Shkedy, Hasselt University, Belgium. –Second edition.
pages cm
Includes bibliographical references and index.
ISBN 978-1-118-35633-3 (cloth)
1. Protein microarrays–Statistical methods. I. Cabrera, Javier. II. Shkedy, Ziv. III. Title.
QP624.5.D726A45 2013
572′.636–dc23

2013013975

Printed in the United States of America

10 9 8 7 6 5 4 3 2 1

To our families in
America, Sri Lanka,
Spain, and Israel

Contents

Preface

In August 1999, at the Joint Statistical Meetings in Baltimore, two of us [DA & JC] were invited to present a paper on "The Analysis of DNA Microchip Data." This was the first presentation in any Joint Statistical Meetings on the topic of DNA microarrays, as they are now called. In just a few years, the field has exploded and, in each of the recent Joint Statistical Meetings, there have been over a hundred presentations related to DNA microarrays!

The Baltimore paper outlined many of the issues that are still being discussed today, including intensity-dependent normalization, the use of methods that are robust to outliers, improving the sensitivity of the analysis by borrowing strength across genes, and interpretation of results in a way that is germane to the overall objectives of a study. However, there have been many developments since then, and this book represents our effort at organizing this material into a semicoherent whole.

ACKNOWLEDGMENTS

We would like to thank several bioinformaticians, scientists, and statisticians at Johnson and Johnson and elsewhere who patiently helped to educate us about genomics and microarrays and in writing this book. We would particularly like to acknowledge Jim Colaianne, Luc Bijnens, Hinrich Gohlmann, Peter Ghazal, Michael McMillian, Nandini Raghavan, Zhenya Cherkas, Albert Lo, Kwok Tsui, David Tyler, Birol Emir, Alicia Nieto Reyes, Chin-Ray Yu, Yung-Seop Lee, Volha Tryputsen, Willem Talloen, An de Bondt, Hugo Ceulemans, Tomasz Burzykowski, Tim Davison, Jackson Wan, Xuejun Liu, Harindra Abeysinghe, Gordon Pledger, Sepp Hochreiter, Adetayo Kasim, Martin Otava, Willem Talloen, Suzy Van Sanden, Dan Lin, Nolen Joy Perualila, Tatsiana Khamikova, Pushpike Thilakarathne, and Dani Yekutieli. We would also like to note that numerous graduate students at Rutgers University and Universiteit Hasselt assisted us in our research.

Ziv Shkedy gratefully acknowledge support from the Belgian IUAP/PAI network "Statistical techniques and modeling for complex substantive questions with complex data." And last, but not least, we would like to thank Gayatri Amaratunga and Maria Drelich, who helped in various ways.

DHAMMIKA AMARATUNGA
JAVIER CABRER
ZIV SHKEDY

CHAPTER 1

A Brief Introduction

Data analysis has, quite suddenly, begun to assume a prominent role in the life sciences. From being a science that generally produced relatively limited amounts of quantitative data, biology has, in the space of just a few years, become a science that routinely generates enormous amounts of it.

To a large part, this metamorphosis can be attributed to two complementary advances. The first is the successful culmination of the Human Genome Project and other genome sequencing efforts, which have generated a treasure trove of information about the DNA sequences of the human genome and the genomes of several other species, large and small. This has resulted in a huge number of genes being newly identified and biologists are now confronted with the daunting, but exhilarating, task of ascertaining their functions.

This is where the second advance, the emergence of modern experimental technology, such as microarray technology, comes in. Currently, the most widely used form of this technology is the DNA microarray, which offers scientists the ability to monitor the behavior patterns of several thousands of genes simultaneously, allowing them to study how these genes function and follow how they act under different conditions. Another form of microarray technology, the protein array, provides scientists the capability of monitoring thousands of proteins simultaneously, for similar purposes. And this is just the beginning. Emerging technical innovations, such as bead-based arrays, have the potential to increase throughput much more.

These developments have ushered in a thrilling new era of molecular biology. Traditional molecular biology research followed a "one gene per experiment" paradigm. This tedious and inherently exhausting approach was capable of producing only limited results in any reasonable period of time. Although it has, without question, logged a series of remarkable achievements over the years, this approach does not allow anything close to a complete picture of gene function and overall genome behavior to be readily determined.

Exploration and Analysis of DNA Microarray and Other High-Dimensional Data, Second Edition.
Dhammika Amaratunga, Javier Cabrera, Ziv Shkedy.

The advent of microarray technology has created an opportunity for doing exactly this by fast-tracking research practice away from a "one gene" mode to a "thousands of genes per experiment" mode and allowing scientists to study how genes function, not just each on their own, but jointly as well.

In fact, the way microarray technology is revolutionizing the biological sciences has been likened to the way microprocessors transformed the computer sciences toward the latter part of the twentieth century (through miniaturization, integration, parallel processing, increased throughput, portability, and automation) and the way the computer sciences, in turn, transformed many other disciplines just a few years later. Microarray technology has been brought into play to characterize genomic function in genome systems spanning all the way from yeast to human.

Microarray experiments are conducted in such a manner as to profile the behavior patterns of thousands of nucleic acid sequences or protein simultaneously. Plus, they are capable of being automated and run in a high-throughput mode. Thus, they can, and do, generate mountains of data at an ever increasing pace. Thus, the proper storage, analysis, and interpretation of this data have turned out to be a major challenge.

Our focus is on the analysis part. After all, data by itself does not constitute knowledge. It must be first be analyzed and relationships and associations studied and confirmed, in order to convert it into knowledge. By doing so, it is hoped that a complete picture of the intermeshing patterns of biomolecular activity that underlie complex biological processes, such as the growth and development of an organism and the etiology of a disease, would emerge.

One issue is that the structure of the data is singular enough to warrant special attention. The raw data from a DNA microarray experiment, for example, is a series of scanned images of microarrays that have been subjected to an experimental process. The general plan for analyzing this data involves converting these images into quantitative data, then preprocessing the data to transform it into a format suitable for analysis, and, finally, applying appropriate data analysis techniques to extract information pertinent to the biological question under study. Application of statistical methodology is feasible as these experiments can be run on replicate samples, although, by and large, the amount of replication tends to be limited. Thus, a complexity is that, while there is data on thousands and thousands of genes, the information content per gene is small. As a result, there is a sense that much of the data collected in microarray experiments remains to be fully and properly interpreted.

It should, therefore, not be a surprise that statistical and computational approaches are beginning to assume a position of greater prominence within the molecular biology community. While these quantitative disciplines have a rich and impressive array of tools to cover a very broad range of topics in data analysis, the structure of the data generated by microarrays is sufficiently unique that, either standard methods have to be tailored for use with microarray data, or an entirely fresh set of tools have to be developed specifically to handle such data. What has happened, of course, is a confluence of the two. The purpose of this book is to present an extensive, but, by no means, exhaustive, series of computational, visual, and statistical tools that are being used for exploring and analyzing microarray data.

1.1 A NOTE ON EXPLORATORY DATA ANALYSIS

Early statistical work was essentially enumerative and exploratory in nature. Statisticians were concerned with developing effective ways of discerning patterns in quantitative data. Then, from about a fourth of the way into the twentieth century, mathematics-driven confirmatory techniques began to dominate the field of statistics, driving data exploration into the background. The focus began to be the development of optimal ways to analyze data rigorously, but under various sets of fairly restrictive assumptions.

Fortunately, toward the latter part of the twentieth century, data exploration began to make a comeback as an imperative aspect of statistics, having been revitalized almost single-handedly by Tukey (1962, 1977, 1986), who likened it to detective work. Exploratory data analysis (EDA), as the modern incarnation of statistical data exploration is called, is an approach for data analysis that employs a range of techniques (many graphical), in a strategic manner, in order to

- gain insight into a data set;
- discover systematic structures, such as clusters, in the data;
- flag outliers and anomalies in the data;
- assess what assumptions about the data are reasonable.

The last of these guides the data analyst to an approach or a model that should be suitable for a more formal phase in the analysis of the data. This confirmatory data analysis (CDA) phase, which may involve inferential procedures such as confidence interval estimation and hypothesis testing, allows the data analyst to probabilistically model the uncertainties of a situation to assess the reproducibility of the findings. By doing so, CDA ensures that chance patterns are not mistaken for real structure. Even at this phase, however, EDA stresses the importance of running diagnostic checks to assess the validity of any underlying assumptions (e.g., Anscombe and Tukey, 1963; Daniel and Wood, 1971).

EDA is particularly well suited to situations where the data is not well understood and the problem is not well specified, such as screening. Because of this, EDA techniques have found their way into the world of data mining (Fayyad, Piatetsky-Shapiro, and Smyth, 1996). In such situations, broad-based methods that have the ability to discover and illustrate essential aspects of the data are of most value. Proper data visualization tools, for instance, are highly effective both at revealing facets of the data that otherwise may not have been apparent and at challenging assumptions about the data that otherwise may have been taken for granted.

It could be argued that EDA is as much an attitude or a philosophy about how a data analysis should be conducted as an assortment of techniques. The EDA approach suggests strategies for carefully scrutinizing a data set: how to examine a data set, what to look for, and how to interpret what has been observed. The key is that EDA permits the data itself to reveal its underlying structure and model without the data analyst having to make too many possibly indefensible assumptions.

Over the years, the popularity of EDA has been boosted by a number of noteworthy publications by Tukey and his students and colleagues, such as Mosteller and Tukey (1977), Velleman and Hoaglin (1981), Hoaglin (1982), Hoaglin, Mosteller, and Tukey (1983), Chambers et al (1983), Tukey (1986), Miller (1986), Brillinger, Fernholz, and Morgenthaler (1997), Fernholz, Morgenthaler and Stahel (2001), and Cabrera and McDougall (2002), and has gained a large following as the most effective way to seek structures in data. Hoaglin, Mosteller, and Tukey (1983) is an excellent introduction to EDA.

That is not to forget CDA. Tukey (1980) argues that exploratory and confirmatory analyzes must both be components of a good data analysis. This is the approach we will take in this book.

1.2 COMPUTING CONSIDERATIONS AND SOFTWARE

The data analyst must have access to computing resources, both hardware and software, that are capable of dealing with the huge amounts of data that must be analyzed. Holloway et al. (2002) is a review of some of the issues related to this topic.

A number of software packages offer the data analyst powerful tools for EDA and CDA, including interactive graphics and a large collection of statistical procedures. Two that are commonly used in the analysis of microarray data are `R` (Ihaka and Gentleman, 1996) and `SPLUS`. Other statistical packages that are good for EDA include SAS, JMP, DataDesk, Matlab, and MINITAB.

In addition, libraries of routines specially designed for analysis of microarray data have begun to spring up. Some of these are in the public domain, others are only available commercially. A couple are listed below.

- DNAMR (URL: `http://www.rci.rutgers.edu/cabrera/DNAMR`), which stands for "DNA Microarray Routines," is a collection of `R` programs developed by the authors of this book and their collaborators. Implementations of many of the procedures described in this book are available in the DNAMR package and can be downloaded from the book's web page.
- Bioconductor (URL: `http://www.bioconductor.org`) is a collection of software packages for the analysis and interpretation of DNA microarray and other high-dimensional data. It is free, open source, and open development. While it is also based primarily on `R`, it does contain contributions in other programming languages.

Care must be taken that software is not used blindly—using the wrong methods to analyze data from an experiment could produce meaningless "findings" and miss signals of potential interest. Unfortunately, few, if any, off-the-shelf packages offer a comprehensive data handling system that integrates all the data-related needs, such as data acquisition, storage, extraction, quality assurance, and analysis, that are essential for even a moderate-sized microarray laboratory.

1.3 A BRIEF OUTLINE OF THE BOOK

This book will mainly focus on the analysis of data from microarray experiments. However, the concepts underlying the methods presented here, if not the methods themselves, can be used in other settings that generate high-dimensional or megavariate data. Such settings are becoming more and more commonplace in biomedical research with the advent of new high-throughput technologies such as protein arrays, flow cytometry, and next-generation sequencing, in addition to microarrays. All these technologies generate large complex high-dimensional data sets from individual experiments. The complexity of this data highlights the importance of implementing proper data management and data analysis procedures as this will significantly impact the reproducibility or nonreproducibility of any findings from these experiments.

EDA and CDA techniques can be applied to microarray data (and other high-dimensional data) to

- assess the quality of a microarray;
- determine which genes are differentially expressed;
- classify genes based on how they coexpress;
- classify samples based on how genes coexpress.

Following this, the investigator will generally try to

- connect differentially expressed genes to annotation databases;
- locate differentially expressed genes on pathway diagrams;
- relate expression levels to other cell-related information;
- determine the roles of genes on the basis of patterns of coexpression.

Hopefully, this process will culminate in an insight of interest.

Figure 1.1 shows, schematically, the path of a typical microarray data analysis. Readers may find it useful to periodically refer to it. In this book, we will present a collection of techniques for analyzing microarray data as per the first set of bullets. Before we embark on our journey, a brief road map of where we are going may be helpful.

Chapter 2 is a brief introduction to molecular biology and genomics. Chapter 3 describes DNA microarrays, what they are, how they are used, and how a typical DNA microarray experiment is performed. Chapter 4 outlines how the output of a DNA microarray experiment, the scanned image, is processed and quantitated and

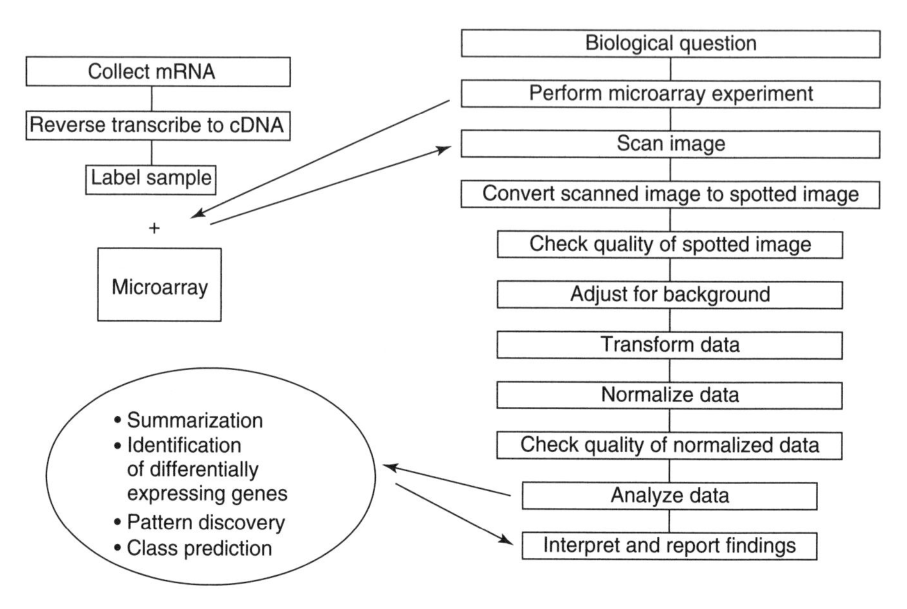

Figure 1.1 Schematic of a typical microarray data analysis.

how image and spot quality checks are done. Chapter 5 discusses preprocessing microarray data, which typically involves transforming the data and then applying a normalization. Chapter 6 discusses summarization of data across replicates. Chapter 7 describes statistical methods used for analyzing the simplest comparative experiments, those involving just two groups. Chapter 8 discusses more complex experiments and issues related to their design. Chapter 9 discusses methods for analyzing gene sets. The next two chapters deal with multivariate methods: Chapter 10 discusses unsupervised classification methods and Chapter 11 discusses supervised classification methods. Chapter 12 describes protein arrays; a typical protein array experiment is outlined and methodology for analyzing protein array data is described.

1.4 DATA SETS AND CASE STUDIES

The following data sets are used at various points in this book.

1.4.1 The Golub Data

The Golub data first appeared in a seminal publication (Golub et al., 1999) which demonstrated that gene expression profiling could be used to classify malignancies. The study involved profiling the expression of several thousand genes in bone marrow from 38 patients with acute leukemia, consists of 27 with the acute lymphoblastic leukemia (ALL) and 11 with the acute myeloid leukemia (AML). In the original analysis, 50 genes whose expression levels differed most between AML and ALL cells were found to be able to correctly classify which patients had AML and which had ALL in a blinded new cohort of 36 acute leukemia patients. The data set has gene expression measurements for 3051 genes for the original 38 tumor mRNA samples and is available in R.

1.4.2 The Mouse5 Data

The Mouse5 data are from an experiment involving 10 pairs of microarrays, C1A, C1B, C2A, C2B, . . . , C10A, C10B. Each pair of microarrays corresponds to a single mRNA sample (labeled C1, C2, . . . , and C10), which was taken from a mouse following treatment and hybridized to two separate microarrays (labeled A and B). The two microarrays in each pair are technical replicates as they were exposed to the same biological sample. The five mice from which samples C1–C5 were drawn are controls, so they are biological replicates, while each of the other five was treated with one of five drugs. There were 3300 genes arrayed on the microarrays.

1.4.3 The Khan Data

The Khan data set contains gene expression measurements, obtained using cDNA microarrays, from four types of pediatric small round blue cell tumors (SRBCTs): neuroblastoma (NB), rhabdomyosarcoma (RMS), the Ewing family of tumors (EWS), and Burkitt lymphomas (BL), a subtype of non-Hodgkin's lymphoma. The four cancer types are clinically and histologically similar, yet their response to treatment is markedly different, making accurate diagnosis essential for proper therapy. The purpose of the study was to classify, as accurately as possible, a cell as being one of these four types using gene expression information. The microarrays measured the expression levels of 6567 genes. This data was filtered to remove any gene that consistently expressed below a certain minimum level of expression, leaving expression data for 2308 genes. A total of 88 cells were analyzed. Data for 63 of these cells (23 EWS, 20 RMS, 12 NB, 8 BL) were used as a training set, while the data for the remaining 25 cells (6 EWS, 5 RMS, 6 NB, 3 BL, 5 non-SRBCT) were set aside to make up a blind test set.

1.4.4 The Sialin Data

The Sialin data are from an experiment in which the gene expression profiles of mice whose Slc17A5 gene (which is responsible for the production of Sialin) was knocked out were compared to the gene expression profiles of wild-type mice (i.e., "normal" mice). In the experiment, RNA samples from total brain were derived from newborn and 18-day-old mice for each of the two groups: Slc17A5 knockout and wild type. There were six biological samples in each group for a total of 24 samples. Microarray experiments were performed on the RNA samples using Affymetrix Mouse430-2 GeneChips; the expression levels of 45,101 genes were profiled.

1.4.5 The Behavioral Study Data

This case study was obtained from a preclinical behavioral experiment, in which 24 male experimentally naive Long-Evans rats from Janvier (France) were randomized into two treatment groups with 12 rats per group. The first group of rats received placebo, while the second group was treated with a novel antipsychotic compound. Animals were tested in a large open field. Rat behavior data parameters were recorded systematically. In particular, the parameter of primary interest to the study investigators was the total distance traveled by the rats. Active response to the treatment was expected to increase this distance. In addition, microarray data, measuring the gene expression of 5644 genes, were obtained. Further details of the experiment can be found in Lin et al. (2012).

1.4.6 The Spiked-In Data

The Affymetrix HGU-133A Spiked-in data set is publicly available for the purpose of determining the sensitivity and specificity of various methods for the analysis of microarray data. The data set has an advantage over real-life data sets because the true number of differentially expressed genes is known. It contains known genes that are spiked-in at 14 different concentrations ranging from 0 to 512 pM, arranged in a Latin squared design. There are 42 arrays and 42 spiked-in probe sets equally distributed over the 14 concentrations. In addition to the original spiked-in transcripts, McGee and Chen (2006) discovered 22 additional probe sets that have similar characteristics as the spiked-in probe sets. Thus, the HGU-133A spiked-in data set contains 64 spiked-in probe sets out of the 22,300 probe sets.

1.4.7 The APOAI Study

This data set is from a cDNA experiment which compared the gene expression profiles of eight apolipoprotein AI (APOAI) knockout mice with the gene expression profiles of eight wild-type mice. Target mRNA was obtained from the liver tissue of each mouse and labeled using a Cy5 dye. The RNA from each mouse was hybridized to a separate microarray. Common reference RNA was labeled with Cy3 dye and used for all the arrays. This data has been employed by a number of authors to illustrate normalization methods for cDNA data. The data is available in `R`.

1.4.8 The Breast Cancer Data

A time course microarray data set. This data set comes from a breast cancer cell line microarray study. Data are available in six time points: 1, 4, 12, 24, 36, and 48 h after treatment. At each time point, eight replicate arrays are available, consisting of 1900 genes. For more details about the data, we refer to Lobenhofer et al. (2002) and Peddada et al. (2003).

1.4.9 Platinum Spike Data Set

The Platinum Spike data set consists of 18 Affymetrix GeneChip Drosophila Genome 2.0 microarrays, divided into two groups (A and B). The 2189 RNAs are spiked in so that the number of up- and downregulated transcripts between the two conditions is balanced. Moreover, 3426 transcripts were spiked in at the same concentrations for both conditions. The spiked-in transcripts are measured by 5615 probe sets, whereas the 13,337 probe sets are empty and not expected to carry any signal. In each group, there were three samples synthesized and for each sample, three technical replicates were used for the microarray analysis. For more details about the data, we refer to Zhu et al. (2010).

1.4.10 Human Epidermal Squamous Carcinoma Cell Line A431 Experiment

The data come from an oncology experiment designed to better understand the biological effects of growth factors in human tumor. Human epidermal squamous carcinoma cell line A431 was grown in Dulbecco's modified Eagle's medium, supplemented with L-glutamine (20 mM), Gentamicin (5 mg/ml,) and 10% fetal bovine serum. The cells were stimulated with growth factor EGF (R&D Systems, 236-EG) at different concentrations (0, 1, 10, and 100 ng/ml) for 24 h. RNA was harvested using RLT buffer (Qiagen). All microarray-related steps, including the amplification of total RNAs, labeling, hybridization, and scanning, were carried out as described in the GeneChip Expression Analysis Technical Manual, Rev.4 (Affymetrix, 2004). The collected data were quantile normalized in two steps: first within each sample group, and then across all sample groups obtained (Amaratunga and Cabrera, 2000, 2003; Bolstad et al., 2002). The resulting data set consists of 12 samples, 4 dose levels, and 3 microarrays at each dose level, with 16,998 probe sets.

1.4.11 Note: Public Repositories of Microarray Data

Bioconductor, ArrayExpress, and Gene Expression Omnibus (GEO) are large repositories of DNA microarray and other high-dimensional data.

CHAPTER 2

Genomics Basics

It is useful to review the basic concepts of modern molecular biology before fully immersing ourselves in the world of microarrays. We are sure that readers who have had limited exposure to this fast-developing field would appreciate this review, others may skip ahead. Genomics is a fascinating subject; after all, it is the story of life, and can occupy a multivolume book just by itself. In the interest of space, of course, it is necessary that we confine our discussion to those topics that are essential to an understanding of the science underlying microarrays, leaving other topics for interested readers to explore on their own. Some excellent general references that we, not being trained as molecular biologists ourselves, have found useful are listed at the end of the chapter.

2.1 GENES

From ancient times, it was suspected that there existed some sort of a hereditary mechanism that carried information from parent to child. It is because of this mechanism that family members tend to exhibit similar characteristics or *traits*. For example, they tend to resemble each other in terms of appearance and physical characteristics such as skin color; they tend to be predisposed toward certain diseases such as diabetes, cancer, and heart disease; and so on. However, inheritance is clearly not a perfect copying process. For example, a child of brown-eyed parents could turn out to be blue-eyed. Despite the efforts over the years of many leading scientists and thinkers to understand the hereditary mechanism, its precise nature remained an intriguing mystery until quite recently.

Following centuries of speculation and research, the existence of discrete hereditary units, which we now call *genes*, has been firmly established. Each gene, either by itself or in combination with some other genes, provides a clear and

Exploration and Analysis of DNA Microarray and Other High-Dimensional Data, Second Edition.
Dhammika Amaratunga, Javier Cabrera, Ziv Shkedy.

unambiguous set of instructions for producing some property of its organism. The complete set of genes in an organism, essentially the master blueprint for that organism, is referred to as its *genome*. This blueprint contains all the hereditary instructions for building, operating, and maintaining the organism, and for passing life in like form on to the next generation of that organism.

Until the twentieth century, there was hardly any concrete information as to what genes were and how they operated. Then, a panoply of innovative research work and pathbreaking discoveries over (roughly) the first half of the twentieth century gave genes a chemical (molecular) existence. This culminated in the pivotal realization that genes are made of *deoxyribonucleic acid* (DNA).

2.2 DEOXYRIBONUCLEIC ACID

A DNA molecule consists of two long strands wound tightly around each other in a spiral structure known as a *double helix*. The structure has been likened to a twisted ladder, whose sides are made of sugar and phosphate and whose rungs are made of bases.

Each strand of the DNA molecule (i.e., each side of the ladder once it has been untwisted and straightened out) is a linear arrangement of repeating similar units called *nucleotides*. Every nucleotide has three components: a sugar (deoxyribose), a phosphate group, and a nitrogenous base. The base is one of *adenine* (A), *thymine* (T), *guanine* (G), or *cytosine* (C). The bases on one strand are paired with the bases on the other strand according to the *complementary base pairing rules* (also called the *Watson–Crick base pairing rules*): adenine only pairs with thymine, guanine only pairs with cytosine. The pairs so formed are called *base pairs* (bp); they form the coplanar rungs of the ladder. The force that holds a bp together is a weak hydrogen bond. Even though each individual bond is weak, their cumulative effect along the strands is strong enough to bind the two strands tightly together. As a result, DNA is chemically inert and is a stable carrier of genetic information.

The sequences of bases along each of the two strands of DNA are complementary to each other as they are matched by the *complementary base pairing rules*. This complementary sequencing has an important consequence. It was recognized from very early on that, whatever the entity was that was a hereditary unit, it must be able to self-replicate so that information could be passed on from generation to generation. At the time that the structure of DNA was deduced, there was a lot of excitement, as it was clear that the complementary structure of the DNA molecule would allow every DNA molecule to create an exact replica of itself, thus fulfilling this requirement.

The DNA replication process is, in principle, quite straightforward. First, the DNA molecule unwinds and the "ladder" unzips, thereby disrupting the weak bonds between the bps and allowing the strands to separate. Then, each strand directs the synthesis of a brand new complementary strand, with free nucleotides matching up with their complementary bases onto each separated strand, a process that produces two descendant DNA molecules. Each descendant consists of one old and one new DNA strand. The constraints imposed by the complementary base pairing rules ensure that each new strand is an exact copy of the old one with the order of the bases along the strands being faithfully preserved.

The preservation of the base order is crucial. The particular order of the bases arranged along any one strand, its DNA sequence, is the mechanism that specifies the exact genetic instructions required to create the traits of a particular organism.

Many genes are located along each long DNA molecule. A gene is a specific contiguous subsequence of the DNA *sequence* whose A-T-G-C sequence is the *code* required for constructing a *protein*. Proteins are giant complex molecules made of chains of amino acids and it is they that are actually both the building blocks and the workhorses of life. Proteins also regulate most of life's day-to-day functions; in fact, even the DNA replication process is mediated by *enzymes*, proteins whose job is to catalyze biochemical reactions.

2.3 GENE EXPRESSION

An organism's DNA is located in its cells. *Cells* are the fundamental units of all living organisms, both structurally and functionally. A cell is a microscopic, yet extraordinarily complex, structure that contains a heterogeneous mix of substances essential to life.

There are many substructures within a cell. The most prominent one is a highly protected subcompartment called the *nucleus*, in which resides the organism's DNA. Enclosing the nucleus is the *nuclear membrane*, the protective wall that separates the nucleus from the rest of the cell, which is called its *cytoplasm*. The entire cell is enclosed by the *plasma membrane*. Embedded within this membrane is a variety of protein structures that act as *channels and pumps* to control the movement of molecules into and out of the cell.

The set of protein-coding instructions in the DNA sequence of a gene resembles a computer program. A computer program must first be compiled and executed in order for anything to happen. In much the same way, a gene must be *expressed* in order for anything to happen. A gene expresses by transferring its coded information into proteins that dwell in the cytoplasm, a process called *gene expression.*

The transmission of genetic information from DNA to protein during gene expression is formulated by the *central dogma of molecular biology*, which can be stated in oversimple terms as "DNA → mRNA → protein." This postulates that the protein-coding instructions from a gene are transmitted indirectly through *messenger RNA* (mRNA), a transient intermediary molecule that resembles a single strand of DNA. There are a few differences between mRNA and DNA, three being that mRNA is single stranded, its sugar is ribose, and it has the base *uracil* (U) rather than the base thymine.

When a gene is expressed, the DNA double helix splits open along its length. One strand of the open helix remains inactive, while the other strand acts as a template against which a complementary strand of mRNA forms (a process called *transcription*). The sequence of bases along the mRNA strand is identical to the sequence of bases along the inactive DNA strand (except that mRNA has uracil where DNA has thymine). The mRNA strand then separates from the DNA strand and transports out of the nucleus, across the nuclear membrane, and into the cellular cytoplasm. There it serves as the template for protein synthesis, with consecutive (nonoverlapping) triplets of bases (called *codons*) acting as a code to specify the particular amino acids that make up an individual protein. The sequence of bases along the mRNA is thus converted into a string of amino acids that constitutes the protein molecule for which it codes (a process called *translation*).

Each possible triplet of mRNA bases codes for a specific amino acid, one of the twenty amino acids that make up proteins. For example, GCC codes for alanine, CAC for histidine, AUC for isoleucine, and GAG for glutamic acid—the complete list is referred to as the *genetic code*. As there are four possible bases, there are $4^3=64$ possible triplets, but only 20 possible amino acids. This means that there is room for redundancy: for example, GCU, GCC, GCA, and GCG, all code for alanine. This redundancy is a valuable feature of the genetic code as it provides a safeguard against small errors that might occur during transcription.

In addition, the genetic code has specific triplets to signal the start and the end of a coding sequence. The *start codon*, AUG, is the triplet of mRNA bases that signals the initiation of a sequence that is to be translated, while the stop codon is a triplet of mRNA bases, UGA, UAG, or UAA, that signals the termination of a coding sequence. The sequence of mRNA bases in between and including these two is called an *open reading frame* (ORF). All sequence information of coding interest lies in ORFs (but not every ORF codes for a gene). As the codes for the start and stop codons are known, given an mRNA sequence, it is a simple matter to read off all of its ORFs.

Scientists involved in gene expression research usually find it easier to work with *expressed sequence tags* (ESTs) instead of the whole gene. An EST is a unique short subsequence (only a few hundred bps long), generated from the DNA sequence of a gene, that acts as a "tag" or "marker" for the gene. An advantage of ESTs is that they can be back translated into genetic code that is coded for or expressed as an exon as opposed to an intron or other noncoding DNA. A short (typically 5–50 bp long) fragment of single-stranded DNA, not necessarily associated with a gene, is called an *oligonucleotide* (*oligo*, for short).

Although every cell in an organism has a copy of the exact same genome (more or less), not all cells express the same genes, which is why different cells perform different functions. For instance, genes that are expressed in a brain cell may not be expressed in a stomach cell. In addition, even within the same cell, different genes will be expressed at different times, and perhaps at different levels, depending on the phase of the cell and perhaps as a response to different stimuli. There are, however, a few exceptions: these are genes, called *housekeeping genes*, that are in constant use to maintain basic cell functions.

2.4 HYBRIDIZATION ASSAYS AND OTHER LABORATORY TECHNIQUES

Two single-stranded DNA molecules whose sequences are complementary to each other will exhibit a tendency to bind together to form a single double-stranded DNA molecule, a process known as *hybridization*. Two DNA strands (or one DNA strand and one mRNA strand) will hybridize with each other, irrespective of whether they originated from a single source or from two different sources, as long as their bp sequences match according to the complementary base pairing rules. Even when the sequences on the two strands do not match perfectly, as long as there is sufficient similarity, it is likely that some base pairing will occur and that a hybrid DNA molecule will be formed.

The tendency of DNA strands of complementary sequence to hybridize preferentially is exploited in *hybridization assays*. In these assays, a probe consisting of a homogeneous sample of single-stranded DNA molecules, whose sequence is known, is prepared and labeled with a reporter chemical, usually a radioactive or fluorescent substance. An immobilized target, usually a heterogeneous mixture of single-stranded DNA molecules of unknown composition is challenged by the probe. As the probe will hybridize only to sequences complementary to its sequence, DNA sequences in the target that are complementary to the probe DNA sequence can be identified by the presence of reporter molecules.

This concept is applied in blotting techniques. In Southern blotting, the target DNA is separated by electrophoresis (see below) and transferred onto a filter, where it is exposed to the probe. Northern *blotting* is a variant in which the target is mRNA instead of DNA. As mRNA is the intermediary molecule in gene expression, Northern blotting provides a means of studying the expression patterns of specific genes. DNA microarrays can be regarded as a massively parallel version of Northern blotting.

In *in situ hybridization*, denatured DNA (DNA in which the two strands are unwound and separated) is kept in place in the cell and is then challenged with mRNA or DNA extracted from another source and labeled with a reporter chemical, usually a fluorescent substance. By retaining the DNA in the cell, the specific chromosome containing the DNA sequence of interest can be identified by observing, under a microscope, the location of the fluorescence.

Besides hybridization assays, there are several laboratory techniques that have had, and continue to have, an enormous impact on progress in genomics research. As they play an important role in microarray experiments, we shall outline them briefly.

Electrophoresis is a method of using an electric field to separate large molecules, such as DNA, RNA, and proteins, from a mixture of similar molecules. An electric current is passed through a porous medium containing the mixture, usually a gel. The different kinds of molecules separate as different molecules will travel through the medium at different rates, depending on their electrical charge and size (e.g., small molecules typically travel farther through the medium than large molecules).

Cloning is the process of using specialized DNA technology to produce multiple, exact copies of a single gene or other segment of DNA to obtain enough material for further study. These clones can be grown in bacteria to produce multiple copies and large amounts of a given DNA molecule. The resulting cloned collections of DNA molecules are called *clone libraries*.

Polymerase chain reaction (PCR) is a rapid and versatile procedure for generating multiple copies of (in other words, for *amplifying*) virtually any fragment of DNA. The number of copies is limited only by rate-limiting factors such as the number of cycles and the amount of enzymes, bases, and other reagents required.

PCR is a cyclic process that involves repeating three basic steps multiple times. The three basic steps are as follows. First, the two strands of the target DNA are unwound and separated by heating (a process called *denaturing*). Next, primers, short strands of single-stranded DNA that match the sequences at either end of the target DNA, are bound to their complementary bases on the now single-stranded DNA (a process called *annealing*). Finally, DNA is synthesized by a *polymerase*, an enzyme that is present in all organisms and whose job is to copy and, where necessary, repair genetic material. Starting from the primer, the polymerase reads a template strand and matches it with free complementary bases. This produces two descendant DNA strands, each of which consists of one old and one new DNA strand. As in DNA replication, the complementary base pairing rules ensure that each new strand is an exact copy of the old one. Cycling through these three basic steps over and over generates more and more copies of the target DNA. The amount of DNA grows exponentially as it doubles with every cycle. As each cycle takes only a few minutes, a laboratory scientist can generate millions of copies of the target DNA in less than an hour. For this reason and because of its specificity, its versatility and its easy automatability, PCR has had a major impact on molecular biology and many related sciences in less than two decades.

Reverse transcription is a procedure for reversing, in a laboratory, the process of transcription. It is accomplished by isolating mRNA, which is unstable and subject to degradation, and using it as a template to synthesize a *complementary DNA* (cDNA) strand, which is stable and is not easily degraded. cDNA is so called because its sequence is complementary to the original mRNA sequence. This process utilizes the enzyme *reverse transcriptase*. The resultant single-stranded cDNA molecule is considerably shorter than the parent DNA sequence, as it will have only its coding exon sequences; the noncoding intron sequences would have been excised during the formation of the original mRNA. Incidentally, as far as is known, the process of translation cannot be reversed.

The cDNA generated by reverse transcription can, if needed, be amplified by PCR. The process is then called *reverse transcriptase polymerase chain reaction* (RT-PCR). RT-PCR is the one of the most sensitive techniques for detecting and quantifying target mRNA sequences. Among other uses, RT-PCR can be utilized to provide information regarding gene expression.

Recently, *RNA sequencing technologies* (such as RNA-seq) have become popular. These technologies use high-throughput sequencing techniques to measure the RNA content of a sample. In addition, they provide information that allows for improved mapping of exons and introns and better understanding of splice variants.

2.5 THE HUMAN GENOME

A few words now about our own genome. DNA in the human genome is made up of roughly three billion bps and is partitioned into 46 molecules, each of which resides in a threadlike cellular structure called a *chromosome*. *Chromosomes* come in pairs (except for the sex chromosomes): one of these is one of the father's two corresponding chromosomes, the other is one of the mother's two corresponding chromosomes. The two members of a pair of chromosomes are called *homologous chromosomes*.

Chromosomes range in length from about 50 to 250 million bp. Each chromosome contains many genes. In total, the human genome is estimated to contain somewhere around 40,000 genes. Genes vary widely in length, from a few hundred bp to several thousand bp. Only a tiny percentage of human DNA includes exons, the protein-coding sequences of genes. Interspersed within many genes are *introns*, sequences that have no coding function and that are excised during transcription. In between many genes are other noncoding regions whose functions remain largely obscure.

Every single human being has almost the exact same genome. In fact, at the genome level, we are 99.9% identical! However, genomes do vary slightly from person to person, a phenomenon known as *genome variation* (or *genetic variation*). It is this subtle variability in our genomes that is responsible for the evolution and diversity of the human race. Some genome variations are unique to a person, while others are passed on generation through generation via reproductive cells.

The existence of genome variation means that some genes will differ slightly from person to person. When this happens, each alternate version of a gene is called an *allele*. In fact, every person carries two alleles of each gene, one in each of a pair of homologous chromosomes. When both alleles are the same, the person is said to be *homozygous* for that gene; otherwise, the person is said to be *heterozygous* for that gene. In the latter case, only one of the alleles (called the *dominant allele*) may be expressed, while the other one (called the *recessive allele*) may not be. The presence of two versions of each gene is another protective mechanism provided by nature; if one copy should happen to be defective, the other copy is there to compensate.

Besides physical characteristics, a familiar example of genome variation is blood type. We are all of us classified as being A, B, AB, or O. The ABO gene that controls the blood group has three alleles, which are designated as A, B, and O. All three alleles have generally the same DNA sequence except for differences at a few nucleotides. Alleles A and B, which code for proteins A and B respectively, are codominant. Everyone is assigned a blood type according to which two alleles of the ABO protein he or she is carrying. Anyone who has AA or AO (and therefore has protein A only) is said to have blood type A. Anyone who has BB or BO (and therefore has protein B only) is said to have blood type B. Anyone who has AB (and therefore has both proteins) is said to have blood type AB. Anyone who has OO (and therefore has neither protein) is said to have blood type O.

As everyone has almost the exact same genome and any person-to-person genome variation is relatively minor, it is reasonable to try to establish a *consensus* human genome sequence; in other words, to *sequence* the entire human genome. This, in fact, is exactly the stated goal of the much-publicized massive international undertaking known as the *Human Genome Project*. A near-complete catalog of the human genome is now available and a complete catalog is only a few years away.

2.6 GENOME VARIATIONS AND THEIR CONSEQUENCES

Most genome variations are small and simple, and involve only a few bases—for example, one person might have a G where another has a C, or one person might be missing a T that another person has. Such genome variations are due to *mutations and polymorphisms*, alterations in a DNA sequence. The following are some common alterations: one base being replaced by another (substitution), a base being excised (*deletion*), a base being added (insertion), a small subsequence of bases being removed and then reinserted in the opposite direction (*inversion*), and a small subsequence of bases being removed and then reinserted in a different place (*translocation*).

A genome variation may be inherited or acquired. An inherited genome variation is present in the DNA of almost all of the organism's cells and could be passed on to the next generation of that organism. Acquired genome variations are mutations that occur spontaneously during DNA replication or are caused by an external environmental factor such as exposure to a toxic substance. Such variations will only be present in the DNA of the affected cells and their direct descendants. Thus an acquired mutation will be passed on to the next generation of that organism only if it affects a reproductive cell, in which case a new line of hereditary gene mutation would be initiated.

In practice, the terms "mutation" and "polymorphism" tend to be used interchangeably, but, technically, a polymorphism is a genome variation in which every possible sequence is present in at least 1% of people, whereas a mutation refers a genome variation that is present in less than 1% of people. Thus a location in a DNA sequence where 95% of people have an A and 5% have a T is a polymorphism, while a T in a location in a DNA sequence where 99.5% percent of people have an A and only 0.5% have a T is a mutation. The common and properly functioning version of a gene is referred to as its *wild-type allele*; a version with a mutation is called a *mutant allele*.

Many genome variations do not produce any noticeable effects, even at the cellular level. An obvious way for this to happen is for a variation to occur outside the genome's coding regions. What may be somewhat surprising is that it can happen even when a variation occurs within a coding region. This is because of the redundancies in the genetic code that allow the same protein to be produced from two slightly different sequences. In addition, if that is not enough, cells have mechanisms that are capable of repairing certain types of damaged DNA.

A small percentage of genome variations do produce noticeable effects, some deleterious, some beneficial. This is the genetic basis of biological diversity and the evolutionary process.

Many polymorphisms that produce noticeable effects are, in general, harmless; if not, they would not survive the natural selection process. However, this is not a hard and fast rule. For example, people with blood type O are more susceptible to peptic ulcers and cholera than others, yet the trait did not die out (in fact, almost half the world's population has this blood type), perhaps because they also are less susceptible to malaria and certain types of cancer.

Certain mutations can be harmful with no obvious beneficial features. They could either cause a disease or increase a person's susceptibility to a disease or even lead to death. For example, mutations in the p53 gene, which, in its wild type, codes for a protein that suppresses abnormal cell proliferation, may cause it to lose its ability to block abnormal cell growth, leading to cells dividing uncontrollably and forming tumors. Not surprisingly, mutations in the p53 gene have been found to be strongly associated with cancer.

It has been conjectured that most human genome variation may be attributable to *single nucleotide polymorphisms* (SNPs), polymorphisms that involve just one nucleotide. Blood grouping is an example: the only difference between the genes for blood types A and O is that the gene for the former has a G base that has been deleted in the gene for the latter. SNPs are frequent in our genomes: it has been estimated that, on average, about one in every one thousand nucleotides is an SNP.

Many scientists believe that SNPs underlie the susceptibility of certain people to certain diseases. An often-cited example is the association between the apolipoprotein E gene (ApoE) and Alzheimer's disease. ApoE has three alleles (called *E2*, *E3*, *E4*), each of which differs from any other by an SNP (there are two SNPs in all). It appears that those who have at least one copy of the E4 allele have a greater risk of developing Alzheimer's disease (and earlier on in life), whereas those who have at least one copy of the E2 allele have a lesser risk of developing Alzheimer's disease.

Given a specific DNA sequence, there are, in theory, a huge number of possible combinations of SNPs. However, SNPs are not randomly scattered along a chromosome. Instead, many of them occur in groups, called *haplotypes*, and relatively few of the countless number of theoretically possible haplotypes are observed with any significant frequency. The SNPs defining a haplotype tend to be inherited together over generations and serve as more reliable genetic markers for diseases and other traits, than any of the individual SNPs.

As research progresses, the genomic basis of health and disease is being better and better understood. Clearly, the central theme of this effort is the better elucidation of *genotype–phenotype* relationships, such as the association between ApoE and Alzheimer's disease. Genotype refers to the genetic makeup of an individual. Phenotype refers to the outward characteristics of the individual. They are, naturally, connected, as the phenotype essentially results, functions, and develops on the basis of the information provided by and encoded in the genotype. Despite this, the association between the genotype and the phenotype is, by no means, perfect. Environmental effects and other external factors tend to appreciably modify the actual manifestation. Statistical procedures that measure association play a significant role in analyzing these complex relationships.

2.7 GENOMICS

Genomics is the branch of biology that studies the structure and function of genes. Much progress has been made in the area of *structural genomics*. Structural genomics refers to the application of sequencing technologies to establish representative genome sequences for different organisms, particularly humans. Nowadays, the term is increasingly being used to also refer to methods for determining protein structures as a primary tool for discovering the biological functions of genes and proteins and their interrelationships.

The other key area is *functional genomics*, which, as its name implies, is the study of the functions of genes. It seeks to understand the behavior of all the genes in a genome (for all genomes). It is important to realize that just knowing the sequence of a gene does not imply that its function is also known. In addition, genes do not function in isolation. Instead, genes (and proteins) operate collectively in *pathways*, as coordinated sequences of genetic and molecular activities. Such pathways underlie all cellular processes. Therefore, studying each gene as a separate discrete entity tells only part of a story, like a still from a film. On top of that, a plethora of external factors can alter or disrupt a pathway. This constant interplay between genes, proteins, and external factors makes functional genomics a complex subject, one that was almost intractable until technologies, such as microarrays, emerged that allowed large numbers of molecular entities (perhaps even entire genomes) to be studied simultaneously.

The following are among the important questions in functional genomics:

- Which genes are expressed in which tissues? How is the expression of a gene affected by extracellular influences? Which genes are expressed during the development of an organism? How does gene expression change during development and differentiation? What is the effect of misregulated expression of a gene? What patterns of gene expression cause a disease or lead to disease progression? What patterns of gene expression influence response to treatment?

The past decade has seen a great deal of progress in all the various branches of genomics and it is likely that this trend will continue to be the case for decades to come, to the benefit of medicine, agriculture, and everyday life.

2.8 THE ROLE OF GENOMICS IN PHARMACEUTICAL RESEARCH AND CLINICAL PRACTICE

The immediate benefits of the progress in genomics will be seen in the discovery and development of novel pharmaceutical products (Debouck and Goodfellow,

1999, Lennon, 2000). For example, much can be learnt from studying general genotype–phenotype relationships and how these, in turn, affect drug response. This is the key aspect of pharmacogenomics, the study of pharmacologically relevant genes. Research in pharmacogenomics attempts to elucidate how these genes manifest their variations, how these variations interact to produce phenotypes, and how these phenotypes and environmental factors combine to affect drug response.

That genome variation does contribute to different individuals experiencing different pharmacological and toxicological reactions to medication has been amply demonstrated. For example, variations in the CYP2D6 gene, which codes for an enzyme involved with the metabolism of many commonly prescribed drugs, including analgesics, antiarrhythmics, beta blockers, neuroleptics, and antidepressants, have been found to seriously affect the therapeutic response to these drugs. Severe adverse drug reactions have also been associated with these variations. The wild-type allele of this gene is referred to as CYP2D6*1. Two variant alleles are CYP2D6*3 and CYP2D6*4. Both are due to SNPs: the CYP2D6*3 polymorphism is a deletion, the CYP2D6*4 polymorphism is a substitution. Both truncate the protein that they code for, which results in functional CYP2D6 protein being absent. Those who have inherited two copies of variant alleles in any combination are likely to be poor metabolizers. Drugs such as codeine, which need CYP2D6 for activation, will not be effective in these patients. Other drugs, such as lidocaine, are known to cause serious side effects, even heart failure, in these patients. On the other hand, those who have one wild-type allele and one polymorphic allele are likely to be fast metabolizers, in whom the drugs are ineffective or unsafe.

The fact that it is now possible to gather this sort of knowledge has led to the hype that the ultimate goal of pharmacogenomics will be "personalized medicine," the ability to target a drug specifically to a patient on the basis of his or her genotype, so that he or she will have maximal response with maximal safety. Needless to say, if pharmacogenomics ever lives up to this promise, medicine would be revolutionized, as most currently available drugs are fully effective in only about half the patients to whom they are prescribed, and, moreover, a subset of these patients will experience undesirable side effects. Still, personalized medicine is a long way off and, to be realistic, it is uncertain as to whether it is even possible, given that environmental factors, diet, age, lifestyle, life history, and state of health, all have the potential to influence an individual's response to medication.

Thus the true long-term promise that pharmacogenomics offers is likely to be the ability to stratify patients and diseases on the basis of genotype and to develop better strategies for therapy and prevention based on these stratifications. An example of a potential genotype-based therapy is pravastatin, which appears to be more effective in lowering cholesterol levels in people with the B1B1 variant of the CETP gene than in other people. An example of potential genotype-based prevention is tamoxifen, which appears to prevent breast cancer among women with BRCA1 and BRCA2 gene mutations.

Clearly, such knowledge is useful for the development of novel pharmaceutical products. Therefore, it is hardly surprising that the pharmaceutical industry has embraced genomics and greatly expanded their investment in genomics-related research. The greatest impact has been on the drug discovery process. Genomics has begun to play a pivotal role in drug discovery, particularly through pharmacogenomics and through improving the processes of *target identification* and *target validation*.

A drug target is typically a protein that is intimately associated with a disease process and that is the intended site of drug activity. For example, the protein, immunoglobulin or IgE, is a target for allergy, it having been established that the allergy response is mediated by it. Information obtained from studying correlations between genome variations and disease information and from studying correlations between gene expression differences and disease information can be used to identify target molecules that directly underlie the disease processes themselves, rather than just the symptoms. Statistical methods play a significant role in this endeavor.

Once a target has been identified, it must be *validated* to prove that inhibiting the target has the desired pharmacological effect. Gene expression studies can be used to validate a target by demonstrating that target genes are indeed expressed differently in different disease states. A more complex validation approach is to make a *knockout mouse* (a mouse lacking the gene that produces the target) and check whether it shows the desired behavior. For example, an IgE knockout mouse exhibits no allergic reactions, validating IgE as a target. Once an identified target has been adequately validated, an assay can be developed to screen a number of chemicals, perhaps in a high-throughput mode, for potential activity with it.

Protein research can also contribute to better *drug design*. Drugs generally work by binding with a target protein at a particular site on the protein, thereby inhibiting its normal function. If the structure of the target protein were known, it may be possible to construct a drug specifically to interact with it, for example, by using a technology such as X-ray crystallography to examine a three-dimensional protein structure and then designing a small molecule that will be able to fit and bind into the pockets of the structure.

The more specific a target site is, the better. A drug's toxic side effects usually stem from *nonselectivity*, the affinity of the drug to more than just the intended site of activity. Drugs aiming specifically for the molecular differences between diseased and normal cells are likely to be less toxic and, therefore, more useful clinically.

In addition, genomics and modern biotechnologies are expected to be invaluable for the identification of biomarkers. A *biomarker* is "a biological molecule found in blood, other body fluids, or tissues that is a sign of a normal or abnormal process or of a condition or disease" (as defined in 2001 by an NIH working group). Essentially, a biomarker is any parameter of a patient that can be measured, such as a gene expression profile, a protein, a lipid, a scan, or an electrical signal.

Use of disease-related biomarkers for decision making in clinical practice is certainly not a new phenomenon. Familiar examples include (i) blood glucose for diagnosis and management of diabetes, (ii) cholesterol for assessment of cardiovascular risk, and (iii) mammograms for assessment of breast cancer risk.

A biomarker can be used to supplement information to clinical and pathological analyses. It could facilitate screening and detection of a disease, monitoring the progression of a disease, and predicting the prognosis and survival after clinical intervention. A biomarker could also be used to evaluate the process of pharmaceutical development and to improve the efficacy and safety of treatment by enabling physicians to tailor treatment for individual patients.

Biomarkers can be categorized into various types on the basis of their intended purpose.

- A *risk stratification biomarker* can be used to provide information on the likely course of a disease in an individual (such as for assessing whether or not the individual is at risk for developing Alzheimer's disease or for assessing occurrence or recurrence of prostate cancer). Such biomarkers can be used in clinical screens focusing on prevention of disease development.
- A *diagnostic biomarker* can be used to determine the presence of a disease in a patient.
- A *prognostic biomarker* can be used to help estimate the likely outcome of a disease and can be used to establish treatment.
- A *predictive biomarker* can be used to identify subpopulations of patients who are most likely to respond to a given therapy and could form the basis for individualized disease management and for predicting efficacy of a particular therapy in clinical practice.
- A *therapeutic biomarker* can be used for assessing the effectiveness and adverse effects of a treatment and to provide early determination and treatment of recurrent disease.

These are only some of the ways genomics and associated sciences can contribute to pharmaceutical research.

2.9 PROTEINS

All living organisms are composed largely of proteins. Proteins perform and regulate most of life's basic functions. Thus, *structural proteins* form part of a cellular structure, *enzymes* catalyze almost all the biochemical reactions occurring within a cell, *regulatory proteins* control the expression of genes or the activity of other proteins, and *transport proteins* carry other molecules across membranes or around the body.

Structurally, proteins are giant complex chains of amino acids. A protein's sequence of amino acids is determined by the DNA sequence of the gene that produced it. Proteins belong to a class of large compounds that are called *polypeptides* as the amino acids that comprise them are held together by peptide bonds. Polypeptide chains in general and protein chains in particular have a tendency to fold up into complex three-dimensional structures. A protein's particular function in the cell is determined not only by its amino acid sequence but also by the specific structure into which it folds. It is also likely to be affected by other proteins present in the same cell at the same time with which it associates and reacts. Thus, proteins are much harder to study than genes.

Interestingly, there are far more proteins than there are genes. This is partly due to *posttranslational modifications* (proteins, once synthesized at the translation step of gene expression, are subject to a multitude of modifications) and partly due to *alternative splicing* (different ways of splicing the exons together after they are separated during transcription produces different mRNA sequences and thereby different proteins).

The multitude of all proteins generated by a genome of an organism is called its *proteome* and the study of protein structure and behavior, which is getting more and more attention, is called *proteomics*. Proteomics encompasses the identification of proteins in tissues, the characterization of their physicochemical properties (such as their sequences and posttranslational modifications), and the description of their behavior (such as what functions they perform and how they interact with one another and their environment).

2.10 BIOINFORMATICS

As stated in Chapter 1, an inevitable consequence of the modern-technology-driven research effort in genomics and genomics-related sciences is a steadily growing mountain of data, which is neither easy to examine nor straightforward to understand. Given the sequence of the human genome, for instance, it is already an immense task just to identify the individual genes. Ascertaining the function of the many thousands of genes and proteins identified and determining how this constellation of genes and proteins interact among themselves (and under what circumstances) is a mind-boggling task that will challenge those working in this area for many years. Issues lie in data storage, in querying and analysis of this data, in effective communication of these results, and in organizing them to infer functional relationships (see Bassett, Eisen, and Boguski, 1999, for a review of some of the challenges involved in doing this).

The steady influx of genomics information has spawned a new discipline called *bioinformatics* that has become an integral part of genomics research. In bioinformatics, scientists in the biological and computational sciences, together with significant contributions from other disciplines, collaborate to provide insight into biological processes. Statistics is an essential component of many of these activities. As a fledgling discipline, bioinformatics does not yet have a well-defined charter, but some common bioinformatics activities are given below.

Creation and Maintenance of Databases. As a first step, the magnitude and complexity of the data being collected has led to the creation of large relational databases to store, organize, and index such data. At the moment, DNA sequences (and protein sequences derived from them) comprise the majority of such catalogs. Some well-known examples are GenBank (a database that contains the totality of public DNA and protein sequence data), SWISS-PROT (a protein sequence database), and PDB (a database of three-dimensional biological macromolecular structure data).

Analysis of Sequence Information. In parallel with the development of large sequence databases, specialized tools (e.g., BLAST) are being devised to efficiently search, view, and analyze the data in these databases. This includes the development of methods for finding the genes in the DNA sequences of various organisms, clustering sequences into families of related sequences, aligning similar genes and proteins, and examining evolutionary relationships. Probability and statistical techniques, such as hidden Markov models, can efficiently and automatically build representations of related sequences. They form the basis of several of the more sensitive database searching tools. Statistical methodology can also be brought into play to assess the significance of any match found.

Prediction of Three-Dimensional Structure. Knowledge of physics and chemistry and information gathered from similar molecules are being used to deduce the three-dimensional structure of proteins and other large molecules.

Expression Analysis. The analysis of patterns of gene expression data (mostly obtained from DNA microarrays) using statistical and data mining tools is a major effort in bioinformatics.

Modeling Dynamic Life Processes. The ultimate challenge in bioinformatics is to develop ways of putting together the information gathered from all the diverse areas of research in order to understand fundamental life processes.

SUPPLEMENTARY READING

The book by Gonick and Wheelis (1991) is an excellent introduction to genetics presented in an amusing and informal style. The book by Clark and Russell (1997) is a more in depth introduction. More detailed treatment is provided by the molecular biology textbooks by Alberts et al. (1994) and Strachan and Read (1999).

Vingron (2001) argues the importance of applying statistical thinking to bioinformatics. The book by Ewens and Grant (2001) offers an introduction to statistical methods employed in bioinformatics.

EXERCISES

2.1. What are the complementary base pairing rules? Describe their role in (i) DNA replication, (ii) gene expression, (iii) hybridization assays, and (iv) PCR.

2.2. Explain the function of (i) DNA, (ii) mRNA, and (iii) start and stop codons in protein synthesis.

2.3. Explain how a child of parents, both of whom are blood type A, could be blood type O.

2.4. Discuss some ways in which developments in genomics could alter the practice of medicine.

2.5. Please explain the central dogma of molecular biology.

CHAPTER 3

Microarrays

The state of a cell at any given time is governed by which of its genes are expressed at that time. Recall that, according to the central dogma of molecular biology (Section 2.3), the first step in gene expression is transcription, in which expressed DNA sequences are transcribed into mRNA. Thus, it is reasonable to conjecture that knowledge of what mRNAs are present in the cell and in what quantities would enable a scientist to make some inferences regarding the state of that particular cell. This line of reasoning has led to a considerable effort to measure and compare the levels of mRNA in cells in various states. The complete collection of mRNAs (including their alternative splicing variants) is referred to as the organism's *transcriptome.*

It could be argued that it is more pertinent to study the end products of gene expression, the proteins, rather than mRNA, which is an intermediate molecule. After all, it is these proteins that are responsible for most biological activities in the body. However, the function of a protein is determined not only by its amino acid sequence, but also the specific structure it folds up into. Furthermore, proteins are difficult to purify. Thus, an added inducement for working with mRNA levels, in order to investigate cell state, is that they are relatively simple to study with current technology, even in a high-throughput mode, unlike proteins.

The *DNA microarray* (*microarray* or *array*) has now become the most widely used technology for studying mRNA levels. DNA microarrays were developed as a general means of monitoring the expression patterns (or more precisely, the transcription patterns) of large numbers of genes (perhaps even entire genomes) at once, thereby bringing about a tremendous improvement over the tedious "one gene per experiment" paradigm that prevailed until then (Brown and Botstein, 1999).

In brief, a typical DNA microarray experiment proceeds as follows. Take a small glass slide. Suppose that the surface of the slide has been divided into series of imaginary square cells to form a rectangular grid. Onto each square cell, stick a tiny amount of liquid that contains DNA corresponding to a gene of known

Exploration and Analysis of DNA Microarray and Other High-Dimensional Data, Second Edition.
Dhammika Amaratunga, Javier Cabrera, Ziv Shkedy.

sequence. Different cells will have different genes. Separately, prepare a solution that contains a mixture of mRNAs whose sequences are unknown. Add to this solution a substance that fluoresces when excited by light. Pour the solution onto the slide. The mRNA molecules will diffuse over the slide and, wherever they find a matching (i.e., complementary) DNA sequence, for example, one taken from the gene from which the mRNA was transcribed, they will hybridize to each other and the solution will stick to the slide. Without a match, the solution will not stick to the slide and can be washed away. Use a laser scanner to detect and measure the fluorescent signal being emitted at each cell.

In a comparative microarray experiment, different slides containing the same set of genes will be exposed to different mRNA samples. By comparing the intensity levels of the fluorescent signals across the multiple mRNA samples, a scientist will be able to understand how the expression profile of a set of genes differs across the different mRNA samples.

3.1 TYPES OF MICROARRAY EXPERIMENTS

This simple idea has an enormous potential. Microarrays have already been used heavily in biological research to address a wide variety of questions. To motivate our subsequent discussion, we begin by presenting a few examples of some of them. We emphasize that this list is by no means exhaustive and, in fact, represents only a fraction of the types of experiments that a scientist could envision addressing with this technology.

3.1.1 Experiment Type 1: Tissue-Specific Gene Expression

Cells from different tissues perform different functions. Although it is a simple matter to distinguish cells from different tissues by their phenotypes, the details of precisely why cells from one tissue behave differently from cells from another tissue remains a fertile topic for research. As it is the individual proteins, particularly enzymes, within each cell that control all the various intermeshing biochemical reactions within that cell, a cell's functions are determined by which proteins are produced by the cell, and this, in turn, depends on which genes are expressed by the cell. Microarray experiments can be used to identify which genes are preferentially expressed in which tissues. This would enable scientists to gain valuable insight into the mechanisms that govern the functioning of genes and cells.

3.1.2 Experiment Type 2: Developmental Genetics

The genes in an organism's genome express differently at different stages of its developmental process. Interestingly, it has been found that there is a subset of genes involved in early development that are used and reused at different stages in the development of the organism, generally in different order in different tissues, with each tissue having its own combination. Crucial to these processes are growth factors; the same growth factors that can, later in the organism's development, be involved in causing or promoting cancer; these genes are known as *proto-oncogenes*. Microarrays can, in principle, be used to track the changes in the organism's gene expression profile, tissue by tissue, over the series of stages of the developmental process, beginning with the embryo up to, perhaps, the adult.

Supplementary applications of this line of research include deducing evolutionary relationships among species and assessing the impact of environmental changes on the developmental process of an organism.

3.1.3 Experiment Type 3: Genetic Diseases

There are many diseases called *genetic diseases* that are the result of mutations in a gene or a set of genes. A gene that is thus altered is called a *mutant gene*. The result can be a disease as these genes express inappropriately or do not express at all. Cancer, for example, could occur when certain regulatory genes, such as the p53 tumor suppressor gene, are deleted, inactivated, or become constitutively active (i.e., become always transcribed, regardless of any regulatory factors).

Microarray experiments can be used to identify which genes are differentially expressed in diseased cells versus normal cells. This would enable scientists to identify genes associated with the disease process, such as the tumor suppressor genes and the oncogenes (i.e., normal cellular genes which, when inappropriately expressed or mutated, can transform normal cells into tumor cells) associated with the onset of cancer and the genes associated with the development of a cancer form a low-grade malignancy through to a high-grade malignancy. This would enable the development of drugs aimed directly at the difference between diseased and normal cells. Such drugs can be designed to specifically target a particular gene, protein, or signaling cascade and they are therefore less likely to cause undesirable side effects. One way in which this knowledge would be useful is in the development of target assays for screening new compounds in high-throughput mode to assess their potential efficacy as treatments for the disease.

In addition, certain diseases have subtypes that are clinically indistinguishable but are genetically heterogeneous. As they are different subtypes, it is most likely that they will call for different treatments. A case in point is ALL and AML. It is crucial for proper therapy that a correct clinical diagnosis be quickly made. However, this can be extremely difficult due to the clinical similarity of the two diseases. Microarray experiments can be used to identify which genes are differentially expressed in the two different types of cancer patients, thereby creating specific disease profiles by virtue of their gene expression patterns. The information gleaned from these studies could lead to diagnostic procedures.

Sometimes, such experiments may also uncover disease subtypes that were not even known to exist. This would happen, for instance, if, during the course of studying a group of patients thought to be homogeneous, it is found that they exhibit two very distinct gene expression profiles, indicating two different disease subtypes, and perhaps explaining why some patients were responding well to treatment while the others were not.

Thus, these types of experiments will afford scientists the capability of grouping diseases into classes and should eventually enable more precise, but less invasive, clinical diagnosis procedures to be developed.

3.1.4 Experiment Type 4: Complex Diseases

There are many diseases called *complex diseases* that are not caused by an error in genetic information but are caused instead by a combination of small genetic variations (polymorphisms) predisposing an individual to a serious problem. The risk of such an individual contracting a complex disease tends to be amplified by nongenetic factors, such as environmental influences, diet, and lifestyle. Coronary artery disease, multiple sclerosis, diabetes, and schizophrenia are complex diseases where the genetic makeup of the individual plays a major role in predisposing the individual to the disease. The genetic component of these diseases is responsible for their increased prevalence among certain groups, such as within families, within ethnic groups, within geographic regions, and within genders. Microarray experiments can be used to identify the genetic markers, usually a combination of SNPs, which may predispose an individual to a complex disease.

3.1.5 Experiment Type 5: Pharmacological Agents

Some genes alter their expression patterns when the organism is exposed to an external stimulus such as a pharmacological agent or a substance present in the environment. Microarray experiments can be used to identify genes that express differently in response to such exposure. The information obtained from such experiments will be useful for target identification and target validation.

The simplest such experiment is one in which a sample of cells is exposed to the pharmacological agent and permitted to reach a steady state of transcription. The mRNA levels in the treated cells can then be compared to those in a control sample.

A potentially more informative experiment would be a temporal study. A temporal study is an experiment in which a sample of cells is exposed to the pharmacological agent and subsamples of the cell sample are drawn at successive points in time. This allows the scientist to monitor the gradual change in gene expression profiles from the old steady state through to the new steady state. Such temporal studies provide information not only on which genes undergo expression profile changes but also the order in which these changes occur.

Microarrays are also useful as a means of assessing toxicity that evokes changes in gene expression. A toxicologist would expose cells or tissues or a few animals to a class of chemicals whose toxicity is known and, from this, establish a *signature*, a common set of changes in gene expression produced by this class of toxic agents. Then they can expose another set of cells or tissues or animals to a chemical whose toxicity is unknown and match the results against the signature. From this, they should be able to make a prediction regarding the potential toxicity of that chemical. If successful, this procedure could be automated to allow for high-throughput toxicity screening of new molecular entities and should reduce the need for lengthy, expensive, and unpleasant animal testing of potential drugs.

3.1.6 Experiment Type 6: Plant Breeding

For centuries, researchers in plant breeding have been trying, with some success, to improve cultivated plant species and their products. For example, given that crops are heavily influenced by the environmental conditions to which they are continuously exposed, researchers in plant breeding have attempted to induce greater tolerance for environmental stressors such as extreme weather conditions. The following are some other goals of plant breeding: to boost the resistance of plants to infections, to reduce insect predation, to maximize the productivity of plants, to improve the quality of plant products, to increase the nutrition level of foods processed from plants, and to develop characteristics of plant products that are valued by consumers (e.g., fruits that stay ripe for long periods of time).

Microarray experiments can be used to identify the genes responsible for various traits of interest and to determine the conditions under which these traits are expressed. This information would enable scientists to create plant varieties with exact combinations of desirable traits.

3.1.7 Experiment Type 7: Environmental Monitoring

Environmental factors are known to affect gene expression, both as to whether or not a particular gene is expressed, and the degree to which it is expressed if, in fact, it is. Should a normal biological pathway be disrupted as a result of a gene expressing differently, the health of the affected organism could suffer. Thus, it is important to assess the genome-level impact of exposure to environmental stressors, especially contamination of air, food, and water. Microarrays can be used to compare and contrast gene expression patterns across affected versus unaffected organisms, whether they are flora or fauna, taking into account natural effects such as seasonal fluctuations (Gibson, 2002). One goal of these experiments is the characterization of environmental changes that may be a hazard to health.

Another goal of environmental monitoring is the detection of pathogens in food and water. This is generally done by examining the DNA in potentially contaminated samples, as each pathogen possesses a DNA sequence unique to it. The traditional approach tends to be a slow and laborious process, which is highly undesirable in situations where rapid intervention may be critical. Using microarrays, monitors can simultaneously and swiftly screen for several different strains of pathogens. To do this, a microarray containing the DNA of a number of different pathogens would be prepared, DNA would be extracted from an environmental sample, and this DNA would be applied to the microarray. If a pathogen is present in the sample, it will hybridize to the microarray and its presence would be detected. With this information, scientists can assess whether or not there is a hazard to health.

3.2 A VERY SIMPLE HYPOTHETICAL MICROARRAY EXPERIMENT

It is easiest to explain the principle behind microarray experiments with a very simple hypothetical example.

Suppose that we have obtained some cancerous liver tissue and some normal liver tissue from a liver cancer patient and that we want to know which genes are expressed differently in the two. We would begin by extracting mRNA from each tissue, so that we have two mRNA samples. In each sample, only mRNA corresponding to any genes that were expressed (i.e., transcribed) would be present. We would reverse transcribe the mRNA to cDNA and add some fluorescent dye to each sample. These two labeled samples are sometimes called *targets* (Note: sometimes, they are also called probes because they are used to probe the collection of spots on a microarray, but this usage appears to be now less standard—in order to avoid confusion, we shall call them the *labeled samples*).

Now suppose that we have prepared a DNA microarray containing the entire human genome (there is no such microarray as of yet, which is one reason why this example is hypothetical). Suppose that there are 36,000 genes. A DNA microarray for this experiment would be a tiny glass slide on which the 36,000 genes are printed in a, say, 300×120 rectangular array of spots, one gene per spot. Each gene printed on the microarray is called a *probe* (Note: in the confusion about terminology, they are sometimes called *targets*). Two such microarrays are prepared.

We would now flood one of the microarrays with the labeled sample from the cancerous tissue and flood the other microarray with the labeled sample from the normal tissue. We allow enough time for any cDNA in the samples to recognize and hybridize to its complementary sequence in the microarray. Once we are satisfied that this has happened, we wash off any excess labeled sample from the microarrays and dry them.

Each spot on the microarrays where the labeled sample bound to the spot would identify a gene that corresponds to some reverse-transcribed mRNA in the sample. Such spots can be easily recognized, as they are the only ones that will fluoresce. In this way, every spot on the microarray functions much like an independent assay for the presence of a particular mRNA.

We would then scan the microarrays and measure the intensity level of fluorescence at each spot. By comparing these intensities across the two microarrays, we would be able to tell which genes are differentially expressed in cancerous liver tissue versus normal liver tissue.

Example. Let X_g and Y_g denote the intensities measured for the gth gene in the normal liver tissue microarray and cancerous liver tissue microarray, respectively, and let the ratio of these intensities be $R_g = Y_g/X_g$. This ratio is usually called the *fold change*. Figure 3.1a shows a scatterplot of Y_g versus X_g and Figure 3.1b shows a histogram of R_g. It is impossible to discern any structure in these graphical displays because the data are so heavily skewed. However, by taking logs, we are better able to see structure. Figure 3.1c shows a scatterplot of $\log(Y_g)$ versus $\log(X_g)$ and Figure 3.1d shows a histogram of $\log(R_g)$. In Figure 3.1a and c, most genes

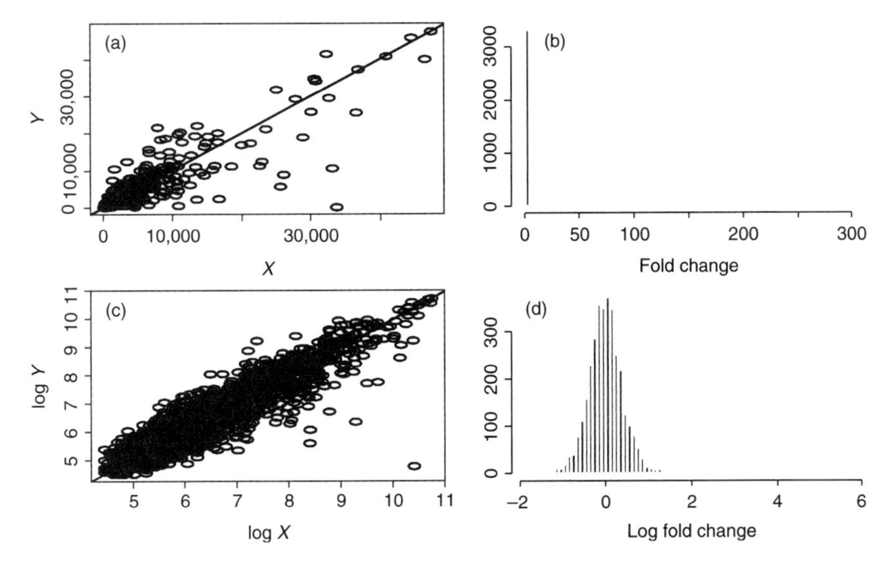

Figure 3.1 Comparing two samples by (a) scatterplot of intensities, (b) histogram of fold changes, (c) scatterplot of log intensities, and (d) histogram of log fold changes.

fall along the $Y = X$ line, indicating that they are expressed to the same degree in both tissues. The differentially expressing genes are those that lie far away from the $Y = X$ line. In Figure 3.1b, most genes have R_g values close to one (and, correspondingly, in Figure 3.1d, most genes have $\log(R_g)$ values close to zero), again indicating that they are expressed to the same degree in both tissues. The differentially expressing genes are those whose R_g is large ($R_g > 2$ say), indicating genes that are overexpressed or upregulated in the cancer cells, and those whose R_g is small ($R_g < 0.5$, say) indicating genes that are underexpressed or downregulated in the cancer cells. Of the 3300 genes in this example, 145 genes are upregulated ($R_g > 2$) and 124 genes are downregulated ($R_g < 2$).

This is the general idea behind microarray experiments.

3.3 A TYPICAL MICROARRAY EXPERIMENT

The very simple hypothetical example that was given above outlined the five basic steps of a typical actual microarray experiment. The five steps are

1. preparing the microarray;
2. preparing the labeled sample;
3. hybridizing the labeled sample to the microarray and washing the microarray;
4. scanning the microarray;
5. interpreting the scanned image.

We shall now describe each of these steps in greater detail.

3.3.1 Microarray Preparation

To start with, we must have a collection of purified single-stranded DNAs. A drop of each type of DNA in solution is placed onto a specially prepared glass microscope slide by a robotic machine called an *arrayer*. This process is called *arraying* or *spotting*. The arrayer can quickly produce a regular grid of thousands of spots in a dime-sized area, small enough to fit under a standard slide coverslip. The DNA in the spots is bonded to the glass to keep it from washing off during the hybridization reaction and subsequent wash. This then is the DNA microarray for the experiment.

The DNA spotted on the microarray may be either cDNA, in which case the microarray is called a *cDNA microarray*, or oligonucleotides, in which case the microarray is called an *oligonucleotide microarray*.

The DNA spotted on cDNA microarrays are cloned copies of cDNA, amplified by PCR, corresponding to whole or part of a fully sequenced gene or putative ORF; ESTs are commonly arrayed. These microarrays are widely applicable as their manufacture requires only that a large library of cDNAs be available as a source of clones. The sequence of the cDNA could be several hundred to a few thousand base pairs long. When only a part of a gene is spotted, the subsequence that is spotted is carefully chosen for maximal specificity.

The DNA spotted on oligonucleotide microarrays are synthesized chains of oligonucleotides corresponding to part of a known gene or putative ORF; each oligonucleotide is usually only about 25 base pairs long. In oligonucleotide microarrays, a gene is represented by several different oligonucleotides; the oligonucleotides are carefully chosen for maximal specificity.

The selection of DNA probes to be spotted on the microarray determines which genes can be studied in the experiment in which it is used. For organisms whose genomes have been completely sequenced, including several bacteria, viruses, and yeast, it is possible to array genomic DNA from every known gene or putative ORF in the organism. For these organisms, enough DNA must be produced to make as many arrays as needed. One way to do this is to amplify each gene or putative ORF from total genomic DNA by PCR. However, one disadvantage of using PCR to make multiple copies for array spotting is that PCR can induce mutations, especially at higher cycles. An alternative is to clone fragment cDNAs and then make large amounts of identical DNA copies by growing them in bacteria, then extracting plasmid and excising out the specific cDNA fragments.

For organisms with larger and more complex genomes, such as the human genome, that have not yet been completely sequenced, a comprehensive array for the entire genome cannot yet be produced. Of course, in the case of the human genome, the location and sequence of a large percentage of human genes is now known, chiefly as a result of the Human Genome Project. Therefore, the same method as above can be used to produce an incomplete but substantial human genome microarray, with a complete one perhaps only a few years away. In addition, there are methods for producing arrayable DNA even for unknown genes.

There are a few different robotic technologies that have been developed for arraying microarrays. One method uses a robotic arm to touch and spot nanoscale droplets of the solution containing the cDNA or oligonucleotide. Another method uses ink jet technology to eject the solution onto the surface of the glass slide without the robot actually touching it. Other technologies concurrently synthesize oligonucleotides on the slide *in situ*, using either photolithography (a proprietary method developed by Affymetrix) or ink jet technology (a method developed by Rosetta Inpharmatics).

The DNA probes arrayed on the microarrays are frequently referred to as *genes* even though this may not be quite accurate.

3.3.2 Sample Preparation

The labeled sample is prepared separately. The first step here is to purify mRNA from total cellular contents. The experimenter must contend with several challenges here: (i) mRNA accounts for only a small fraction (<3%) of all mRNA in a cell; (ii) the more heterogeneous the cells (e.g., the cells of solid tumors), the more difficult it is to isolate mRNA specific to the study; and (iii) captured mRNA degrades very quickly. As far as the latter is concerned, in order to prevent the experimental samples from being lost, the mRNA is immediately reverse transcribed into more stable cDNA (for cDNA microarrays) or cRNA (for oligonucleotide arrays—cRNA is synthetic RNA produced by transcription from a single-stranded DNA template).

Even here, there is a small problem: not all mRNAs are reverse transcribed with the same efficiency. As this effect is gene specific, the fluorescence intensity that is measured for a gene at the end of the study may not be a true reflection of original mRNA level. Consequently, it would not be correct to compare fluorescence intensities for different genes across a single sample. Fortunately, however, it would not be incorrect to compare fluorescence intensities across several samples.

In order to be able to detect which cDNAs are bound to the microarray, the sample is labeled with a reporter molecule that flags their presence. The reporters currently used in microarray experiments are fluorescent dyes, called *fluors* or *fluorophores*, chemicals that fluoresce when exposed to a specific wavelength of light. The labeled sample is the target for the experiment.

The number of fluor molecules that label each cDNA depends on its length and also possibly its sequence composition. This is another reason why fluorescent intensities for different cDNAs cannot be quantitatively compared. However, identical cDNAs from different labeled samples will still be comparable as long as the same number of label molecules is added to the same DNA sequence in each labeled sample.

3.3.3 The Hybridization Step

The labeled sample is poured onto the microarray and allowed to diffuse uniformly all over it. Then it is sealed in a hybridization chamber and incubated at a specific temperature for enough time to allow the hybridization reactions to complete. The experimental conditions should ensure that all areas of the microarray are exposed to a uniform amount of labeled sample throughout this time.

A single-stranded DNA molecule will bind with highest affinity to another single-stranded DNA molecule with a precisely matching sequence and with significantly lower affinity to one with an imperfect match. The stringency of the hybridization depends on experimental conditions such as temperature. If the labeled sample contains a cDNA whose sequence is complementary to the DNA on a given spot on the microarray, that cDNA will hybridize to the spot. Enough incubation time should be allowed for the hybridization reactions to complete.

The microarray is then removed from the hybridization chamber and thoroughly, but carefully, washed to eliminate any excess labeled sample. Finally, the microarray is dried using a centrifuge or by blowing with clean compressed air.

The quality of the hybridization can be assessed experimentally by spotting the probes for a set of hybridization control genes, spiking the labeled sample with a known amount of these controls prior to exposure to the array and verifying that these control genes are, indeed, showing up as having been hybridized.

3.3.4 Scanning the Microarray

Now the microarray is scanned to determine the amount of labeled sample bound to each spot. Recall that the sample was labeled with fluorescent reporter molecules that emit detectable light when stimulated by a laser. The emitted light is captured by a scanner, such as a charge-coupled device or a confocal microscope, which records its intensity. Spots with more bound sample will have more reporters and will therefore fluoresce more intensely.

Although it is only supposed to pick up light emitted by the target cDNAs bound to their complementary spots, the scanner will inevitably also pick up light from various other sources including labeled sample hybridizing nonspecifically to the glass slide, residual (unwashed) labeled sample adhering to the slide, various chemicals used in processing the slide, and even the slide itself. This extra light is called *background*.

Scanner settings can affect both the precision of the intensity measurements as well as the lower and upper threshold intensity levels that can be measured. Intensities outside this range, called the *dynamic range*, cannot be properly quantified and are often set to the corresponding threshold level. When intensities exceed the upper threshold, saturation is said to have occurred. There is a trade-off between the precision and the dynamic range; increasing one will decrease the other and vice versa; a balance must be struck.

3.3.5 Interpreting the Scanned Image

The end product of a microarray experiment is a scanned grayscale image (Figure 3.2) whose intensity measurements range from 0 to 216. The image is usually stored in 16-bit *tagged image file format* (tiff). Image-processing software

Figure 3.2 Single-channel scanned image.

will convert the image into spot intensity measurements, which will then be analyzed for gene expression differences.

Figure 3.2 shows a typical microarray image. The whiter spots are of higher intensity and can be associated with higher hybridization activity. The very dark spots occur at locations where there was little or no hybridization.

3.4 MULTICHANNEL cDNA MICROARRAYS

It has become a common practice among those who use cDNA microarrays to fashion the labeled sample out of two or more mRNA samples mixed together. Each mRNA sample in the mixture is labeled with a different fluorescent dye. At the scanning stage, the slide is scanned as many times as there are samples. Such microarrays are called *multichannel cDNA microarrays*.

Figure 3.3 shows the two scanned images from a two-channel cDNA microarray, in which one of the channels was exposed to a control mRNA sample and the second channel was exposed to a treated mRNA sample. Any spot whose intensity is different between the two channels (e.g., dark in channel 1 and white in channel 2) corresponds to a spot that was differentially hybridized and, by inference, to a gene that was differentially expressed in treated versus control owing to a treatment effect.

Multichannel cDNA microarrays have some advantages that have led them to becoming the standard technology for cDNA microarrays over single-channel cDNA microarrays. For one thing, it is often difficult to tightly control the amount of DNA that is spotted onto the slides and this could vary from array to array for the same gene. The effect of this variation on downstream analysis can be reduced by the natural matching of samples in multichannel microarrays. In addition, some economy is gained as data on expression levels of several mRNA samples can be gathered using just one slide.

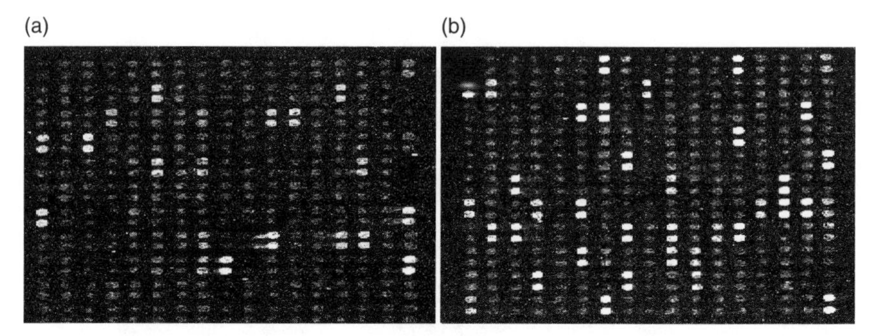

Figure 3.3 Scanned images from a small two-channel microarray. (a) Channel 1 (control) and (b) channel 2 (treated).

However, there are some drawbacks as well: (i) there is an overall dye effect, although this can usually be corrected by normalization (Chapter 5). (ii) If the objective is to compare a large number of mRNA samples, the logistics of setting it up become more complex with multichannel microarrays. (iii) A more serious problem is that some genes may incorporate certain dyes better than other dyes, so that gene-specific dye effects could occur.

3.5 OLIGONUCLEOTIDE MICROARRAYS

The technology for the production of high-density oligonucleotide microarrays (Lockhart et al., 1996; Lipshutz et al., 1999) was pioneered by Affymetrix and remains proprietary to this day. In an oligonucleotide microarray, a gene is represented by a set of 20 or so oligonucleotides, called *perfect match probes* (PM). The multiple oligonucleotides that represent a gene are designed in such a way as to hybridize to different regions of the RNA corresponding to an expressed gene and act as a series of multiple independent detectors for the gene.

Each perfect match probe is paired with an artificially created *mismatch probe* (MM) that is fashioned by changing the middle base of the corresponding perfect match probe to its complementary base. The MM probe is intended to play the role of an internal control for hybridization specificity peculiar to its particular hybridization site. The hybridization to the gene by the perfect match probe represents specific hybridization and should be stronger than any nonspecific hybridization to the MM probe. In addition, if the PM intensities are consistently larger than the MM intensities for a probe set, this global effect is more likely to be indicative of actual presence of mRNA corresponding to that gene in the sample as opposed to being a random chance event. At least, that is the theory—in practice, there is a great deal of controversy about the use of the MM probes.

Affymetrix refers to each PM–MM pair as a *probe pair* and the entire set of probe pairs for a gene is called a *probe set*. High-density oligonucleotide microarrays are manufactured by synthesizing the oligonucleotides directly onto the surface of a silicon chip. The process is highly elaborate and involves defining the exposure sites on the chip with a series of semiconductor-based photolithographic masks and following this with a light-directed chemical synthesis of the oligonucleotides guided by their DNA sequences. The nature of the process is such that a very large number of oligonucleotides can be densely arrayed at the same time.

3.6 BEAD-BASED ARRAYS

New technologies are constantly emerging in an effort to extend the throughput and potential of microarrays. One of the most promising is *bead-based microarray* technology.

A bead-based fiber-optic microarray is a bundle of optical fibers. Microscopic wells are etched onto the end of each fiber. These wells hold the probe DNA sequences in bead form. The array is exposed to the fluorescently labeled sample. Wherever the labeled sample finds a matching (i.e., complementary) DNA sequence on the microarray, hybridization takes place. Without a match, the labeled sample does not hybridize to the probe. The array is illuminated with a lamp. This triggers fluorescence in the tagged samples, which causes a signal to be passed through the optical fiber to a detector, which indicates which probe DNA sequences match some sequence in the labeled sample.

The throughput of three-dimensional bead-based microarrays is a great deal higher than conventional two-dimensional microarrays. In fact, the number of DNA sequences tested could be in the hundreds of thousands, or even, millions range.

3.7 CONFIRMATION OF MICROARRAY RESULTS

Microarray technology is still a dynamic and evolving entity. As such, the reliability of state of the technology at this time is that microarray experimental results could be rather variable. The value of microarray technology as a high-throughput screen for gene expression information is without question, but investigators should interpret any results from microarray experiments with some circumspection (see, e.g., Kothapalli et al., 1992). The analysis approach used to analyze the data should be chosen carefully with both the data and the goals of the experiment in mind (Slonim, 2002). The key is to utilize microarrays as a means of screening and prioritizing a large number of genes, but any findings pertaining to genes of special interest should be independently confirmed. This is generally done on a gene-by-gene basis using methods such as Northern blots or quantitative RT-PCR.

SUPPLEMENTARY READING AND ELECTRONIC REFERENCES

1. *Animations*. The web site
   - `http://www.bio.davidson.edu/courses/genomics/chip/chip.html`

has animations that demonstrate how a DNA microarray experiment is performed.

2. Lander (1999) is a good introductory article on the promise of microarrays. *The Chipping Forecast* (2001), *The Chipping Forecast* II (2002), and The Chipping Forecast III (2005) are special supplementary issues of the journal *Nature Genetics* that carry several excellent review articles by several researchers who either pioneered or significantly advanced the field of DNA microarrays. These are all freely available online.
3. The book by Schena (1999) discusses various aspects of microarray experiments.
4. Nguyen et al. (2002) provides an excellent review of the biological and technological aspects of microarray experiments in a format suitable for data analysts.

EXERCISES

3.1. What is the difference between a genetic disease and a complex disease? How would a microarray experiment to discover the genes involved in a genetic disease differ from an experiment to discover the genes involved in a complex disease?

3.2. What is the advantage of doing a temporal study?

3.3. Outline the various steps of a typical microarray experiment.

3.4. Explain the terms: background, saturation.

3.5. Discuss the advantages and disadvantages of a two-channel microarray versus a single-channel microarray.

3.6. What is (i) a probe pair and (ii) a probe set?

3.7. In what way does quantitative RT-PCR complement microarrays?

CHAPTER 4

Processing the Scanned Image

When microarrays are scanned at the end of an experiment, the result is a series of images, one image per channel. Thus, a one-channel microarray, such as an oligonucleotide array, yields one image per array, whereas a two-channel microarray yields two images per array, one image per channel.

The scanner "reads" a microarray by dividing it up into a very large number of pixels and recording the intensity level of the fluorescence at each pixel. The resulting rectangular array of pixels and their associated intensities constitutes the image of the microarray.

The image must be converted into spot intensities for analysis (see the schematic in Figure 4.2). The purpose of this conversion is to assign to every DNA sequence that was spotted on the microarray an intensity measure, called the *spot intensity*, reflecting the amount of labeled sample that hybridized to it.

Following this, it is generally advisable to perform a series of quality checks on the data and, if necessary, generate warnings about possible problems, such as aberrant spots and defective microarrays, so that the investigator could take appropriate action.

Finally, the spot intensity data should be adjusted for background fluorescence.

4.1 CONVERTING THE SCANNED IMAGE TO THE SPOTTED IMAGE

The task of quantifying a scanned image is often carried out in three steps. First, the location of each spot in the array is defined by assigning coordinates to the center of each spot—this is called *gridding*. Second, the *signal*, the set of pixels that correspond to labeled cDNA hybridizing to its complementary DNA sequence spotted on the microarray, is separated from the *background*, the set of pixels that

Exploration and Analysis of DNA Microarray and Other High-Dimensional Data, Second Edition.
Dhammika Amaratunga, Javier Cabrera, Ziv Shkedy.

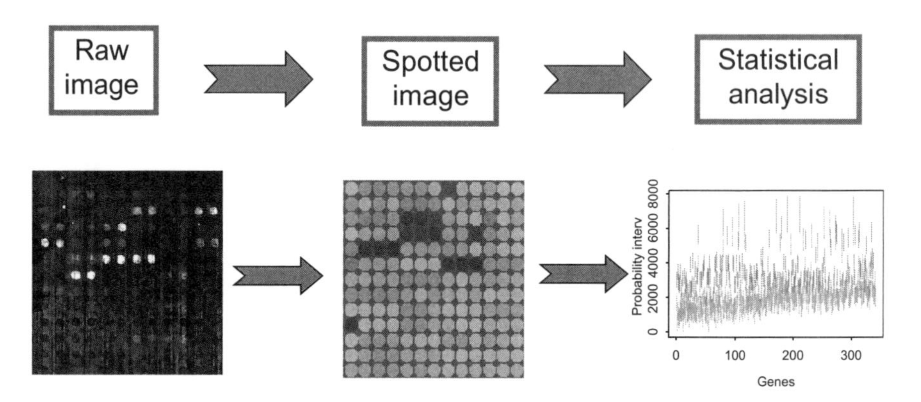

Figure 4.1 Data processing steps starting with the raw image.

correspond to labeled cDNA hybridizing nonspecifically to the microarray—this is called *segmentation*. Third, each spot is assigned an intensity value—this is called *quantification*. We now mention some aspects of each step; Yang et al. (2000, 2001) provide more detailed accounts.

4.1.1 Gridding

If the arraying process arrayed the spots in a perfect rectangular grid, as it should, the task of defining the spots by assigning coordinates to the center of each circular spot would be a simple matter: just overlay an appropriately sized grid on the microarray and move it around until it is properly aligned. In practice, however, the arraying process is not perfect, so that the grid that is actually arrayed tends to be a slightly deformed version of the target regular rectangular grid. As a result, the overlaid grid will need some fine-tuning, which can be done by manipulating the rows and columns of the overlaid grid until it is satisfactorily aligned. Care must be taken that speckles and dust, which can fluoresce as brightly as a spot, do not confuse the procedure.

A somewhat more rigorous method would be to first locally smooth the image using a Gaussian kernel, designate the modes of the smoothed regions as the spot centers, and, then, modify the grid so that the distances from the spot centers to the centers of the rectangular or square regions containing each spot are minimized.

4.1.2 Segmentation

Once the locations of the centers of the spots have been determined, the next step is to separate the spot, that is, the region of the slide on which cDNA was actually arrayed, from the background. This should not be too difficult if all the spots were circular with a well-defined boundary. The procedure would involve either fitting a circle with a constant diameter to all the spots on the image (*fixed circle segmentation*) or fitting circles with different diameters to different spots on the image (*adaptive circle segmentation*).

In practice, neither of these segmentation procedures works particularly well as the spots tend to vary considerably in size, shape and regularity owing to a number of factors, such as the quality of the spotting tip of the arrayer (which degrades with use), how long the tip stays on the slide, the deposition of the cDNA causing a bowl-like depression, the coating on the slide, the surface tension and viscosity of the solution being arrayed, the ambient temperature and humidity, the post-hybridization processing of the microarray, and so on. Work in computer vision has suggested some ways of dealing with this problem.

One such method is the *seeded region growing algorithm*. The algorithm consists of the following steps:

1. *Seed Specification*. To get this algorithm started, a set of pixels called seeds have to be specified. One simple way to do this is to let the seeds for signal be the estimated spot locations from the gridding step and the seeds for background could be the midpoints.
2. *Region Growing*. For each spot we have a seed for a signal region and a seed for a background region. The seeds are then "grown" into regions by allocating the remaining pixels to either signal or background region, depending on their intensity and their closeness to a seeded region. A pixel that is adjacent to an allocated pixel is considered as a candidate for allocation into that region. At each step, among the pixel candidates for all regions, the pixel that is the closest in intensity to the average intensity of the corresponding region is assigned to that region.
3. *Stopping Rule*. This process continues until all the pixels have been allocated to one of the regions.

Another method is *histogram segmentation*. A mask is placed over each spot. The mask should be larger than the spot. The histogram of pixel intensities within the mask is examined to determine a threshold value. Each pixel within the mask is then classified as signal or background depending on whether its intensity is above or below this threshold.

Therneau et al. (2002) discuss a method, based on the EM algorithm (Dempster et al., 1977), for sharpening spots to correct for the bleeding of one spot onto another.

4.1.3 Quantification

At each spot, the average intensity of the pixels is measured. This observation is complemented by a number of other spot-related statistics that allows the quality of the spot to be assessed (see, e.g., Kuklin, Petrov, and Shams, 2001; Wang et al., 2001; also Brown et al., 2001, recommend a pixel-by-pixel analysis of individual spots for two-channel microarrays). The following list outlines some typical spot-related statistics that are reported.

- *The Spot Intensity*. The end product of the conversion process is an array X_{rc} of spot intensities: here X_{rc} denotes the intensity of the spot located at the rth row and cth column of the array. At each spot, the average intensity of the pixels designated as signal is taken to be its spot intensity value. The average used is often the mean, because it should be representative of the number of labeled mRNA molecules hybridizing to the DNA spotted on the array. However, because the distribution of pixel intensities might be irregular, other measures of location, such as the median or trimmed mean or biweight or mode, are also sometimes used.
- *The Spot Background.* This is the average intensity of the pixels around the spot that were designated as background. The average used is often the mean or median. The background intensities are represented as an array B_{rc} of the same dimension as X_{rc}.
- *Pixel Intensity Distribution.* In general, the distribution of pixel intensities in and around a spot does not resemble a normal. Instead, for example, it could be peaked with one or two long tails. This is one reason why the segmentation process can sometimes be imprecise. *Spot cv* and *background cv* are the coefficients of variation of the intensities of the pixels assigned to signal and background respectively. The higher the spot *cv* the more variable the intensities of the pixels that make up the spot and, possibly, the lower the quality of the spot. Moreover, the closer the spot intensity is to spot background or to saturation, the less reliable it is.
- *Spot Morphology.* Measures associated with geometric characteristics of the spot, such as the size of the spot, also provide information regarding the quality of the spot. When seeking circular spots, two other such measures are *circularity*, which is 4π times the area of the spot divided by its perimeter squared and regularity, which is the proportion of pixels designated as background by the segmentation procedure among the pixels falling within the circle designated by the gridding procedure. The closer these measures are to unity, the more circular is the spot.

Owing to its unique technology, the oligonucleotide arrays manufactured by Affymetrix are treated somewhat differently. Unlike the spots on cDNA microarrays, probe cells on these arrays are square in shape rather than circular. A scanner reads an Affymetrix array by dividing each cell into a square array of pixels, recording the fluorescence level at each pixel, then ignoring the border pixels, and returning a summary (e.g., the 75th percentile) of the remaining pixels as the spot intensity of the probe cell.

4.2 QUALITY ASSESSMENT

Once the spotted image and related statistics are obtained, it is advisable to (i) assess the quality of the array and (ii) evaluate the quality of the individual spots

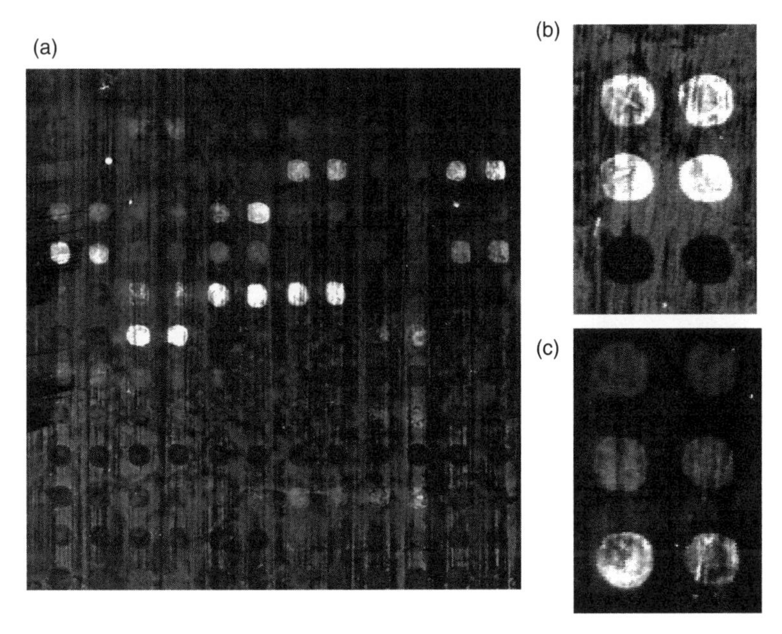

Figure 4.2 Scanned image.

on the array. This is because, sometimes, (i) the array could have a region of generally increased or decreased intensity and (ii) some spots might be defective. Figure 4.2a shows a scanned image that has a few such blemishes. There are some speckles that could be dust. The background seems to be nonuniform. Figure 4.2b shows some spots with high-contrast background effects, and Figure 4.2c shows some defective spots.

Artifacts such as these, introduced, perhaps, by the experimental process or some odd random event (e.g., dust particles settling on the array), could seriously compromise the corresponding spot intensities. If the affected arrays and/or spots are not identified and removed or otherwise adequately downweighted, they could mask true experimental effects. Several steps are involved in assessing the quality of an array and the spots within an array.

4.2.1 Visualizing the Spotted Image

Visual inspection of the data is a first attempt to appraise the quality of the spotted image. This can be done using a typical image plot (referred to as a *heat map* in the computer science literature), in which each image pixel corresponds to a spot. The image plot is then examined and searched for obvious nonrandom patterns that would suggest poor data quality. If none is observed, the image is passed on to the next step.

A basic graph for visualizing a spotted image is shown in Figure 4.3. The graph contains a central panel showing a color image with a color scale underneath. The

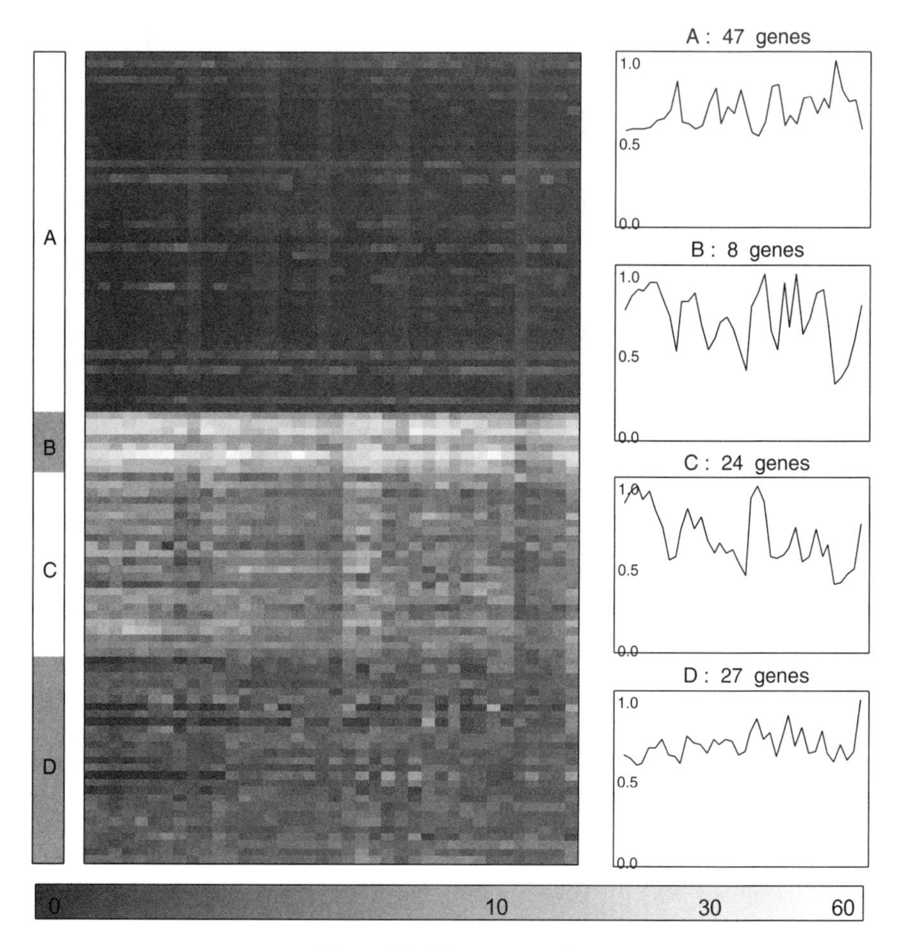

Figure 4.3 Microarray graph.

central panel may be subdivided into groups from top to bottom giving the images of subpanels or clusters with a bar on the left indicating the subgroups. Finally, the right side of the graph shows the average profiles of each of the groups or subpanels. The average profiles are computed by taking the average of the subgroups across the columns and then normalizing each profile by dividing it by its maximum.

4.2.2 Numerical Evaluation of Array Quality

In addition to visual methods for checking for patterns in the spotted image, numerical methods should also be considered. This is because of the following:

- It is possible that some of the more subtle spatial patterns in a spotted image are not visible in the image graph because the variation is small enough not to show on the color scale or the color scale may not be sensitive enough to show the pattern.

- Automated methods are crucial for processing a large number of microarray images, such as those that occur in a high-throughput environment, without the need for tedious individual visual inspection.

4.2.3 Spatial Problems

In order to ensure the integrity of the data, the spot and background intensities, $\{S_{rc}\}$ and $\{B_{rc}\}$, must satisfy some quality criteria related to the spatial distribution of the intensities. The first one is that the background intensities must be uniformly distributed. We expect this to be approximately correct or, at a minimum, we expect that the background intensities will not display clear nonuniform patterns.

A few nonuniform patterns that appear quite often, because they may be related to specific problems with the experimental process, such as hybridization artifacts, inconsistent washing across the slide, and other technical problems that introduce topographical variation, are discussed below:

- Case 1: A large smudge covering a substantial part of the area of the background image. These smudges are areas of the array that show higher or lower intensities compared to the rest of the image.
- Case 2: Vertical or horizontal strips on the background image that show higher or lower intensities.
- Case 3: Diagonal strips again showing higher or lower background intensities.
- Case 4: A gradient in the background intensities going across the array.
- Case 5: A row or column effect such as an edge effect.
- Case 6: Bleeding in the spotted image, that is, a series of consecutive spots that are blurred together forming a horizontal or vertical line.

In order to detect patterns such as the above, Amaratunga and Cabrera (2003b) proposed a method that separates pixel intensities into high and low and separates them using only the two coordinates: row number and column number. If the separation is successful, the array has a spatial problem and should be discarded, otherwise the array is accepted. The steps of the algorithm they proposed are as follows:

- Step 1: Split the image into high-intensity and low-intensity spots. This is a binary split similar to the ones performed by a regression tree algorithm at a single node. The CART procedure (Breiman et al., 1984) does this by identifying the cutoff that minimizes the within-group sum of squares. However, this split is not robust against outliers. A simple alternative that is resistant to outliers is to set the cutoff to the midpoint between to quantiles (say 5% and 95% quantiles). Then define the response at the spot at row r and column c: $Y_{rc} = 1$ for high-intensity spots and $Y_{rc} = 0$ for the rest.

- Step 2: Fit a quadratic discriminant function (see Section 10.3) to the binary response $\{Y_{rc}\}$ using the spot coordinates (r, c) on the microarray as predictors. Suppose that Z_{rc} are the predicted responses by the discriminant function. In order to assess the goodness of the fit, calculate the proportion π of correctly predicted spots, that is, the proportion of spots with $Y = Z$. The null distribution of the π-statistic can be simulated by randomizing the images. To do this, generate a large number (say, 300) of images by random permutations of the spot intensities and calculate the value of π for each image, resulting in the set $\{\pi_1, \ldots, \pi_{300}\}$. Estimate the p-value as the proportion of π_i greater than the observed π. This p-value measures the performance of the quadratic discriminant analysis and is used to determine the overall quality of the microarray.

The outcome of the above procedure could be summarized in an image quality graph such as the one shown in Figure 4.4. The figure consists of a central panel showing a color image and a set of four graphs on the right side of the figure. The main panel displays an image representing the background intensities that are being analyzed. The color or grayscale corresponding to the main panel is shown on a narrow horizontal strip below the main panel. The right side of Figure 4.4 shows a column of four graphs:

- The two graphs at the top of the right side show the average profiles of the rows and columns of the main panel, respectively.
- The third and fourth graphs show the image graphs of the arrays $\{Y_{rc}\}$ and $\{Z_{rc}\}$, respectively.

4.2.4 Spatial Randomness

Another way of assessing whether any part of an array is emitting higher signals compared to the rest of the array is to check whether the "outliers" in either the signal or background are randomly scattered throughout the array or clustered together or distributed according to some pattern. In the algorithm in Section 4.2.3, this check could be used as Step 2. The assessment could be made using a simple test of complete spatial randomness, such as that proposed for a problem in ecology by Clark and Evans (1954).

Suppose that the array has G spots, r of which are "outliers." For the ith "outlier," let d_i be the distance to the "outlier" closest to it, so that

$$\overline{d} = \sum_{i=1}^{G} \frac{d_i}{G}$$

is the average nearest neighbor distance between the "outliers." The test statistic for complete spatial randomness is $\overline{d}$ or its standardized form

$$T_{\text{CSR}} = \frac{\overline{d} - 1/(2\sqrt{\rho})}{\sqrt{(4 - \pi)/4G\pi\rho}},$$

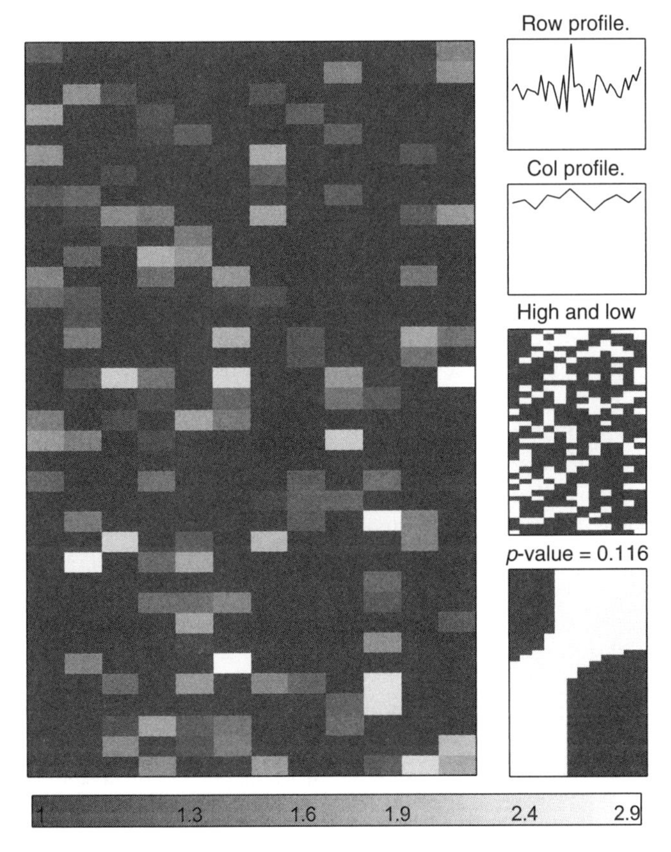

Figure 4.4 Image quality graph.

which has a standard normal distribution under complete spatial randomness. The parameter ρ can be estimated as $\hat{\rho} = r/G$. Note that two aspects of the data are being ignored in doing this test: nonindependence of some nearest neighbor distances and edge effects. More complex tests that adjust for these aspects of the data have been developed in the spatial data analysis field.

This method is fast and would produce good results for arrays where the outliers appear in small clusters, such as the bleeding spots, case 6 in the list in Section 4.2.3. If the smudge covers a large part of the array, then it would help to smooth the image, but it may be harder to detect with this approach.

4.2.5 Quality Control of Arrays

Rigorous quality assurance ensures that the accuracy and precision of an experimental process is maintained over time. Besides continuously making sure that the quality of the various individual steps of the microarray experimental protocol is being preserved, the experimenter should use the data being collected to monitor the stability, consistency, and overall performance of the experimental process as a whole.

Microarray experiments are usually performed over time. It is important to take this temporal effect into account because experimental conditions tend to be affected by time. For example, the sample could vary (perhaps degrade) over time, operators of varying ability may run the experiment over several days, various day effects (such as temperature and humidity) could affect the materials and the results, and so on. All these could potentially have a significant impact on experimental results. Therefore, such effects should be monitored carefully. Some of these effects, if reasonably small, may be accounted for at the modeling stage of the analysis. However, it is useful to be able to detect when an experiment may be going "out of control" in the early stages of an experiment or a series of experiments as it is being run, so that the experimenter can intervene immediately and address any experimental problems.

The process of data acquisition starts with the outcome of the experiment, that is, the microarray. The microarray is then scanned and the scanned raw image is processed to generate the spotted image. The spotted image is stored in the database.

A simple quality control procedure can be established at the moment when the spotted image is stored in the database by running a procedure that produces the following items.

1. An image quality graph, such as the one shown in Figure 4.4, could be used to detect specific problems with the array.
2. A side-by-side display of boxplots of the sequence of arrays that have been observed up to this point, or a set of summaries based on them, could be used to check whether there are any changes from the previous arrays to the current one.

This quality control process requires that the process of data acquisition be automated as much as possible, in order to avoid unnecessary delays on the experimental side. Figure 4.5 shows an experiment where a change in operator produced a shift in the scale of the observations in the last four arrays.

4.2.6 Assessment of Spot Quality

Once an array is deemed to be of satisfactory quality to be included in an analysis, the quality of the individual spots should be assessed. Actually, spot quality assessments could be done at two different stages of an analysis:

1. At the image-processing stage, the quality of a spot can be assessed by studying the properties of its pixel intensity distribution or its spot morphology (see Section 4.1.3). As it is unlikely that a single quantity could capture everything that could go wrong with a spot or a spot intensity measure, some composite index must be formed from the above quality metrics to flag suspect spots. These flagged spots can then be individually examined visually, if necessary.

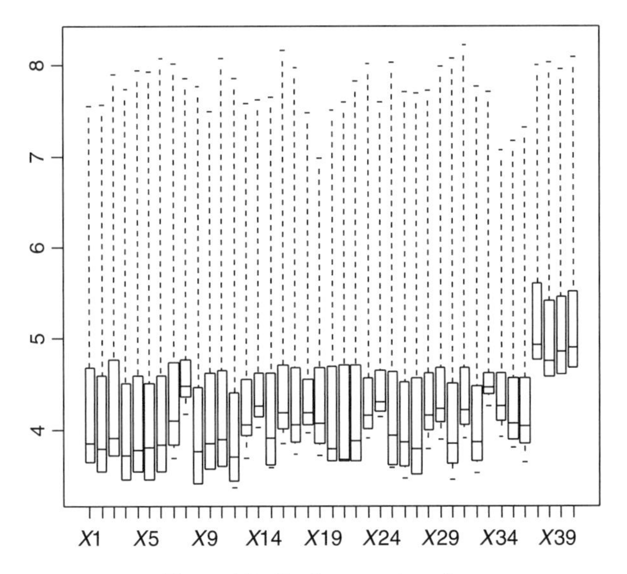

Figure 4.5 Quality control graph.

2. At the post-normalization stage, if replicates are available, each set of replicate spots can be analyzed to check whether any value in the set is markedly different from the others (this is described in Section 5.7). The replicates may be repeated spots on an array, technical replicates, or biological replicates. Exclusion or downweighting of spots that are considered low quality is likely to improve downstream analyses.

4.3 ADJUSTING FOR BACKGROUND

In principle, the intensities of those pixels not corresponding to spots should be zero. However, this never happens. Instead, because of various reasons such as nonspecific binding of the labeled sample to the array substrate and substrate fluorescence, these pixels emit a low, but not insubstantial, level of fluorescence, which may vary with location.

This leads to the concern that the spot intensities might also contain a certain amount of this nonspecific fluorescence, called the *background fluorescence*. It is customary, therefore, to estimate a background intensity from data and, assuming that the spot signal intensity is an additive combination of the true spot intensity and the background, subtract the background from the raw spot intensity values to yield a set of background-adjusted spot intensity values.

4.3.1 Estimating the Background

There are a few different ways in which the background is estimated.

Global Background Adjustment. A very simple estimate of the background is the average intensity of all the pixels not belonging to spots. However this naive approach is rarely effective, because the background often tends not be uniform over the entire microarray.

Example. Figure 4.6 is an image graph of the background intensities for a microarray of 140 rows and 24 columns. The left side of the graph shows the row and column medians, while the right side shows an image plot of the background. Clearly, there is some topographical variation across the slide. The intensities decrease moderately from the left to right along the columns and a few rows on the bottom of the array have higher intensities than the rest.

Spot Background Adjustment. The spot background can be subtracted from the spot intensity value to yield a *spot-background-adjusted spot intensity values*. However, the segmentation process, which separates spot from background, is usually imperfect and the spot background often contains a contribution from the signal. This manifests itself as a nonzero correlation between spot intensity and background intensity; spots with high intensity tend to have high spot local background, whereas spots with low intensity tend to have low spot background. In this case, it is evident that subtracting the spot local background would not be the right idea.

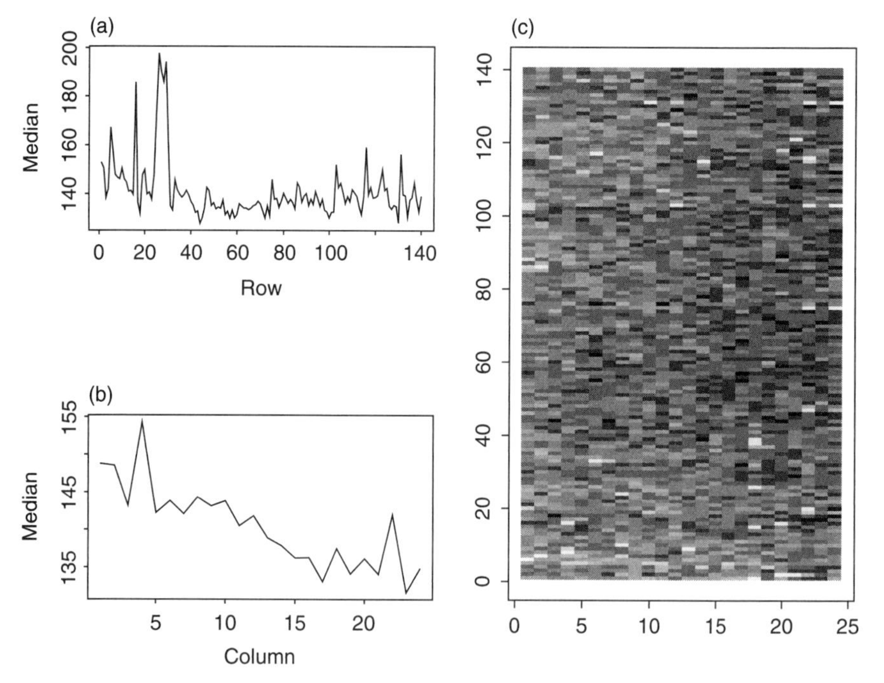

Figure 4.6 (a,b) Line graphs of background showing the row and column medians. (c) Image plot of the background.

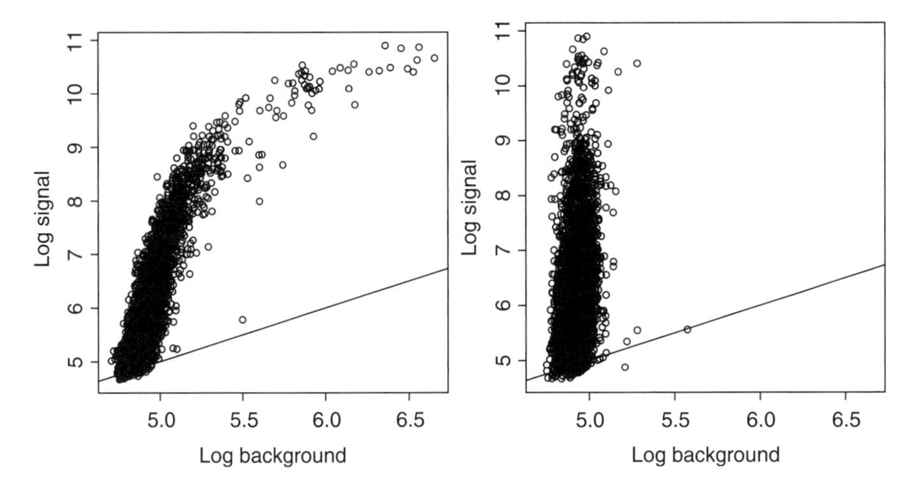

Figure 4.7 Scatterplots of signal versus background before and after local smoothing.

Example. Figure 4.7a shows a scatterplot of spot intensity versus background intensity, both on a log scale. The Spearman's correlation coefficient (see Section 5.6) is 0.92, indicating a strong monotone relationship.

Smoothed Background Adjustment. The true variation in background across an array should be smooth as it is due to experimental effects, such as hybridization artifacts, the washing process, and scanning variation, that vary gradually across the slide. The background may be smoothed by running a simple smoothing procedure through the array. For example, one simple smoothing procedure is to take the median of the 49 values in the 7×7 subgrid surrounding a spot as the smoothed background value at the spot. Yang et al. (2000) describe a more sophisticated smoothing procedure called *morphological opening*.

Example. Figure 4.7b shows a scatterplot of spot intensity versus smoothed background intensity, both on a log scale. The smoothed background values are now uniformly distributed across the spot intensity values. Nevertheless, certain spatial features, notably the left-to-right gradient and the rows of high intensities in the bottom rows still remain, as shown by Figure 4.8, which is the smoothed background analog of Figure 4.6. In other words, while the sporadic high background intensities that were associated with the high signal spots have been dampened by the smoothing, the background is not uniform throughout the slide.

Zonal Background Adjustment. Affymetrix uses a variation of smoothed background adjustment called *zonal background adjustment* for its oligonucleotide microarrays. This approach can also be used with cDNA microarrays.

First, the microarray is split up into K rectangular zones, Z_k, $k = 1, \ldots, K$ (Affymetrix uses the default $K = 16$). For each zone, a low percentile of the spot intensities, S_{Ig}, is chosen as the background, B_k, for that zone (Affymetrix uses the

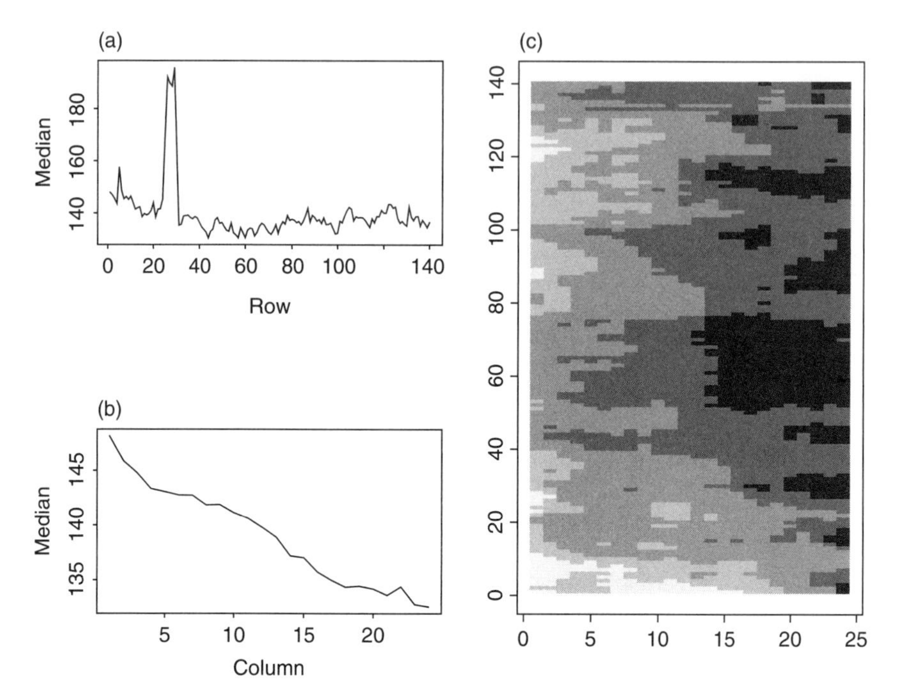

Figure 4.8 (a,b) Line graph of locally smoothed background showing the row and column medians. (c) Image plot of the smoothed background.

second percentile as its default; this is the value such that 98% of spot intensity values are larger than it and 2% are smaller).

If we were to just use B_k as the background for zone Z_k, there could be a sharp transition in background estimates when crossing a zone. As this is unlikely to reflect reality, a smoothed version of these background estimates is used instead. The background for a given spot is then a weighted sum of all the B_k values, where the weights are inversely proportional to how far the spot is from the various zone centers; that is, if the distance between the gth spot and the center of Z_k is d_{gk}, the gth spot would be assigned a weight $w_{gk} = 1/d_{gk}^2$. In practice, a small positive factor, d_0, is added to the denominator to ensure that it will never be zero, so that $w_{gk} = 1/(d_{gk}^2 + d_0)$. The background, BI_g, for the gth spot is then the weighted sum

$$BI_g = \frac{\sum_{k=1}^{K} w_{gk} B_k}{\sum_{k=1}^{K} w_{gk}}.$$

4.3.2 Adjusting for the Estimated Background

Most arrays generally have a background that, even after smoothing, is not spatially uniform. This background could be sizable enough to affect the spot intensity distribution and therefore any downstream analysis. Therefore, it is generally removed from the spot intensities before formal analysis.

Suppose that the spot intensity at the gth spot is SI_g and the background intensity was estimated to be BI_g. The *background-adjusted spot intensity value*, AI_g, is obtained by shifting the spot intensity down by the background intensity:

$$\mathrm{AI}_g = \mathrm{SI}_g - \mathrm{BI}_g.$$

In principle, SI_g should be larger than BI_g. However, either due to some problem or perhaps purely due to random variability, this may not always be the case and BI_g could exceed SI_g, leading to a negative value for AI_g. As this is not desirable, sometimes a small additional adjustment may be made.

One very simple way to do this is to set a threshold. For example, if T is a low percentile of the SI_g values (e.g., the 5th percentile), take the *background-adjusted threshold spot intensity value*, AI_g, to be

$$\mathrm{AI}_g = \max(\mathrm{SI}_g - \mathrm{BI}_g, T).$$

While all these suggestions are reasonable, how to properly adjust for spatially nonuniform background still appears to be an open research problem.

4.4 EXPRESSION-LEVEL CALCULATION FOR TWO-CHANNEL cDNA MICROARRAYS

Let the adjusted spot intensities for the two channels of a two-channel array be $\{\mathrm{AI}_{gR}\}$ and $\{\mathrm{AI}_{gG}\}$, where the letters R and G refer to the colors, red and green respectively, that are typically used to label the channels. If channel G is a reference channel, then the expression level of the gth gene in channel R is usually stated as *a gene expression ratio*:

$$R_g = \frac{\mathrm{AI}_{gR}}{\mathrm{AI}_{gG}}.$$

Usually, however, there is a systematic effect due to the use of two different dyes that needs to be removed from $\{\mathrm{AI}_{gR}\}$ and $\{\mathrm{AI}_{gG}\}$ by normalization before calculating these ratios (see Section 5.5.4).

4.5 EXPRESSION-LEVEL CALCULATION FOR OLIGONUCLEOTIDE MICROARRAYS

In high-density oligonucleotide microarrays, such as those manufactured by Affymetrix, a gene is represented by a probe set, which is a set of twenty or so oligonucleotides called the *perfect match probes*, along with a set of paired mismatch probes. The expression level for a gene, which Affymetrix refers to as the gene's *signal*, is therefore not directly measured, but rather obtained by combining the perfect match and mismatch intensities of the probe set for the gene in some way. There are several ways in which a composite value can be calculated.

4.5.1 The Average Difference

Let PM_{gi} and MM_{gi} denote the (untransformed) background-adjusted spot intensity measurements for the ith perfect match probe and mismatch probe respectively for gene g ($i = 1, \ldots, m_g$, $g = 1, \ldots, G$). Noting that $Y_{gi} = \mathrm{PM}_{gi} - \mathrm{MM}_{gi}$ functions as a measure of the hybridization level of the gth gene's ith probe, the most natural estimate of the signal, S_g, for the gth gene is

$$S_g = \frac{\sum_{i=1}^{m_g} (\mathrm{PM}_{gi} - \mathrm{MM}_{gi})}{m_g} = \frac{\sum_{i=1}^{m_g} Y_{gi}}{m_g}.$$

In other words, S_g is the arithmetic mean of the Y_{gi} values. One of Affymetrix's early approaches was exactly this, with one modification: in order to lessen the impact of gross outliers on this estimate, any Y_{gi} value further than three standard deviations away from the mean is discarded from the calculation of S_g. Affymetrix called this estimate the *average difference* (an older version used a trimmed mean, which Affymetrix referred to as *Olympic scoring*). However, recognizing problems with this estimator, Affymetrix has recently modified their algorithm.

4.5.2 A Weighted Average Difference

One problem with the average difference is that, even though the mismatch probes are placed on the array to provide probe-specific estimates of any stray signal due to nonspecific hybridization that may affect the perfect match probe, it could happen that MM_{gi} also contains some portion of the true target signal. Thus a nonlinear relationship between the PM_{gi} and MM_{gi} intensities can often be detected. Therefore, each MM_{gi} value may have to be adjusted to give an ideal mismatch value, IM_{gi}, before subtracting it from its corresponding PM_{gi}.

If PM_{gi} exceeds MM_{gi}, Y_{gi} represents a possible measure of the true hybridization level for the ith probe for the gth gene and IM_{gi} is usually set to MM_{gi}. On the other hand, if MM_{gi} exceeds PM_{gi}, which could happen either due to some biological or physical effect or due to random variability, Y_{gi} is negative and no longer represents a possible measure of the hybridization level. In this case, Affymetrix recommends using an algorithm they developed for calculating a value for IM_{gi} that satisfies $0 < \mathrm{IM}_{gi} < \mathrm{PM}_{gi}$ on the basis of the behavior of the totality of probes in the gth probe set (the Affymetrix web site offers details).

Once this is done, S_g is calculated as an average of the Y_{gi} values, where now $Y_{gi} = \mathrm{PM}_{gi} - \mathrm{IM}_{gi}$ (and all $Y_{gi} > 0$). However, as the Y_{gi} values may contain outliers, instead of merely taking their arithmetic mean as above, they are log transformed (let $X_{gi} = \log(Y_{gi})$), then averaged using their one-step biweight mean, and, finally, exponentiated back to the original scale, that is,

$$S_g = \exp(T_{\mathrm{biwt}}\{X_{gi}\}).$$

The log transformation reduces the skewness of distribution of $\{Y_{gi}\}$ and the use of the one-step biweight mean reduces the influence of outliers on the final estimate.

The *one-step biweight mean* is a weighted mean that offers both efficiency as well as resistance to outliers. It is calculated as follows. Let M_g and MAD_g denote, respectively, the median and the MAD (median absolute deviation from the median) of the $\{X_{gi}\}$. For each observation, X_{gi}, calculate $u_{gi} = (X_{gi} - M_g)/\tau\mathrm{MAD}_g$, which indicates how "unusual" it is, then assign it a weight w_{gi} based on the *biweight weighting function*: $w(u) = (1 - u^2)^2$ if $|u| < 1$ and $w(u) = 0$ otherwise. The weighting process is such that observations relatively close to the center of the data will be assigned high weights, while if there are any observations relatively far from the center of the data, that is, outliers, they will be assigned low weights. The *tuning constant*, τ determines the amount of efficiency and resistance desired. The larger τ is, the more efficient the estimator is if the $\{X_{gi}\}$ are normally distributed, but the more vulnerable it is to being affected by outliers. The smaller τ is, the less efficient the estimator is if the $\{X_{gi}\}$ are normally distributed, but the less influenced it is by outliers. A compromise between these two extremes offers both high efficiency at the normal distribution and resistance should the data contain outliers. The one-step biweight mean is the weighted mean:

$$T_{\mathrm{biwt}}(\{X_{gi}\}) = \frac{\sum_{i=1}^{m_g} w_{gi} X_{gi}}{\sum_{i=1}^{m_g} w_{gi}}.$$

Various other averaging methods have been proposed. For instance, Efron et al. (2001) explored the possibility of averaging $\{\log(\mathrm{PM}_{gi}) - c \log(\mathrm{MM}_{gi})\}$, with a preference for the compromise value for c of 0.5.

4.5.3 Perfect Matches Only

Concerned that MM_{gi} contains too much target signal to function as a true measure of nonspecific hybridization, some investigators prefer to avoid utilizing them altogether (e.g., Naef et al., 2001). These investigators calculate S_g as an average of the PM_{gi} values. However, as the distribution of $\{\mathrm{PM}_{gi}\}$ is usually skewed, instead of merely taking their arithmetic mean as in Section 4.5.1, it is better to log transform them before averaging, and use as signal either

$$S_g = \exp\left(\frac{\sum_{i=1}^{m_g} \log\ (M_{gi})}{m_g}\right),$$

or the one-step biweight mean described in Section 4.5.2 with $\text{IM}_{gi} = 0$.

4.5.4 Background Adjustment Approach

Irizarry et al. (2003) examined the distribution of $\{\text{MM}_{gi}\}$ on an array and, observing that it was consistent with a mixture of low background intensities and high signals caused by probes mistakenly hybridizing to some transcript, concluded that the mode of this distribution constituted a natural estimate of background for the array. Estimating the mode using a density kernel estimate and using it as the background, an average of the background-adjusted perfect match values is then the estimate of signal:

$$S_g = \exp\left(\frac{\sum_{i=1}^{m_g} \log\ (M_{gi} - \text{mode}(\log\ (\text{MM}_{gi})))}{m_g}\right),$$

4.5.5 Model-Based Approach

Li and Wong (2001b) proposed a model-based approach. Their model

$$Y_{gi} = \text{PM}_{gi} - \text{MM}_{gi} = \theta_g \phi_{gi} + \varepsilon n_{ij},$$

postulates that the perfect match to mismatch difference is, except for random error, $\varepsilon_{gi}\quad N(0, \sigma_g^2)$, the product of a model-based expression index θ_g, whose estimate functions as S_g, and a probe-specific sensitivity index ϕ_{gi}. The model parameters are estimated using maximum likelihood and S_g is estimated as a weighted mean:

$$S_g = \exp\left(\frac{\sum_{i=1}^{m_g} \phi_{gi}(\text{PM}_{gi} - \text{MM}_{gi})}{m_g}\right),$$

The Li and Wong model is most useful when several replicates are available (see Section 6.2).

4.5.6 Absent–Present Calls

The availability of several PM_{gi} and MM_{gi} intensities for a probe set allows the reliability of the measurement of the signal corresponding to that probe set to be assessed. The rationale behind the procedure is that a probe set whose probe pairs consistently exhibit PM_{gi} intensities greatly exceeding their corresponding MM_{gi} intensities is more likely displaying a reliable signal than one whose PM_{gi} intensities are all close to their corresponding MM_{gi} intensities.

On the basis of this rationale, Affymetrix reports, for each gene on the array, an *absolute call*, which indicates whether the transcript (mRNA) for that gene was likely to have been present, absent or marginal in the sample. A *present call* (P, for short) indicates a gene for which there was enough transcript in the sample to quantify the abundance of that transcript to an acceptable degree of reliability. In most cases, the genes that are so designated can be considered to be expressed. On the other hand, an *absent call* (A, for short) indicates the exact opposite. This does not necessarily imply that the transcript was absent in the sample but rather that the amount of transcript could not be established reliably. A *marginal call* (M, for short) indicates that the detectable level of transcript for that gene was close to negligible.

One simple way to assign an absolute call is to calculate the t-statistic (see Chapter 7):

$$T_g = \frac{S_g}{\mathrm{se}(S_g)},$$

and check whether it exceeds a specific cutoff.

Affymetrix's algorithm is based on a rank-based statistic. For probe set g, each probe pair, i, is assigned a score R_{gi}:

$$R_{gi} = \frac{\mathrm{PM}_{gi} - \mathrm{MM}_{gi}}{\mathrm{PM}_{gi} + \mathrm{MM}_{gi}}.$$

A probe pair whose PM_{gi} intensity greatly exceeds its MM_{gi} intensity will have an R_{gi} score close to unity, whereas a probe pair whose PM_{gi} and MM_{gi} intensities are roughly similar will have an R_{gi} score close to zero. The scores for a probe set are then ranked from 1 to m_g according to their distance from r, a specified low threshold (e.g., 0.15). The sum, R_{g+}, of the ranks of all probe pairs whose R_{gi} exceeds r is the *one-sided Wilcoxon's signed rank test* statistic for testing whether the R_{gi} scores are consistently below r. The p-value, p_a, associated with this statistic can be obtained. A probe set that has many R_{gi} scores near unity and is therefore considered more reliable will have a large R_{gi} and, therefore, a low (more significant) p-value, whereas one with many R_{gi} scores near zero will have a small R_{gi} and, therefore, a high (less significant) p-value. An absolute call is then made based on this p-value, for example, if $p_a < 0.04$, a present call is made, if $0.04 < p_a < 0.06$, a marginal call is made, if $p_a > 0.06$, an absent call is made.

Absolute calls are often used for gene filtering purposes.

SUPPLEMENTARY READING

The ScanAlyze user manual written by Eisen, available online at `http://www.microarrays.org/software.html` user manuals of other image processing software, such as Genepix, QuantArray, Genespring, and Imagene, and the Affymetrix white papers, available online at `http://www.affymetrix.com/index.affx` provide useful information about the topics covered in this chapter.

SOFTWARE NOTES

`DNAMR 2.0`

This package implements the data visualization dianostic plots producing the graphs in this chapter.

`www.rci.rutgers.edu/~cabrera/DNAMR.`

EXERCISES

Use the data set `p4.txt` that is found in the book web site. This data set consists of 432 genes by 14 columns. The first two columns are labeled row and column representing the positions of the spots on the slide. The next 12 columns are labeled $S1, \ldots, S6, B1, \ldots, B6$, representing data from six microarrays. The column labeled $S1$ is the signal data and the column labeled B1 is the background data for microarray number 1. In the same way, S_i and B_i correspond to the ith microarray for $i = 1, \ldots, 6$. Each microarray is made of 36 rows and 12 columns that correspond to the positions of the spots on the chip.

4.1. Extract the data and place it in 12 separate arrays of dimension 36×12, 6 for signal arrays and 6 for background arrays. Verify that the array rows and columns are correctly placed by manually checking a few individual spots. As a check of the quality of the arrays, explore the individual arrays using image plots and compare the intensities and backgrounds using scatterplots. Try to evaluate the data quality with the information that you have collected at this stage.

4.2. Some of the six background images in the data set may show that the corresponding sample is defective, from the point of view that each one may have one or more of the nonrandom patterns listed in Section 4.2. Identify the samples that you think are defective and which appear to pass the quality check. Note: If you use `R` or `SPLUS` the functions for performing, several quality checking routines are available in the DNAMR package.

4.3. Use the complete spatial randomness (CSR) criterion to check for nonrandom arrays among the set and compare the results of the test to the results that you obtained in Problem 4.2.

4.4. Perform a background correction of the six arrays in two ways:

(a) Take the difference between the signal and background and take the ratio between signal and background. Which one gives the most reasonable results?

(b) Draw pairwise scatterplots of the microarrays before and after you remove the background and use the graph to justify whether or not to adjust and which way is better.

4.5. Another way to remove the background is to smooth the background using a spatial smoother. You may use the function provided for this purpose in our `R/SPLUS` library DNAMR.

(a) Once the background intensities have been smoothed, repeat the same tasks as in Problem 4.4, but using the smoothed background.

(b) Write a brief summary of the results of both problems. State which background correction method appears to work best and why.

CHAPTER 5

Preprocessing Microarray Data

Once the experiment has been run and the spot intensity data have been collected, it is necessary to preprocess this data before formally analyzing it. Preprocessing is needed to address several data-related issues:

1. to transform the data into a scale suitable for analysis,
2. to remove the effects of systematic sources of variation,
3. to identify discrepant observations and arrays.

Preprocessing can greatly enhance the quality of any downstream analyses. We will now discuss each of these issues in turn.

Example. The methods in this chapter are illustrated using the Mouse5 data, which is from an experiment involving 10 pairs of microarrays, C1A, C1B, C2A, C2B, ..., C10A, C10B. Each pair of microarrays corresponds to a single mRNA sample (labeled C1, C2, ..., C10), which was taken from a mouse following treatment and hybridized to two separate microarrays (labeled A and B). The two microarrays in each pair are technical replicates as they are exposed to the same biological sample. The five mice from which samples C1–C5 were drawn are controls, so they are biological replicates, while each of the other five was treated with one of five drugs. There were 3300 genes arrayed on the microarrays.

5.1 LOGARITHMIC TRANSFORMATION

Often, spot intensity data are initially transformed by a *logarithmic transformation*, $X \rightarrow \log(X)$, for analysis. It is preferable to work with logged intensities rather than absolute intensities for a number of reasons: the variation of logged intensities

Exploration and Analysis of DNA Microarray and Other High-Dimensional Data, Second Edition.
Dhammika Amaratunga, Javier Cabrera, Ziv Shkedy.

tends to be less dependent on the magnitude of the values, taking logs reduces the skewness of highly skewed distributions, and taking logs improves variance estimation.

Moreover, it facilitates visual inspection of the data. The raw data are often very heavily clumped together at low intensities followed by a very long tail. More than 75% of the data may lie in the lowest 10% in the range of intensities. The details of such configurations are impossible to discern. After a log transformation, the data are spread out rather more evenly, making it easier to examine visually.

Often, logarithms base 2 are used. Other simple *power transformations* (i.e., transformations of the form $X \to X^{\beta}$ for some $\beta > 0$) have been found to be useful for certain data sets (e.g., Amaratunga and Cabrera, 2001a, 2001b use a square root transformation, $X \to \sqrt{X}$, and Tusher, Tibshirani, and Chu, 2001, use a cube root transformation, $X \to X^{1/3}$), but the log transformation is, by far, the most widely used.

Example. Figure 5.1 shows a histogram and normal probability plot of the data for C1A before and after log transformation. It is clear that the transformation greatly reduced the skewness of the distribution, but it did not eliminate it altogether. We use the log-transformed data in the remainder of this chapter.

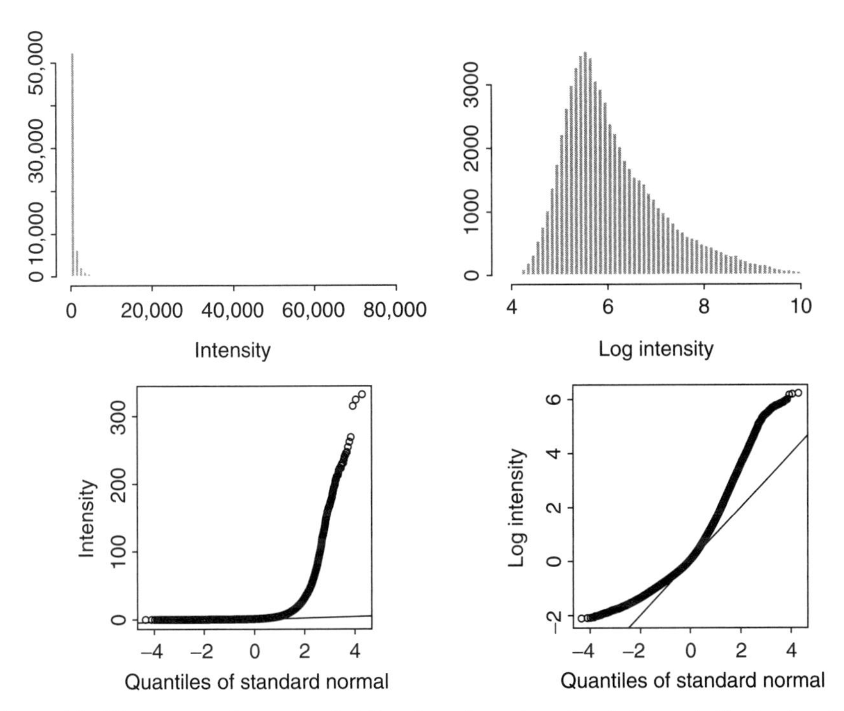

Figure 5.1 Histograms and normal probability plots of spot intensities before and after log transformation. The straight lines in the normal probability plots are identity lines.

5.2 VARIANCE STABILIZING TRANSFORMATIONS

Several data analysts observed that more complex transformations, such as the *started log transformation*, $X \to \log\,(X + c)$, appeared to better achieve the dual objective of symmetrizing the spot intensity data and stabilizing their variances (e.g., Sapir and Churchill, 2000, use such a transformation).

The rationale for this was investigated in greater detail by Rocke and Durbin (2001) using data from experiments involving arrays with replicate spots. In analogy with models used for estimating the actual concentration of an analyte in a sample for a given response, they found that it was appropriate to model spot intensity data as

$$X = \alpha + \mu^{\eta} + \varepsilon,$$

where α is the mean background, μ is the true expression level, and the terms η and ε represent normally distributed error terms with mean zero and variances σ_η^2 and σ_ε^2, respectively. Spot intensity data often manifest the distributional features implied by this model:

- At very low expression levels, where μ is close to zero, the measured spot intensity is dominated by the first term in the model, so that $X \cong \alpha$ and X is approximately normally distributed with mean α and variance ε.
- At very high expression levels, where μ is large, the measured spot intensity is dominated by the second term in the model, so that $X \cong \mu e^{\eta}$ and X is approximately lognormally distributed with variance, $\mu^2 S_\eta^2$, where $S_\eta^2 = \exp\,(\sigma_\eta^2)(\exp\,(\sigma_\eta^2 - 1)$. Thus, the variance of X varies linearly with μ^2. However, on the log scale, $\log\,(X) \cong \log\,(\mu) + \eta$, indicating that the variance of $\log\,(X)$ is constant.
- At moderate expression levels, the measured spot intensity is in between the above two extremes and behaves as a mixture of a normal and log normal distribution with variance $\mu^2 S_\eta^2 + \sigma_\eta^2$, which, again, varies with μ.

Durbin et al. (2002) showed that the *generalized log transformation*

$$X \to \left((X - \alpha) + \sqrt{(X - \alpha)^2 + \frac{\sigma_\varepsilon^2}{\sigma_\eta^2}} \right),$$

stabilizes variance in that the transformed data has constant variance equal to S_η^2. A similar transformation was suggested by Huber et al. (2002).

In order to apply this transformation, the parameters α, σ_η^2, and σ_ε^2 must be estimated from the spot intensity data. If replicate blanks or negative controls are available, the background parameters, α and σ_ε^2, can be estimated as their mean and variance. If not, they can be estimated as the mean and variance of a set of unexpressed genes. The parameter σ_η^2 can be estimated as the mean and variance of a set of highly expressed genes. Details of the procedure are provided by Rocke and Durbin (2001).

Unfortunately, by using the generalized log transformation, the convenient interpretation of log ratios as log fold changes (see Chapter 7), which is possible with an ordinary log transformation, is lost. Rocke and Durbin (2002) demonstrate that the started log transformation, $X \rightarrow \log(X + c)$, with $c = \sigma_\varepsilon^2 / S_\eta^2$, is a reasonable compromise.

5.3 SOURCES OF BIAS

The complexities and intricacies of the microarray experimental process often introduce systematic effects into the intensity measurements. These effects can be substantial enough to dilute the effects that the experimenter is trying to detect. Systematic effects have been attributed to, among other sources of variability:

- the concentration and amount of DNA placed on the microarrays, arraying equipment such as spotting pins that wear out over time, mRNA preparation, reverse transcription bias, labeling efficiency, hybridization efficiency, lack of spatial homogeneity of the hybridization on the slide, scanner settings, saturation effects, background fluorescence, linearity of detection response, and ambient conditions.

In addition, *dye bias* is present in almost all multichannel experiments. Generally, the Cy5 (red) intensities tend to be higher than the Cy3 (green) intensities, but the magnitude of the difference generally depends on the overall intensity. The reason for the imbalance between the channels is the difference between the physicochemical properties of the dyes, the labeling efficiencies, the scanning properties of the dyes, and the scanner settings.

Some of these sources of variability can be controlled to a limited extent with due diligence on the part of the experimenter. However, few can be completely eliminated.

Because systematic variation will generally affect different microarrays to different extents, in order to be able to make valid comparisons across microarrays, we need to try and remove the effects of such systematic variations and bring the data from the different microarrays onto a common scale.

5.4 NORMALIZATION

Early microarray researchers noticed substantial differences in intensity measurements even among microarrays that were treated exactly alike. Differences still persist despite huge improvements in the technology, but their magnitude is not as high as in the early days. The differences can generally be traced to systematic effects as described in Section 5.3 above. The purpose of *normalization* is to remove, by data processing, as much as possible, the effects of any systematic sources of variation. Normalization can be regarded as a sort of calibration process that improves the comparability among microarrays treated alike.

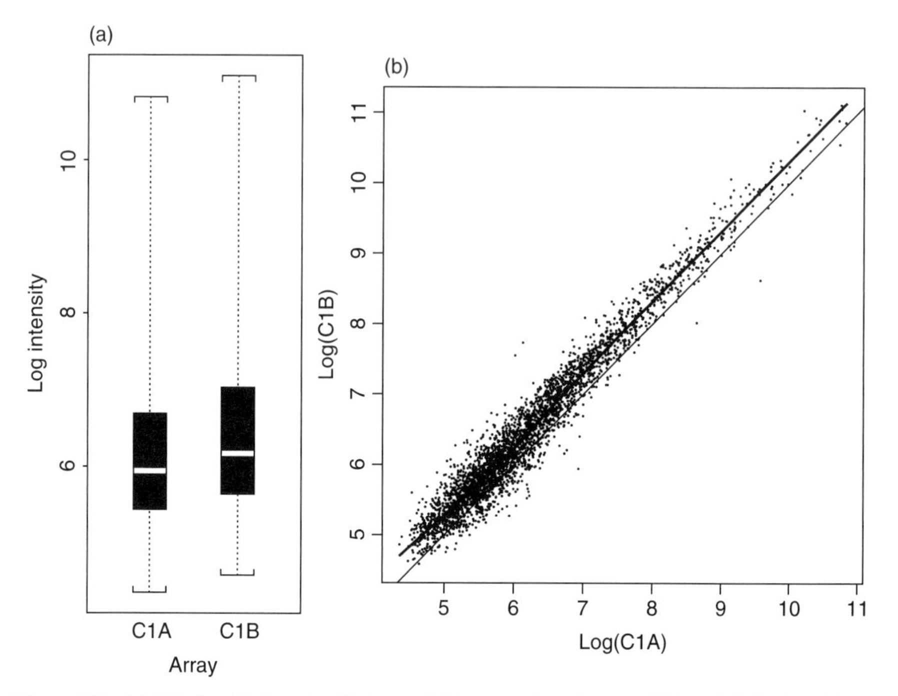

Figure 5.2 (a) Side-by-side boxplot display and (b) scatterplot of arrays C1A and C1B. The thinner line on the scatterplot is the identity line and the thicker line is a smooth of the plot.

Example. In Figure 5.2, the data from microarrays C1A and C1B are plotted against one another. Even though both were hybridized to the same sample, it is clear that the intensities are systematically higher in microarray C1B compared to microarray C1A. In Figure 5.3, the data from microarrays C1B and C5B are plotted against one another. These microarrays were hybridized to different samples, but, because the samples were taken shortly after treatment, it is highly unlikely that more than a few genes would be differentially expressed in the two. Yet the plot shows most of the intensities are generally higher in microarray C1B compared to microarray C1A.

Early efforts at normalization used simple methods. One such method is *normalization by the sum*. In this method, the sums of the intensities of the k microarrays being normalized are forced to be equal to one another. The rationale for doing this is that the total mRNA content should be roughly the same across samples. Suppose that the k original sums were $X_{1+}, \ldots, X_{k+}$. If we divide all the observations in the ith microarray by X_{i+}, their sum will be 1. Doing this for all the microarrays would make all the sums equal (to 1), as desired.

Example. Figure 5.4 shows the data from microarrays C1A and C1B plotted against each other after normalization by the sum. Now the observations are more in agreement.

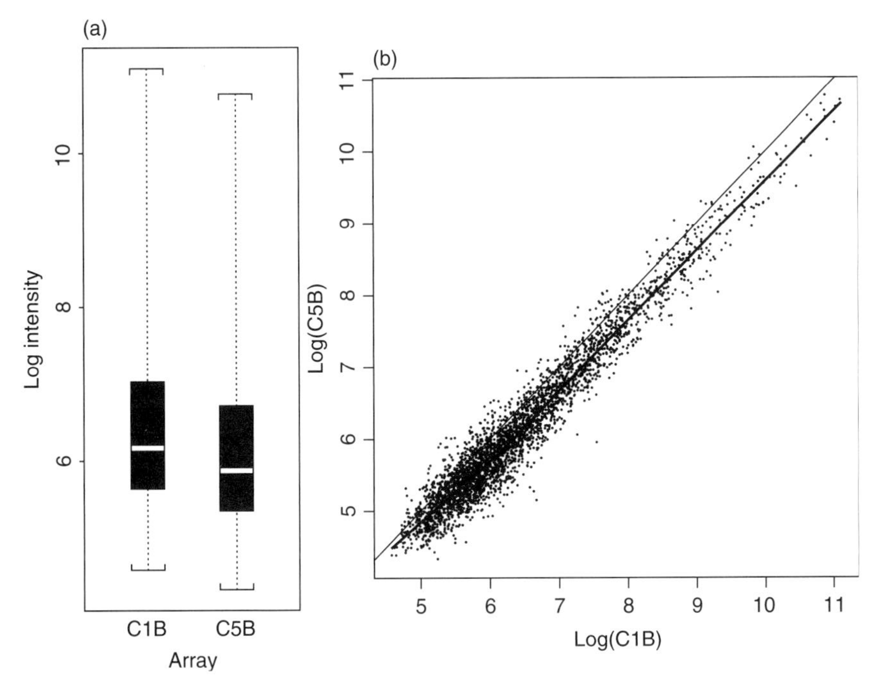

Figure 5.3 (a) Side-by-side boxplot display and (b) scatterplot of arrays C1A and C5B. The thinner line on the scatterplot is the identity line and the thicker line is a smooth of the plot.

An entirely equivalent method is *normalization by the mean*, in which the arithmetic means of the microarrays are equated. A similar, but not equivalent, idea is *normalization by the median*, in which the microarray medians are equated. *Q3 normalization*, in which third quartiles are equated, is on the same lines and is reasonable when it is expected that about half the genes are unexpressed and the third quartile is then roughly the median intensity of the expressed genes.

All these are examples of *global or linear normalization* schemes. The common feature of these normalization schemes is that they assume that the spot intensities on every pair of arrays being normalized are linearly related with no intercept, so that the lack of comparability can be corrected by adjusting every single spot intensity on any microarray by the same amount, called the *normalizing factor*, regardless of its intensity level.

5.5 INTENSITY-DEPENDENT NORMALIZATION

The relationship between the spot intensities in Figure 5.2 is clearly nonlinear. It suggests that the factor necessary to adjust low-intensity measurements should be different from that of high-intensity measurements. In other words, an *intensity-dependent normalization* method, a normalization scheme in which the normalizing

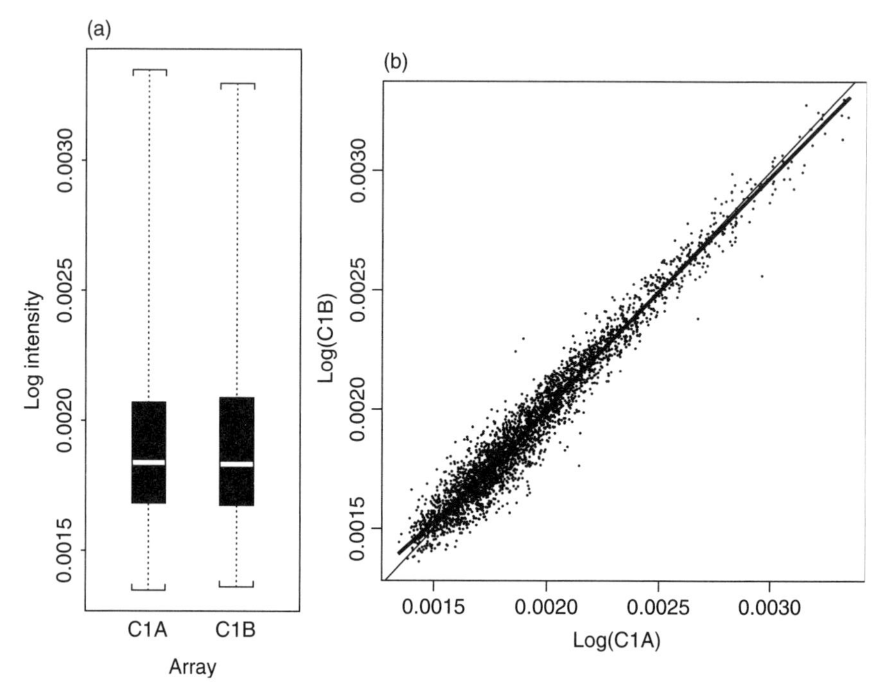

Figure 5.4 (a) Side-by-side boxplot display and (b) scatterplot of arrays C1A and C1B after mean normalization. The thinner line on the scatterplot is the identity line and the thicker line is a smooth of the plot.

factor is a function of intensity level, should be preferable to any global normalization method. In intensity-dependent normalization, the transformed spot intensity data is normalized using a *nonlinear normalization function*: $X \to f(X)$.

As it arises naturally by studying plots such as Figure 5.2, the need for intensity-dependent normalization was recognized independently by a number of different data analysts, including Amaratunga and Cabrera (1999, 2001a, 2001b), Dudoit et al. (2002), Li and Wong (2001a), Schadt et al. (2000, 2001), and Yang et al., (2001). Other papers on this topic include Astrand (2003), Bolstad et al. (2002), Colantuoni et al. (2002), Hoffmann et al. (2002), Irizarry et al. (2003), Quackenbush (2002), Tseng et al. (2001), and Yang et al. (2002). Hoffmann et al. (2002) and Yang et al. (2002) demonstrated that normalization could have a profound effect on downstream analysis.

For an intensity-dependent normalization, there must be a *reference or baseline* microarray to which all the microarrays are normalized. In the absence of a universal standard against which the arrays can be calibrated, this is usually some sort of average microarray, a mock array fashioned out of the averages of the arrays being normalized. One possibility is the *median mock* array. If X_{gi} denotes the transformed spot intensity measurement for the gth gene ($g = 1, \ldots, G$) in the ith microarray ($i = 1, \ldots, I$), the median mock array will have as its gth observation:

$$M_g = \text{median}\{X_{g1}, \ldots, X_{gI}\}.$$

Before constructing the reference microarray, it is generally a good idea to first perform a median or Q_3 normalization, so that all the microarrays are brought to a common overall level to start with and each can contribute to the construction of the reference microarray.

One key issue for any normalization is the selection of an *invariant gene set*, the subset of genes that will be used to estimate the normalization functions. This set of genes should exhibit the following characteristics:

1. Their expression levels should remain constant across the arrays being normalized, so that they can be used to estimate the normalization functions.
2. Their expression levels should span the entire range of expression levels observed in the experiment, so that it will not be necessary to extrapolate the estimated normalization functions.
3. The normalization relationship for these genes should be representative of the normalization relationship for all the genes, so that they can be used to normalize all. The invariant gene set could be

- *Control genes.* A small number of DNA sequences could be specially arrayed onto the microarray specifically for normalization purposes. Synthetic or cross-species DNA sequences have been used for this purpose. Then, if necessary, DNA sequences complementary to these sequences would be spiked into the probe at a known concentration. One concern with this procedure is whether characteristic (3) is satisfied.
- *Housekeeping genes.* A small number of housekeeping genes could be arrayed onto the microarray. If it can be assumed that these genes express at about the same level across the set of arrays being normalized, these genes will form an invariant gene set. However, a number of the more commonly used housekeeping genes have been found to express differentially across various samples, so whether they satisfy characteristic (1) is debatable. If they are all low to moderate expressing genes, they also may not adequately satisfy characteristic (2).
- *Unchanging genes.* Metrics from the raw data could be used to select a subset of genes that appear to be the least likely to be differentially expressed. One way to do this is to rank the spot intensities on each array, including the reference microarray, from smallest to largest, and then to select those genes whose ranks across the microarrays are the least different from the reference microarray as the invariant gene set. If the gene set is not carefully chosen, characteristics (1) and (2) may not be adequately satisfied.
- *All the genes on the array.* If it is reasonable to expect that only a very small percentage of the genes would be differentially expressed across the arrays being normalized, as is the case with many microarray experiments, then the

entire set of genes on the microarray can be used as the invariant gene set because most normalization schema are robust to small perturbations. This assumption will be more realistic (and characteristic (1) more likely to be satisfied), the larger the number of genes on the arrays and the smaller the percentage of genes differentially expressed across the arrays being normalized.

As with global normalization, intensity-dependent normalization can be performed in several different ways.

5.5.1 Smooth Function Normalization

In smooth function normalization, each microarray is normalized as follows. First, the inverse, $g_i = f_i^{-1}$, of the monotone normalization function, f_i, for the ith microarray, is estimated by fitting the model

$$X_{gi} = g_i(M_g) + \varepsilon_{gi},$$

where ε_{gi} is a random error term, to the $(X_{gi},\ M_g)$ data for the invariant gene set. The normalized values for the ith microarray are then obtained from

$$X'_{gi} = f_i(X_{gi}).$$

In *spline normalization*, the function g_i is a smooth but flexible function such as a cubic spline with a small number (e.g., 7) of degrees of freedom; the smaller the degrees of freedom, the smoother the fit. In *lowess normalization*, the function g_i is estimated by fitting a lowess smooth (Cleveland, 1979) to the invariant gene set. The lowess smooth is essentially a series of locally linear fits, each fitted robustly so as to limit the influence of outliers. A user-specified parameter, span, denotes the fraction of data (e.g., span $= 1/3$) used for smoothing at any data point; the larger it is, the smoother the fit. Note that neither of these methods is affected by a small percentage of outliers. Alternative smoothers such as a multilinear continuous function, a piecewise running median or kernel-based methods may also be used.

Example. Figure 5.5 shows the data from microarrays C1B and C5B plotted against each other after spline normalization. As these are biological replicates and, other than natural variability, no differential expression was expected between the two, all 3300 genes were used as the invariant gene set. The observations are now in good agreement.

5.5.2 Quantile Normalization

Quantile normalization was first introduced by Amaratunga and Cabrera (1999, 2001a, 2001b) under the name of quantile standardization and the name was changed to quantile normalization by Irizarry et al. (2003). The objective of quantile normalization is to make the distributions of the transformed spot intensities, $\{X_{gi}\}$, as similar as possible across the microarrays, or, at least as similar as

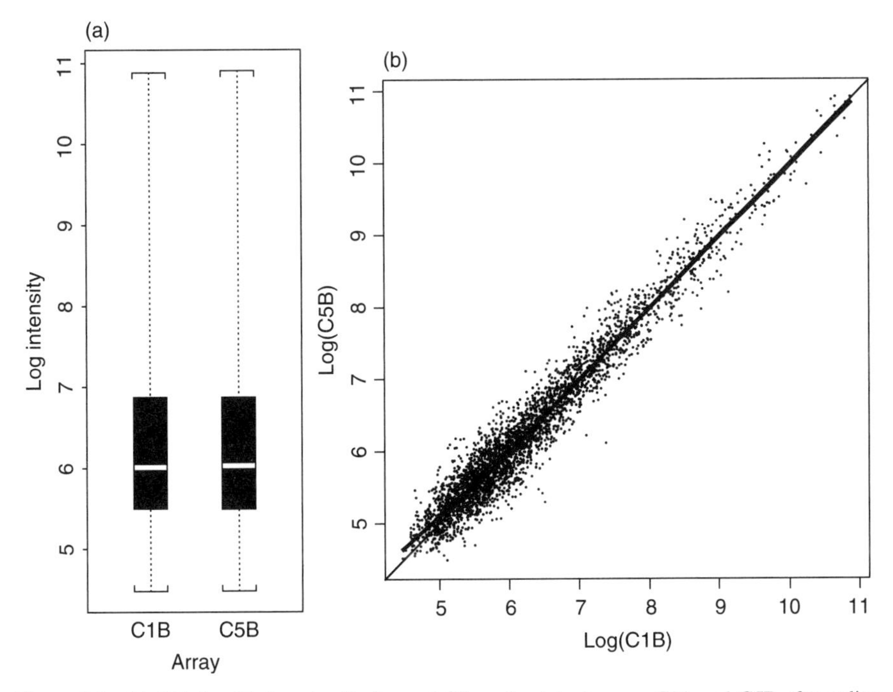

Figure 5.5 (a) Side-by-side boxplot display and (b) scatterplot of arrays C1A and C5B after spline normalization. The thinner line on the scatterplot is the identity line and the thicker line is a smooth of the plot.

possible to the spot intensity distribution of the median mock array. Either a subset of quantiles or all the quantiles may be equated.

To equate a subset of quantiles, say the percentiles, or all quantiles, as in Amaratunga and Cabrera (1999, 2001b), calculate the percentiles $(Q_{i0}, \dots, Q_{i100})$ of the ith array and the percentiles $(Q_{M0}, \dots, Q_{M100})$ of the median mock array. For any value $\{X_{gi}\}$, find the interval, $[Q_{ih}, Q_{i(h+1)}]$, to which it belongs and obtain its normalized value, X'_{gi}, by linearly interpolating between the pair of points: (Q_{Mh}, Q_{ih}) and $(Q_{M(h+1)}, Q_{i(h+1)})$.

Bolstad et al. (2002) give the following algorithm to equate all the quantiles: Arrange the transformed spot intensity $\{X_{gi}\}$ into a GxN matrix $\mathbf{X}$. Sort each column of $\mathbf{X}$ to give $\mathbf{X}_{sort}$. Take the means across the rows of $\mathbf{X}_{sort}$ and assign this mean to each element in the row to get $\mathbf{X}_{*sort}$. Obtain the normalized version $\mathbf{X}'$ of $\mathbf{X}$ by rearranging each column of $\mathbf{X}_{*sort}$ to have the same ordering as the original $\mathbf{X}$. Medians could be used instead of means in this algorithm to improve resistance to outliers.

Quantile normalization is useful for normalizing across a series of conditions where it is believed that a small but indeterminate number of genes may be differentially expressed, yet it can be assumed that the distribution of spot intensities does not vary too much.

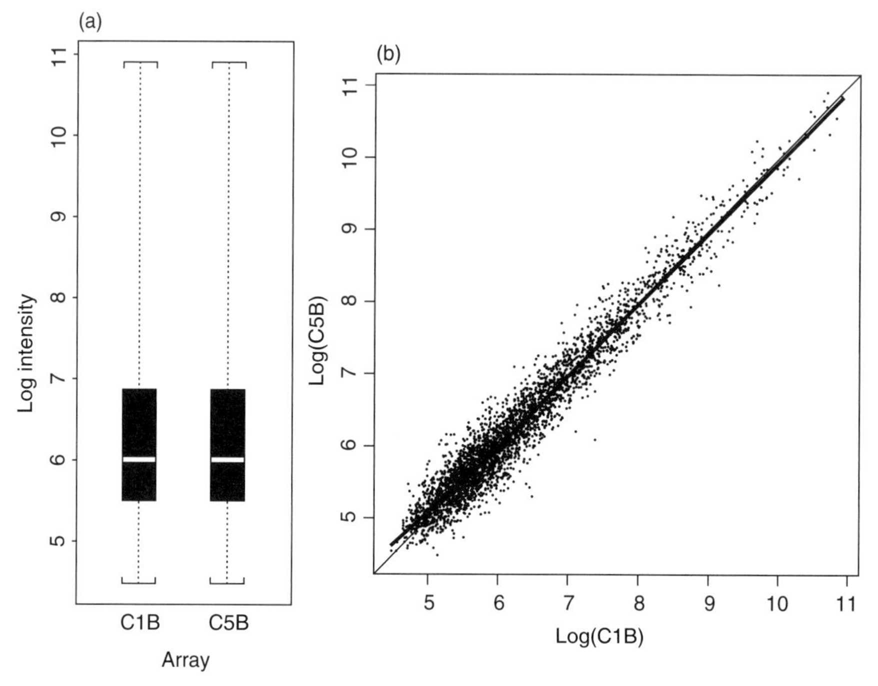

Figure 5.6 (a) Side-by-side boxplot display and (b) scatterplot of arrays C1A and C5B after quantile normalization. The thinner line on the scatterplot is the identity line and the thicker line is a smooth of the plot.

Example. Figure 5.6 shows the data from microarrays C1B and C5B plotted against each other after quantile normalization with, again, all the genes used as the invariant gene set. As with spline normalization, the observations are in agreement. In fact, both methods appear to perform similarly.

One concern with quantile normalization is that the median array may not look similar to any of the arrays and it may have shorter tails than any of the arrays in the data set. This issue is addressed by Nieto and Cabrera (2013) by applying a new method based on functional depth to obtain the median array, which is one of the samples. Then normalization proceeds by equating the quantiles of the other arrays to the median array.

Another concern arises when the number of genes is not large, the median array is very variable and may not be adequate for normalization. In this case, Cabrera and Emir (2013) propose to use the Fisher–Yates rank transformation to normalize the data to a normal distribution. Using the Fisher-Yates transformation is the same as setting the median array to $\{\Phi^{-1}(\frac{1}{G+1}), \ldots, \Phi^{-1}(\frac{G}{G+1})\}$, where $\Phi(t)$ is the normal distribution function and then the quantile normalization algorithm is applied.

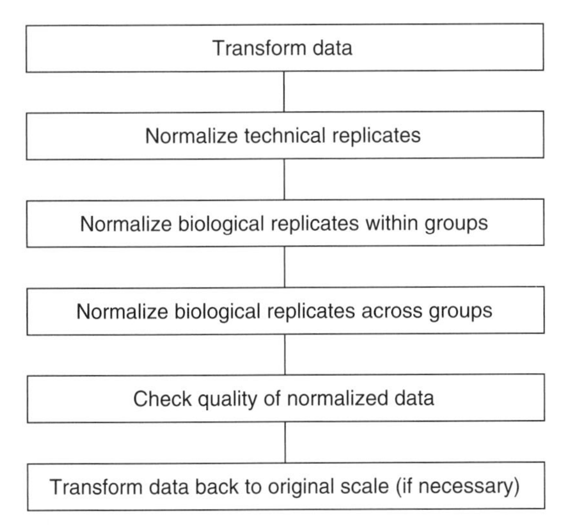

Figure 5.7 Schematic of a stagewise normalization.

5.5.3 Stagewise Normalization

When the data include both technical replicates as well as biological replicates, it is most effective to carry out the normalization in stages. The technical replicates can be normalized using smooth function normalization, and the biological replicates can be normalized using quantile normalization. If the biological replicates fall into groups, such as treatment groups, each group can be normalized separately using quantile normalization and then all the arrays in all the groups can be normalized across all the arrays using quantile normalization. Figure 5.7 is a schematic of a stagewise normalization.

Example. Figure 5.8 shows the results of a stagewise normalization. Figure 5.8a shows a side-by-side boxplot display of the data before any normalization is done (S0). Figure 5.8b is the data after normalizing the technical replicates via spline normalization (S1). Figure 5.8c is the data after normalizing the control biological replicates via quantile normalization (S2). Figure 5.10d is the data after normalizing across all 20 microarrays via another quantile normalization (S3).

5.5.4 Normalization of Two-Channel Arrays

Consider the log transformed spot intensities, $\{X_{gR}\}$ and $\{X_{gG}\}$, for the channels of a two-channel array, where the letters R and G refer to the colors, red and green respectively, that are typically used to label the channels. If there is no systematic dye bias, the data points on a scatterplot of X_{gR} versus X_{gG} should generally lie along the $Y = X$ line. If this is not the case, then it is necessary to normalize the two channels. Yang et al. (2002) argue that it is easier to assess this with an

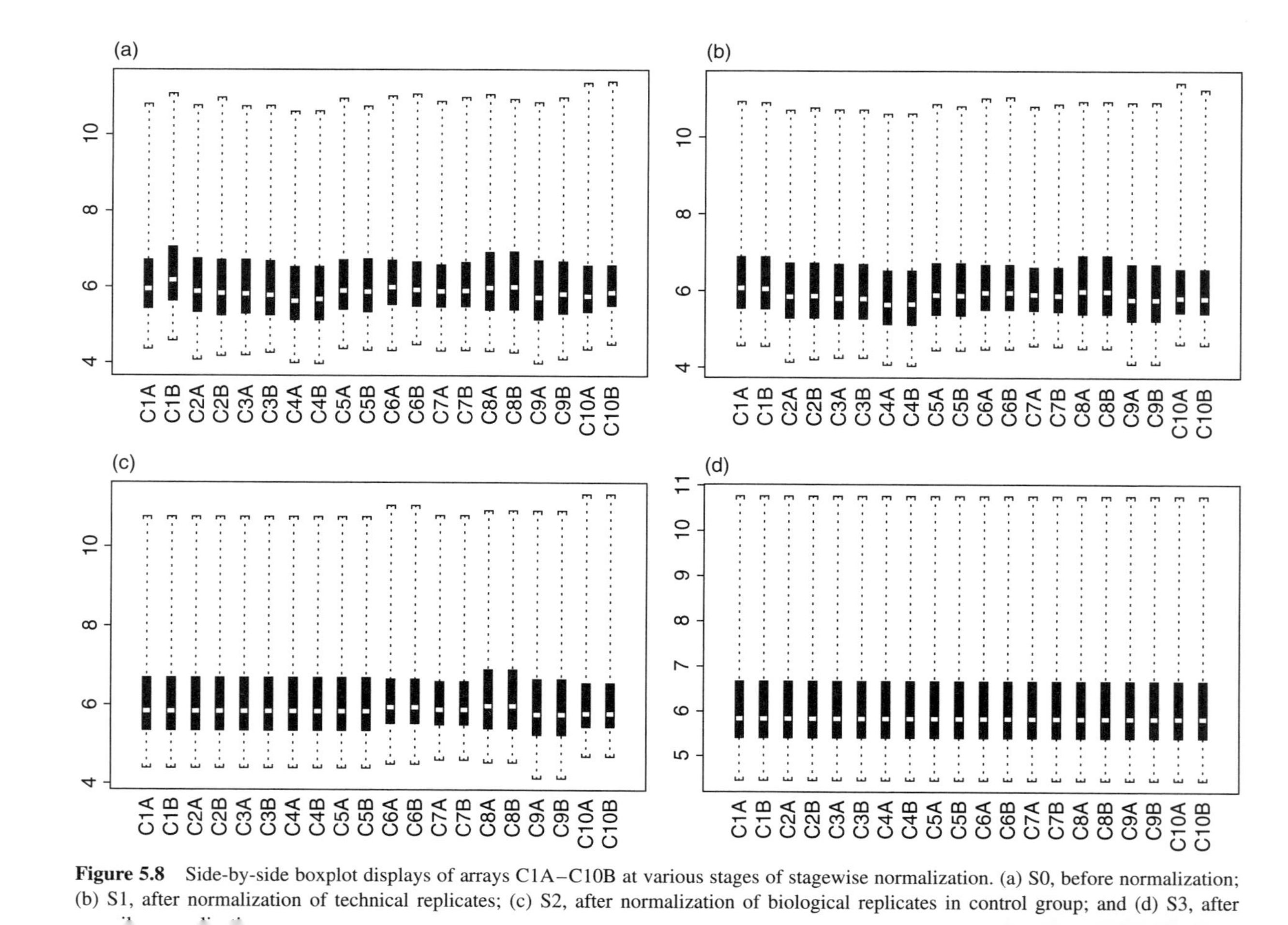

Figure 5.8 Side-by-side boxplot displays of arrays C1A–C10B at various stages of stagewise normalization. (a) S0, before normalization; (b) S1, after normalization of technical replicates; (c) S2, after normalization of biological replicates in control group; and (d) S3, after

MVA plot (or MA plot), a scatterplot of M_g versus A_g, where $M_g = X_{gR} - X_{gG}$ and $A_g = (X_{gR} + X_{gG})/2$. Here, $\{A_g\}$ is analogous to the median mock array that was used as the reference array above. If there is no systematic dye bias, the points on the MVA plot would be scattered around the $M = 0$ line. Otherwise, normalization can be done using any of the methods described above.

For an intensity-dependent normalization, the normalization function is fitted to the MVA plot, the fitted values, which function as the normalization adjustments, are calculated. The normalized values are taken to be $X'_{gR} = X_{gR} - \hat{M}_g/2$ and $X'_{gG} = X_{gG} + \hat{M}_g/2$. Here, $\hat{M}_g$ is the predicted values obtained from the normalization model. After normalization, the expression ratios, $R_g = \exp(X'_{gR} - X'_{gG})$, should be scattered around unity.

Park et al. (2003) generalize the normalization methods discussed in the previous sections a number of normalization methods and suggest choosing the appropriate method according to the nature of the data. In particular, Park et al. (2003) consider three main normalization models,

$$M_g = \begin{cases} \beta_0 & \text{global normalization,} \\ \beta_0 + \beta_1 A_g & \text{linear normalization,} \\ f(A_g) & \text{nonlinear normalization.} \end{cases}$$

Here, f is the smooth normalization function such as the spline normalization function or the lowess normalization function discussed in Section 5.5.1. Note that, as discussed above, both the linear and the nonlinear normalization models are intensity-dependent models, while the global normalization model is intensity independent. Dudoit et al. (2002) present a print-tip-dependent normalization method, where they use a lowess smoother fitted for each print-tip. They showed that there might be a strong print-tip or spatial effect and that it seems preferable in certain cases to normalize per print tip and not for the whole array at once.

Example. Figure 5.9A shows the red and green (Panel a) intensities for array C1 in the APO AI (apolipoprotein AI) experiment discussed in Chapter 1 (see also Yang et al. 2002) and the MA plot (Panel b) for that array. As we mentioned above, the goal of the normalization step is to remove all systematic structure from the data. Panel c in Figure 5.9B shows the data before and after global normalization (Figure 5.9B, panels a and b). We can see that the global normalization model results in a shift of the location of M_g but the structure remained in the data.

Figure 5.9B shows the MA plot after nonlinear (by print tip) normalization. Note how in this MA plot data are distributed symmetrically around zero (although the variability is not constant). Figure 5.10a shows that the MA plots by print tip for the normalized data (with a lowess smoother). After a print-tip lowess normalization, the normalized data are distributed symmetrically around zero and the lowess smoother for the print-tip-specific MA plots results in a flat line (except the last two print tip).

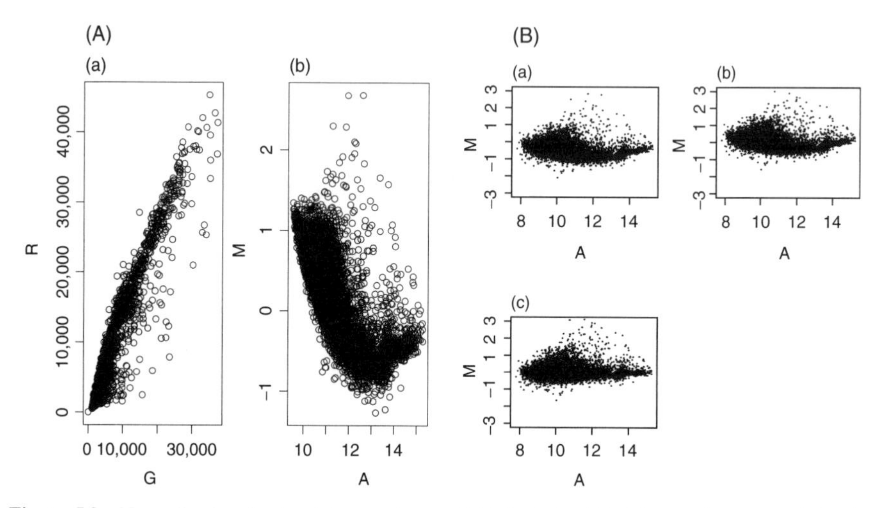

Figure 5.9 Normalization for the C1 array in the APO AI study. (A) MA plot for array C1 for the nonnormalized data in the APO AI experiment. (a) R versus G. (b) M versus A. (B) (a) MA plot for the nonnormalized data. (b) Normalized data with global normalization with median. (c) Normalized data with lowess normalization (print-tip normalization).

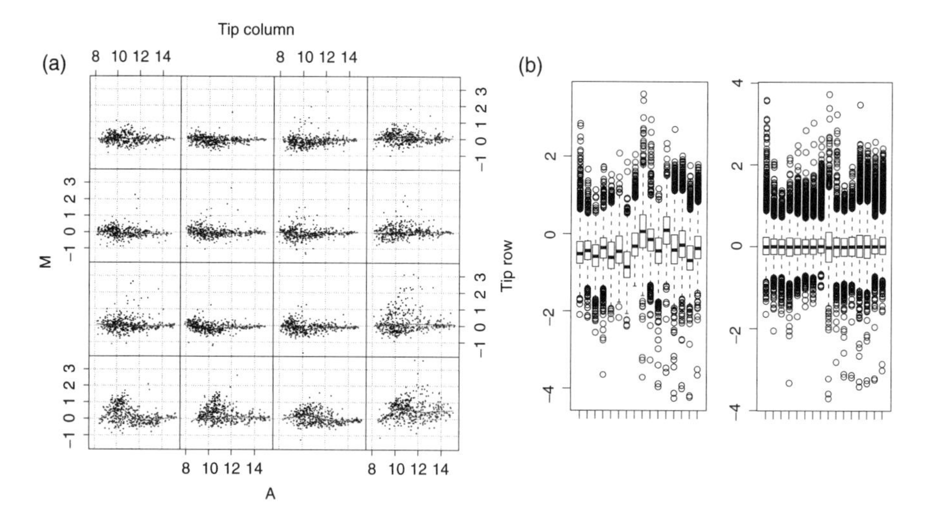

Figure 5.10 Print-tip normalization for the APO AI data. (a) MA plots for array C1 by print tip for the normalized data (with lowess normalization). (b) Boxplot for the arrays in APO AI before and after print-tip (nonlinear) normalization.

The normalization process discussed above implies that the location effect was removed from the data and the normalized data are centered around zero as can be seen in Figure 5.10b. However, we can see that the variability is not constant across the arrays. In order to overcome this problem, Yang et al. (2002) proposed a within array *scale* normalization models. The underlying assumption is that the variability of ith print tip is equal to $a_i\sigma^2$, where a_i is the print-tip-specific factor and σ^2 is the common factor across the print tip in the array. Yang et al. (2002) proposed the following estimate for a_i

$$\hat{a}_i = \frac{\sum_{j=1}^{n_j} M_{ij}^2}{\sqrt{\prod_{k}^{I} \sum_{j=1}^{n_k} M_{kj}^2}}.$$

Here, M_{ij} is the log of the intensity ratio in the ith print tip. A robust estimate for a_i is given by

$$\hat{a}_i = \frac{MAD_i}{\sqrt{\prod_{i}^{I} MAD_i}}.$$

Example. Figure 5.11 shows the boxplot for arrays intensities after location normalization (Fig. 5.11a) and after location and scale normalization (Fig. 5.11b).

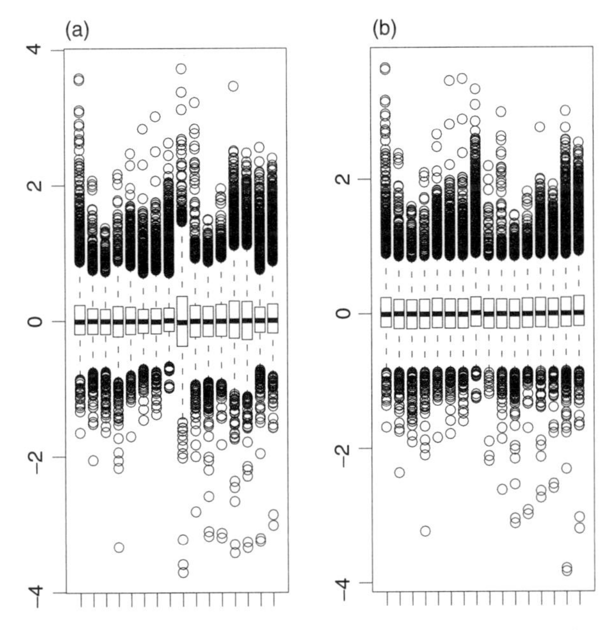

Figure 5.11 Location (a) and location and scale (b) normalization for the APO AI experiment.

Notice how the variability across the arrays changed when scale normalization was used as expected.

5.5.5 Spatial Normalization

Sometimes the arraying equipment or the experimental conditions can introduce systematic spatial effects within a single slide. In such cases, a within-slide normalization should be considered (Colantuoni, et al., 2002; Schuchhardt, et al., 2000; Yang, et al., 2001). This can be done by subdividing the slide into a grid. A natural grid is the grid determined by the print tip of the arrayer. Normalization across the subsections of the grid can be done using any of the methods described above. Care must be taken not to normalize out array defects and other artifacts.

5.5.6 Normalization of Oligonucleotide Arrays

Oligonucleotide arrays can be normalized using any of the methods described above. Normalization can be carried out either at the probe level or at the signal level. Using data from a spike-in experiment, Irizarry et al. (2003) demonstrate that probe-level normalization is the more effective, as it reduces bias and variability with the benefits carrying over to the expression level.

Example. *Normalization of the Platinum data.* Figures 5.12 and 5.13a show the *PM* intensities plots for the Platinum data before and after quantile normalization. Note that after quantile normalization all the densities are overlaid as expected. Figure 5.13b shows the MA plots for arrays 8, 9, and 18. In contrast with cDNA arrays, in which the MA plot is related to one array, the MA plot for oligonucleotide arrays corresponds to a specific pair of arrays i and j. Although the normalization

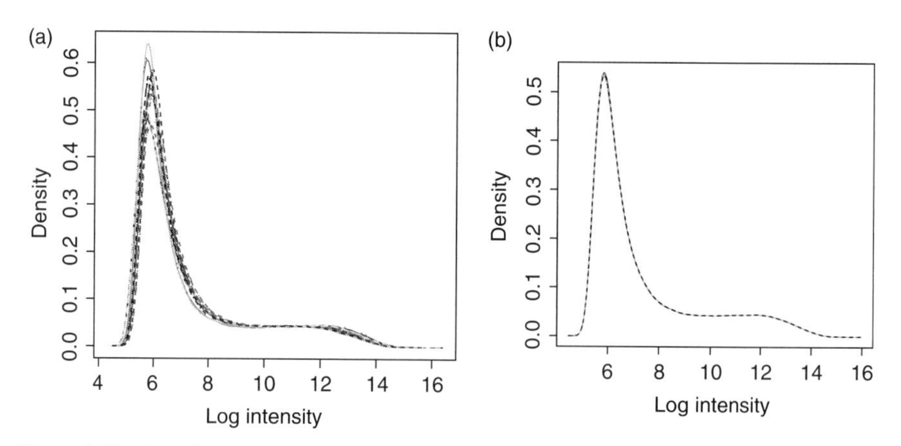

Figure 5.12 Quantile normalization for the platinum data (I). (a) Density estimates for PM intensities in the platinum data before normalization. (b) Density estimates for PM intensities after quantile normalization.

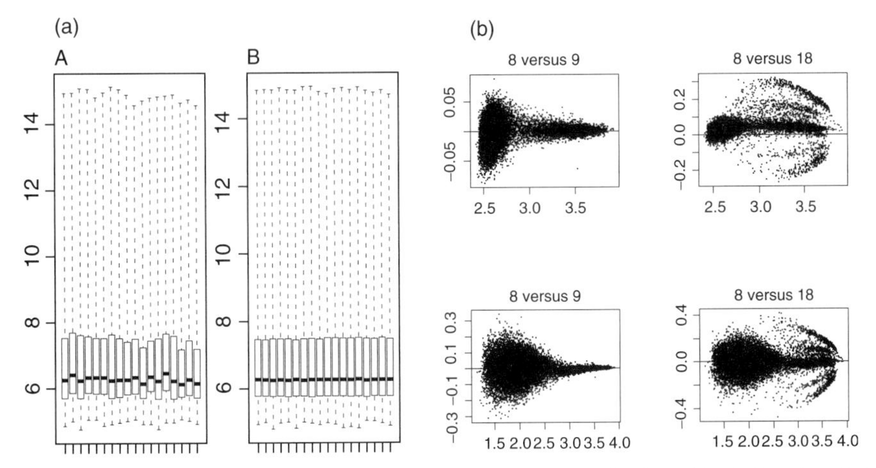

Figure 5.13 Quantile normalization for the platinum data (II). (A) PM intensities before (panel a) and after (panel b) quantile normalization for the platinum data. (B) M versus A plots for arrays 8, 9, and 18.

was done at the probe level, Figure 5.13b shows the MA plot for the summarized data (i.e., the intensity of the gene is a summary of the probes' intensities, see also Chapter 6). The ratios between the expression levels for the gth gene are defined as follows: $M_g = \log_2(X_{ig}/X_{jg})$ and $A_g = 1/2 \log_2(X_{ig}X_{jg})$. The upper panels in Figure 5.13b presents the MA plots for the nonnormalized but summarized data, while the lower plot present the MA plot after quantile normalization. Note how the point clouds are centered around the value of $M = 0$ after the normalization, which implies that the normalization removed systematic bias from the data. An elaborate comparison between different probe-level normalization methods is presented in Bolstad et al. (2002). Summarization methods of oligonucleotide arrays will be discussed in Chapter 6.

5.6 JUDGING THE SUCCESS OF A NORMALIZATION

Consider the normalization of two arrays, whose log-transformed spot intensities are $\{Y_{g1}\}$ and $\{Y_{g2}\}$. A normalization based on a monotone normalizing procedure (as those described in Section 5.5) will be truly successful in bringing them into agreement only if they are, more or less, monotonically related to each other. Whether this holds for $\{Y_{g1}\}$ and $\{Y_{g2}\}$ can be assessed by calculating their *Spearman's rank correlation coefficient*:

$$\hat{\rho}_S = \frac{12 \sum_{g=1}^{G} \{R_{g1} - \frac{1}{2}(G+1)\}\{R_{g2} - \frac{1}{2}(G+1)\}}{G(G^2-1)},$$

where R_{gi} is the rank of Y_{gi} when the $\{Y_{gi}\}$ are ranked across the genes from 1 to G.

Spearman's rank correlation coefficient is a measure of monotone (not necessarily linear) association between two variables. The value of $\hat{\rho}_S$ lies in between -1 and $+1$, with values close to $+1$ indicating that the two sets of values are positively associated to each other, values close to -1 indicating that the two sets of values are negatively associated to each other, and values close to 0 indicating that the two sets of values are not associated with each other. Thus, if $\hat{\rho}_S$ is high (i.e., close to 1), it is likely that a normalization of the sort described above would be able to bring the two sets of values into agreement, whereas, if $\hat{\rho}_S$ is low (i.e., much lower than 1), it is unlikely that a normalization of the sort described above would be able to bring the two sets of values into agreement.

The value of Spearman's rank correlation coefficient is unchanged by a monotone normalization procedure. Therefore, while it is a good measure of whether a normalization would be successful, it cannot be used to judge the success of a monotone normalization procedure.

Instead, once a normalization has been performed, the degree of success of the normalization can be assessed via the *concordance correlation coefficient* (Lin, 1989), an index that quantifies the degree of agreement between two sets of numbers. The concordance correlation coefficient, $\hat{\rho}_c$, is defined as

$$\hat{\rho}_c = \frac{2s_{12}}{s_1^2 + s_2^2 + (\overline{Y}_1 - \overline{Y}_2)^2},$$

where

$$\overline{Y}_c = \Sigma_{g=1}^G Y_{gc}/G \quad \text{and} \quad s_c^2 = \Sigma_{g=1}^G \frac{(Y_{gc} - \overline{Y}_c)^2}{G}$$

are, respectively, the mean and variance of the cth microarray ($c = 1, 2$) and

$$s_{12} = \frac{\Sigma_{g=1}^G (Y_{g1} - \overline{Y}_1)(Y_{g2} - \overline{Y}_2}{G},$$

is the covariance. ρ_c is a standardized measure of $E[(Y_{g1} - Y_{g2})]^2$ and $\rho_c = 1$ if and only if $\{Y_{g1}\}$ and $\{Y_{g2}\}$ are in perfect agreement. Otherwise, $\rho_c < 1$. Spearman's rank correlation coefficients and concordance correlation coefficients can be used together to assess the need for normalization:

- If, for a pair of arrays, $\hat{\rho}_c$ is very high (as a rough rule of thumb, greater than 0.99), normalization may not be necessary.
- On the other hand, if $\hat{\rho}_c$ is not very high and $\hat{\rho}_S$ is high (as a rough rule of thumb, greater than 0.8), indicating a monotone, but not strongly concordant relationship, normalization is very likely to highly beneficial.
- When both $\hat{\rho}_c$ and $\hat{\rho}_S$ are low, indicating that the relationship between the arrays is not strong, it may be worth looking further to see whether there was a problem with either of the arrays before doing any normalization.

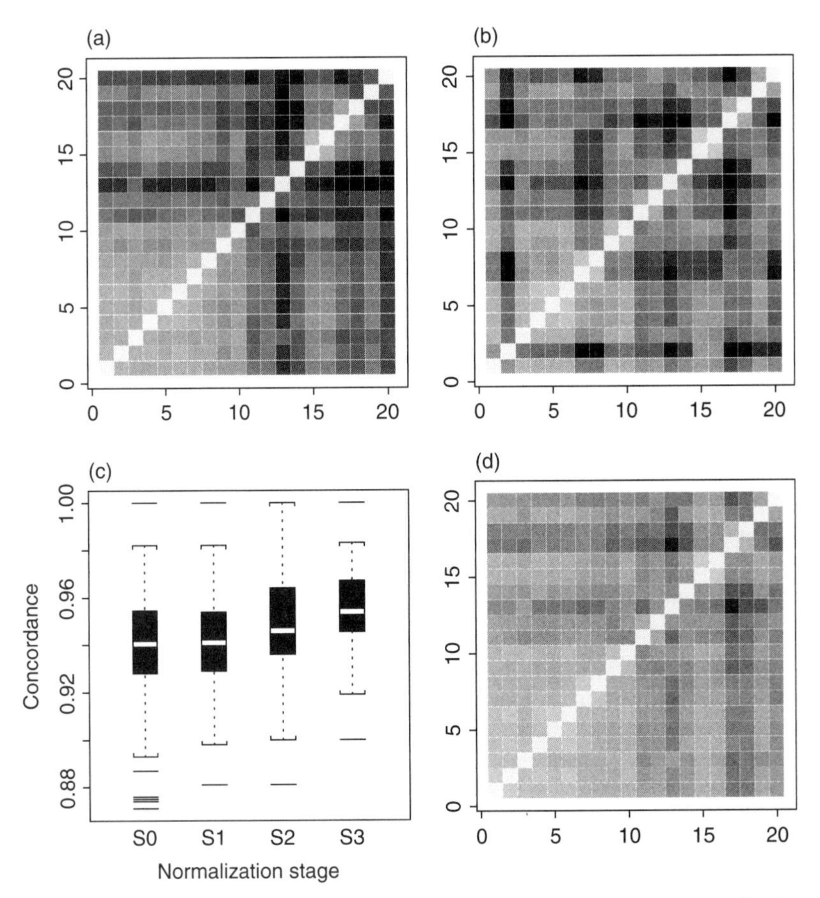

Figure 5.14 The Mouse5 data. (a) Spearman map, (b) concordance map before normalization, (c) concordance correlation coefficients at various stages of normalization, and (d) concordance map after normalization (on gray scale, low to high correlations go from black to white).

When normalizing across a series of arrays, it is instructive to display, on image plots, the pairwise Spearman's rank correlation coefficients (the resulting display is called a *Spearman map*) and the pairwise concordance correlation coefficients (the resulting display is called a *concordance map*).

Example. Figure 5.14 shows a Spearman map of the Mouse5 dataset. It shows a strong monotone relationship among the 10 control replicates and also among 2 other technical replicate pairs. All the Spearman's rank correlation coefficients are greater than 0.85, indicating that the arrays can be normalized. Figure 5.14b shows a concordance map of the data, with several concordance correlation coefficients below 0.9, showing that there is a need for a normalization. Figure 5.14c shows a side-by-side boxplot display of the concordance correlation coefficients after each stage of the stagewise normalization (the stages S0–S3 are defined in Section

5.5.3). Figure 5.14d shows a concordance map after the complete normalization; all the concordance correlation coefficients are now above 0.9. Observe how the concordance improves at each stage, culminating in the substantially higher concordance in the control group after normalization. Some comments regarding various correlation coefficients:

1. If the distributional properties of the values change substantially during a normalization (e.g., the skewness is decreased), it is possible that the concordance correlation coefficients might increase, but this may only be an artificial improvement.
2. The more familiar Pearson's correlation coefficient,

$$\hat{\rho} = \frac{s_{12}}{s_1 s_2}$$

measures how close $\{Y_{g1}\}$ and $\{Y_{g2}\}$ are to linearity rather than to agreement.
3. For a pair of microarrays that have been normalized by equating all the quantiles, the concordance correlation coefficient will equal Pearson's correlation coefficient. This is because, after such a normalization, the quantiles of both microarrays are identical and, therefore, both means are equal, $\overline{Y}_1 = \overline{Y}_2$ as are both variances $s_1^2 = s_2^2$.
4. Spearman's rank correlation coefficient is equal to (i) Pearson's correlation coefficient calculated on the ranks of the data and (ii) the concordance correlation coefficient calculated on the ranks of the data.

5.7 OUTLIER IDENTIFICATION

Outliers are observations that appear to be inconsistent with the majority of the data. When there are replicate arrays, the replicates could be used to identify discrepant spot intensities in the data. Let X_{gi} denote the transformed and normalized spot intensity measurement for the gth gene on the ith array. An outlier is an observation, X_{gj}, that is substantially different from a majority of the other values X_{gi} for that same gene. The same observation may or may not have been discovered as an unusual observation in the spot quality checks performed at the preprocessing stage (see Section 5.2.6).

Many ways of identifying outliers in replicate observations have been suggested. Barnett and Lewis (1994) and Iglewicz and Hoaglin (1993) provide extensive reviews of the vast literature on this topic.

5.8 NONRESISTANT RULES FOR OUTLIER IDENTIFICATION

Some common approaches to outlier identification are as follows:

1. *The z-score rule (Grubbs' test).* Calculate a z-score, z_{gi}, for every observation:

$$z_{gi} = \frac{X_{gi} - X_g}{s_g},$$

where $\overline{X}_g$ and s_g are the mean and standard deviation of the gth gene. Call X_{gj} an outlier if $|z_{gj}|$ is large, say, greater than 5.

2. *The CV rule.* Call the furthest observation X_{gj} from the mean, $\overline{X}_g$, an outlier if the coefficient of variation, $CV = s_g/\overline{X}_g$, exceeds some prespecified cutoff. Neither of these rules is a particularly reliable tool for detecting outliers. Their most serious drawback is that they are based on statistics that are themselves influenced by outliers. For example, if there was a large outlier in the data, both the mean and the standard deviation would be inflated by its influence and both the z-score of the outlier itself and the CV could appear normal. This phenomenon is known as *masking*, an outlier remaining undetected because of being hidden either by itself or by other, usually adjacent, outliers. A related effect is *swamping*, which happens when a normal observation is classified as an outlier because of the presence of an unrelated outlier or outliers.

5.9 RESISTANT RULES FOR OUTLIER IDENTIFICATION

As per the above discussion, it is crucial that an outlier detection method be based on statistics that are resistant to outliers that are uninfluenced by them, such as the median and the MAD (median absolute deviation from the median, scaled to be consistent at the normal distribution), both of which can tolerate up to almost 50% outliers without being affected. Thus a more reliable outlier detection rule is

The resistant z-score rule. Calculate a resistant z-score, z^*_{gi}, for every observation:

$$z^*_{gi} = \frac{X_{gi} - \tilde{X}_g}{\tilde{s}_g},$$

where $\tilde{Y}_g$ and $\tilde{s}_g$ are the median and MAD of the gth gene. Call X_{gj} an outlier if $|z^*_{gj}|$ is large, say, greater than 5 (Iglewicz and Hoaglin, 1993).

One remaining problem is that microarray experiments usually have little replication. With very few replicates, the median and the MAD, in particular the latter, are not dependable estimates of the location and scale of the data. The estimation of the scale can be improved by observing that, with microarray data, there is a relationship between the median and the MAD across all the genes and, assuming that this is a true relationship $\sigma_g^2 = f(\mu_g)$, use it to calculate a smoothed version of MAD, $M\tilde{A}D_g$ that will be more stable as it "borrows strength" from similar expressing genes. To calculate $M\tilde{A}D_g$, first calculate the absolute deviations from the median, $AD_{gi} = \|X_{gi} - \tilde{X}_{gi}\|$; run a smoother, such as a smoothing spline, through the relationship of AD_{gi} versus $\tilde{X}_g$; and use the fitted value, $M\tilde{A}D_g$, as

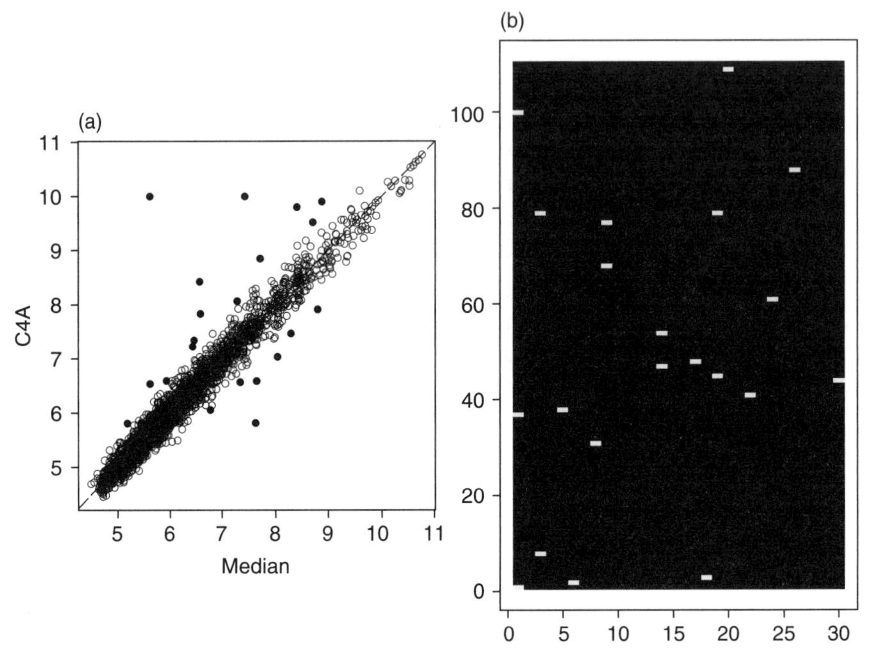

Figure 5.15 (a) Scatterplot of (normalized) array C4A with the outliers plotted as filled circles and (b) an image plot of the array showing, in white, the positions of the outliers.

an estimator of scale for the gth gene. The following revised rule can be used to identify outliers:

The revised z-score rule. Calculate a revised z-score, z_{gi}^{**}, for every observation:

$$z_{gi}^{**} = \frac{X_{gi} - \tilde{X}_g}{\tilde{s}_g\prime}.$$

Call X_{gj} an outlier if $\|z_{gj}^{**}\|$ is large, say, greater than 5.

Example. When the control group data (arrays C1A–C5B) were screened for outliers using the revised z-score rule with a critical value of 5, a total of 119 observations were designated as outliers. None of the arrays had a substantially higher proportion of outliers than the others. Therefore, there is no evidence that any of the arrays is particularly different from the rest. The outliers found on array C4A are shown in Figure 5.15, both on a scatterplot of C4A versus the median mock array and on an image plot of the array. The latter shows that the outliers are randomly scattered through the array. Therefore, there is no evidence that C4A has any spatial problems.

5.10 ASSESSING REPLICATE ARRAY QUALITY

Methods for assessing the quality of a single array or a series of arrays were discussed in Section 4.2. Replicate arrays (such as the set of arrays in the control group in the example) can be also used to judge the array quality by seeing whether any of them is different from the others.

- If the Spearman correlation coefficients between one of the arrays and each of the other arrays is substantially lower than the other Spearman correlation coefficients then that array is suspect.
- When a procedure in Section 5.7 discovers substantially more outliers on one of the arrays more than on any of the other arrays, then that array is suspect.

In addition, when there are groups of arrays, such as one group of arrays hybridized to control samples and another group of arrays hybridized to treatment samples, the extent of the differences can be roughly assessed from a Spearman map or a concordance map (e.g., the lighter 10×10 square area in the lower left quadrant of Figures 5.14a and 5.14d, separating out the control group). The more obvious the separation, the more substantive the difference between groups. However, small and subtle differences between groups would not be evident on these displays.

SOFTWARE NOTES

`DNAMR 2.0`

This package implements some of the methods that are included in this chapter which are (i) MOM (ii) Quantile normalization (iii) Fisher-Yates normalization `www.rci.rutgers.edu/~cabrera/DNAMR`.

`DNAMR`

The DNAMR package contains functions for quantile normalization of microarrays.

`limma`

The normalization of two-color cDNA microarray as discussed in Section 5.5.4 and the graphical output presented in Figure 5.9–5.11 was performed using the bioconductor package `limma`. Different normalization methods are discussed in Dudoit et al. (2002).

`Affy`

The bioconductor `Affy` package contains functions for exploratory oligonucleotide array analysis. In particular, the package can be used for normalization and summarization of oligonucleotide arrays as presented in Figure 5.12. The package includes several methods for smooth function normalization, constant value normalization, and quantile normalization. Comparisons between different normalization methods for Affymetrix microarrays are discussed in Bolstad et al. (2003).

EXERCISES

5.1. A crude, but resistant, estimate of the skewness of a distribution is

$$K = \frac{Q_3 - M}{M - Q_1},$$

where Q_1, M, and Q_3, are the first quartile, median, and third quartile, respectively. Calculate the value of K for the data from C1A in data set E5, before and after transformation by $X \to \log(X - c)$, for $c = 0, 10, \ldots, 50$. Comment.

5.2. Construct an MVA plot for the data from arrays C9A and C9B in data set E5. Normalize the data using a spline normalization and redraw the MVA plot. Compare the gene expression ratios before and after normalization. Comment.

5.3. Consider the data from C1A, C1B, C10A, and C10B in data set E5. Carry out a stagewise normalization for this data. The average expression level in the "control group" can be estimated as the averages of C1A and C1B. The average expression level in the "treated group" can be estimated as the averages of C10A and C10B. Plot these averages against each other before and after normalization. Comment.

5.4. Determine whether there are any outliers in the following:

(a) 10.07 10.11 10.27 10.10 9.88 9.99 10.13 9.76 9.22 10.04
(b) 10.07 10.11 10.27 10.10 9.88 9.99 10.13 9.76 2.22 10.04

using (i) the z-score rule and (ii) the resistant z-score rule.

5.5. Average the data for each mouse, for example, C1 = (C1A + C1B)/2. Identify any outliers in the set of averages for C1, C2, C3, C4, and C5 using (i) the z-score rule and (ii) the resistant z-score rule. Is there any evidence that any of the mice is an outlier?

5.6. Use the postnormalization MVA plot in Problem 5.2 to determine whether there are any discrepant pairs of observations between arrays C9A and C9B.

5.7. The data set SCH contains data from an experiment involving 14 arrays, of which C1–C7 are from tissue samples taken from normal patients (Group 1) and C8–C14 are from tissue samples taken from patients with a certain disease (Group 2). Transform the data using a log transformation. (i) Assess the need for normalization via a boxplot display, a concordance map, and a spearman map. (ii) Perform a stagewise normalization as follows: Normalize arrays C1–C7 using quantile normalization. Normalize arrays C8–C14 using quantile normalization. Finally, normalize all the arrays using quantile normalization. (Use the function `f.qnorm`). (iii) Repeat (i) for the normalized data and assess the improvement. (iv) For each gene g, calculate the standardized log fold change: before and after normalization. Here is the mean of Group 1 for gene g, the mean of Group 2 for gene g, and the pooled standard error (calculated as when doing a two-sample t test) for gene g. (v) Plot the postnormalized t_g values against the pre-normalized t_g values. Pick out the genes with the 10 highest prenormalized $|t_g|$ values and the genes with the 10 highest postnormalized $|t_g|$ values. Are they the same? Comment.

5.8. In 5.7 (ii) Compare the results of performing a quantile normalization with what you get using Fisher-Yates normalization by doing a scatter of the normalized C1 by both methods.

CHAPTER 6

Summarization

Once the spot intensity data have been preprocessed, statistical estimation techniques can be applied to summarize the data across replicates and determine the expression level of each gene.

6.1 REPLICATION

Replication, the execution of an experiment on more than one unit, is an important consideration when performing any experiment (Fisher, 1951) remains a key reference). There is a sound scientific rationale for replication. In the first place, by averaging over replicates, the underlying parameters of interest can be estimated with greater precision, as replication followed by averaging dampens the effect of chance variations on parameter estimates. The higher the number of replicates, the greater the precision. Second, replication provides information that allows the extent of experimental variation to be estimated. This is crucial for evaluating the statistical significance of any findings from the experiment.

Unfortunately, there is often confusion about what constitutes replication in a microarray experiment. This is because there are several types of replication in a microarray experiment, each giving information regarding a different source of variability; for example,

- Spotting a gene several times on an array allows the gene's variability within the array to be assessed.
- Hybridizing a number of microarrays to the same labeled mRNA sample allows the variability across arrays to be assessed. In this case, the microarrays can be regarded as *technical replicates*.

Exploration and Analysis of DNA Microarray and Other High-Dimensional Data, Second Edition.
Dhammika Amaratunga, Javier Cabrera, Ziv Shkedy.

- Hybridizing a number of microarrays to different labeled mRNA samples prepared from the same mRNA sample allows the variability of the labeling and sample preparation procedure to be assessed. Here, again, the microarrays can be regarded as technical replicates, but the source of variability they assess is different from the technical replicates above.
- Collecting several mRNA samples from a number of different but similar subjects allows biological variability (e.g., animal-to-animal or tissue-to-tissue differences) to be assessed. In this case, the replicate microarrays can be regarded as *biological replicates.*

It is important to realize that any type of replication offers information only regarding the particular source of variability associated with that type of replication and no other. Thus, for instance, increasing the number of technical replicates merely because they are less costly than biological replicates will not offer an increase in information about biological variability.

Careful consideration should go into what type of replication to include in an experiment. To increase the overall precision of an experiment, it is most effective to add replication where there is greatest variability and, therefore, least precision. Thus, if there is high subject-to-subject variability and the measurements taken across the technical replicates are very precise, increasing the number of subjects will increase the overall precision of the experiment more than increasing the number of technical replicates. In fact, as the technical aspects of microarray experiments improve, biological variability is likely to constitute the highest percentage of variabilty in an experiment. The drawback is that it is also, usually, the costliest. In any case, the number of biological replicates to include in an experiment should be carefully assessed, as without enough biological replicates, the overall sensitivity of the experiment will be low and reliably extending experimental findings beyond the limited confines of the experiment may prove to be difficult.

Churchill (2002) and Lee et al. (2000) give further guidance regarding replication in microarray experiments.

6.2 TECHNICAL REPLICATES

We first discuss technical replicates. These are used to deal with technical variation, which arises from the handling steps, such as mRNA extraction, amplification, labeling, hybridization, and scanning. This variation introduces uncertainty to the intensity measurements associated with a gene. Using technical replicates and averaging across them allow gene expression levels to be estimated with greater precision. The higher the number of replicates, the greater the precision.

The summarized intensity level of a gene on the microarrays that are exposed to the sample is an average of its intensity levels across the technical replicates. The average could be a simple estimator such as the arithmetic mean or the median or a more sophisticated estimator such as a biweight mean.

Let us examine this in some detail. Let X_{gi} denote the (suitably transformed and normalized) spot intensity measurement for the ith technical replicate of the gth gene, $g = 1, \ldots, G$, $i = 1, \ldots, n$. X_{gi} is a random variable with mean μ_g, which represents the (true) mean expression level of the gth gene, and (true) variance σ_g^2. We write this using statistical notation as $X_{gi} \sim \mathrm{N}(\mu_g, \sigma_g^2)$. The model parameters, μ_g and σ_g^2, are estimated using observed data.

An alternative, and entirely equivalent, formulation is to write this as $X_{gi} = \mu_g + \varepsilon_{gi}$. Here, ε_{gi} is the error introduced by the ith technical replicate for the gth gene. Note that the statistical interpretation of the word "error" differs from its conventional meaning: it is used to denote the difference between an observed value (here X_{gi}) and its value as expected according to a statistical model (here μ_g). The error ε_{gi} is a random variable with mean zero and variance σ_g^2, that is, $\varepsilon_{gi} \sim \mathrm{N}(0, \sigma_g^2)$.

The usual estimators of the model parameters μ_g and σ_g^2 are, respectively, the sample mean, $\overline{X}_g$, and the sample variance, s_g^2, for the gth gene:

$$\hat{\mu}_g = \overline{X}_g = \frac{\Sigma_{i=1}^n X_{gi}}{n},$$

$$\hat{\sigma}_g^2 = s_g^2 = \frac{\Sigma_{i=1}^n (\overline{X}_{gi} - \hat{X}_g)^2}{n-1}.$$

The standard error of $\hat{\mu}_g$ (i.e., the standard deviation of $\hat{\mu}_g$) is $\sigma_g/\sqrt{n}$, which is estimated by $s_g/\sqrt{n}$.

These estimators are all optimal, in many senses, if the underlying distribution of X_{gi}, or equivalently, ε_{gi}, is normal, that is, if $X_{gi} \sim \mathrm{N}(\mu_g, \sigma_g^2)$ or, equivalently, $\varepsilon_{gi} \sim \mathrm{N}(0, \sigma_g^2)$. However, if it is not, they might have undesirable properties. In particular, if X_{gi} contains outliers, as is often the case with microarray data, both $\hat{\mu}_g$ and $\hat{\sigma}_g^2$ will be suboptimal, perhaps seriously so.

It may therefore be preferable to estimate the values of μ_g and σ_g^2 in such a way that the extent to which they are influenced by outliers is limited. Such estimators are said to be resistant. The most resistant reasonable estimators of μ_g and σ_g^2 are the *median* and the *median absolute deviation from the median* (MAD):

$$M_g = \mathrm{median}(X_{gi}),$$

$$\mathrm{MAD}_g = \mathrm{median}\{|X_{gi} - M_g|\}.$$

These estimators are so resistant that almost half the observations have to be bad before the estimators themselves are affected. However, there is a price to pay for so much resistance. These estimators are not very efficient, that is, they tend to have high variability.

It is possible to obtain reasonably high efficiency at the normal distribution coupled with reasonably high resistance should the data contain outliers. Such estimators are said to be *statistically robust*. The price is that they are not 100%

efficient (but the efficiency can exceed 90%) and they come at a slight computational cost. *Biweight means* and *biweight standard deviations* are statistically robust estimators of μ_g and σ_g^2.

The biweight mean is defined as the value $\overline{X}_g$ that maximizes

$$\sum_{i=1}^{n} \rho\left(\frac{X_{gi} - \overline{X}_g}{\tau s_g^o}\right),$$

where the *objective function* ρ is defined by

$$\rho(u) = \begin{cases} \dfrac{(1-(1-u^2)^3}{6} & \text{if } |u| < 1, \\ \dfrac{1}{6} & \text{otherwise.} \end{cases}$$

Note that s_g^o is a resistant estimate of σ_g, and the *tuning constant* τ determines the amount of efficiency and resistance desired. The larger τ is, the more efficient the estimator is if the distribution is truly normal, but the less resistant it is. The smaller the τ is, the less efficient the estimator is if the distribution is truly normal, but the more resistant it is. A compromise between these two extremes offers both high efficiency at the normal distribution and resistance should the data contain outliers.

There is no closed form expression for the biweight mean. This is where the computational cost comes in. The biweight mean has to be calculated using an iterative process. The iteration begun at M_g, the median of the gth gene. For each observation X_{gi}, calculate $u_{gi} = (X_{gi} - M_g)/\tau s_g^o$, which indicates how "unusual" it is, then assign it a weight w_{ig} based on the biweight weighting function: $w(u) = (1-u^2)^2$ if $|u| < 1$ and $w(u) = 0$ otherwise (note $w(u) = \rho'(u)/u$). The weighting process ensures that observations relatively near the center of the data will be assigned high weights, while if there are any observations relatively far from the center of the data, that is, outliers, they will be assigned low weights. Calculate a weighted mean

$$M_g' = \frac{\Sigma_{i=1}^n w_{gi} X_{gi}}{\Sigma_{i=1}^n w_{gi}},$$

using these weights.

These steps can be iterated, now beginning with M_g', until there is, for all practical purposes, no change in M_g'. The resulting estimator is the biweight mean, as desired. However, it has been shown that just doing a single iteration usually produces an estimator that inherits the high resistance of the median and gains substantially in efficiency. Therefore, sometimes, this estimator, called the *one-step biweight mean*, is used instead of the fully iterated version.

The usual choice for s_g^o is MAD_g. This is the natural choice because the estimate of σ_g used here must be resistant but it does not necessarily have to be particularly efficient. However, this choice may not work very well with microarray data. The problem is that the number of technical replicates tends to be very small and the MAD is too unreliable in such instances.

An alternative choice for s_g^o can be obtained by exploiting the fact that σ_g^2 is usually a function of μ_g, that is, $\sigma_g^2 = f(\mu_g)$. This involves first modeling the log (MAD_g) vs log (M_g) relationship using, for example, a spline with a few degrees of freedom; the spline is an estimate of f. Then a value for s_g^o is the value associated with log (M_g) as predicted by the fit.

The biweight mean, originally proposed by Tukey, belongs to a particular class of statistically robust estimators called *M-estimators* (the book by Hoaglin, Mosteller, and Tukey (1983) gives a good review of robust estimation). Other estimators in this class are obtained by using different objective functions with bounded derivatives. Huber proposed

$$\rho(u) = \begin{cases} \dfrac{u^2}{2} & \text{if } |u| < 1, \\ |u| - \dfrac{1}{2} & \text{otherwise.} \end{cases}$$

Hampel proposed

$$\rho(u) = \begin{cases} \dfrac{u^2}{2} & \text{if } |u| < h1, \\ \dfrac{h_1|u| - h_1^2}{2} & \text{if } h_1 < |u| < h_2, \\ h_4 + h_5(h_3 - |u|^2) & \text{if } h_2 < |u| < h_3, \\ h_6 & \text{otherwise.} \end{cases}$$

Andrews proposed

$$\rho(u) = \begin{cases} \dfrac{(1 - \cos(\pi u))}{2} & \text{if } |u| < 1, \\ \dfrac{2}{\pi^2} & \text{otherwise.} \end{cases}$$

Note that the median can be obtained by setting $\rho(u) = |u|$. Finally, it can be observed that the mean corresponds to $\rho(u) = u^2/2$, but because its derivative, $\rho' = u$, is not bounded, it is not, strictly speaking, an M-estimator, as it is the boundedness of the derivative that is the key to the resistance.

The idea of weighting observations according to how distant they are from the center of the data is also used for calculating robust standard deviation estimates. The biweight standard deviation estimate, $\bar{s}_g$, is defined as

$$\bar{s}_g = \frac{\tau_A \text{MAD}_g \sqrt{n}[\Sigma_{i=1}\psi^2(u_i')]^2}{\Sigma_{i=1}\psi^2(u_i')},$$

where τ_A is a tuning constant that determines the resistance and efficiency desired, $u' = (X_{gi} - \overline{X}_g)/\tau_A s_g^o$, with s_g^o set to MAD_g or smoothed MAD_g as before, is a measure of how unusual X_{gi} is, and $\psi(u) = u(1 - u^2)^2$ if $|u| < 1$ and $\psi(u) = 0$ otherwise (note that $\psi(u) = \rho'(u)$). The biweight standard deviation belongs to a particular class of statistically robust estimators of standard deviation called *A-estimators*. Another class of robust variance estimators, with perhaps slightly better properties, are known as *τ-estimators*.

Yet another robust estimator of μ_g is the trimmed mean. The $\alpha\%$ trimmed mean of a set of observations is obtained by ordering the observations from smallest to largest, removing (i.e., trimming) the prespecified percentage, $\alpha\%$, of observations from each end of the ordered list, and taking the mean of the rest. The ordinary mean is, of course, a 0% trimmed mean; the median is something similar to a 50% trimmed mean; the 25% trimmed mean is called a *midmean*.

6.3 BIOLOGICAL REPLICATES

Biological replicates are used to deal with biological variation, which is the natural variability among subjects due to genetic diversity, environmental effects, and other causes. This variation also contributes uncertainty to the intensity measurements associated with a gene. Using biological replicates and averaging across them allows gene expression levels to be estimated with greater biological precision. The higher the number of replicates, the greater the precision.

In this case, the average intensity measurement of each gene can be estimated in an analogous way to the case where there were technical replicates, so we will not go into details here.

6.4 EXPERIMENTS WITH BOTH TECHNICAL AND BIOLOGICAL REPLICATES

In certain experiments, there will be both biological replicates as well as technical replicates.

Example. The first five pairs of microarrays in the MOUSE5 data, discussed in Chapter 1 and 5, C1A, C1B, C2A, C2B, ... , C5A, C5B correspond to five control samples. Each pair of microarrays corresponds to a single mRNA sample (labeled C1, C2, ... , C5), which was taken from a mouse following treatment and hybridized to two separate microarrays (labeled A and B). The two microarrays in each pair are technical replicates as they are exposed to the same biological sample. Samples C1–C5 are biological replicates from five mice. There were 3300 genes arrayed on the microarrays.

In the above example, the number of technical replicates was the same (i.e., two) for every biological replicate. In such cases, the experiment is said to be *balanced* with respect to the replication. If the number of technical replicates was not the same across the biological replicates, the experiment is said to be *unbalanced* with respect to the replication. Balanced experiments have several advantages.

When there are both biological replicates and technical replicates, the estimated average intensity measurement would be subject to both biological variation as well as technical variation and some of the calculations change. In order to study this situation; let X_{gij} denote the intensity of the jth technical replicate within the ith biological replicate for the gth gene. Here, g indexes the genes ($g = 1, \ldots, G$), j indexes the biological replicates ($j = 1, \ldots, a$), and i indexes the technical replicates ($i = 1, \ldots, n$).

The statistical model for this situation shows the presence of both sources of variability:

$$X_{gij} = \mu_g + \alpha_{gi} + \varepsilon_{gij}.$$

In this model, μ_g is the overall (true) mean, α_{gj} is the effect of the jth biological replicate ($\alpha_j \sim \mathrm{F}(0, \sigma^2_{\mathrm{BIOL};g})$, ε_{gij} is the effect of the ith technical replicate within the jth biological replicate ($\varepsilon_{gij} \sim \mathrm{G}(0, \sigma^2_{\mathrm{TECH};g})$, for some generic F, G.

Let $\overline{X}_g = \Sigma_{j=1}^{a} \Sigma_{i=1}^{n} X_{gij}/an$ denote the overall mean and $\overline{X}_{gj} = \Sigma_{i=1}^{n} X_{gij}/n$ denote the mean for the jth biological replicate. The expected value for the overall mean is given by

$$E(\overline{X}_g) = \mu.$$

The mean squared error across biological replicates

$$\mathrm{MS}_g^{\mathrm{BIOL}} = \frac{\Sigma_{j=1}^{a}(\overline{X}_{gj} - \overline{X}_g)^2}{a - 1},$$

measures the variation across biological replicates. It also has a contribution because of the variation across technical replicates as shown by its expected value:

$$E(\mathrm{MS}_g^{\mathrm{TECH}}) = n\sigma^2_{\mathrm{BIOL},g} + \sigma^2_{\mathrm{TECH},g}.$$

The mean squared error across technical replicates,

$$\mathrm{MS}_g^{\mathrm{TECH}} = \frac{\Sigma_{j=1}^{a}\Sigma_{i=1}^{n}(\overline{X}_{gji} - \overline{X}_{gj})^2}{a(n - 1)},$$

measures variation across technical replicates. Its expected value is

$$E(\mathrm{MS}_g^{\mathrm{TECH}}) = \sigma^2_{\mathrm{TECH},g}.$$

We can use the expected values to derive estimators for the model parameters:

$$\hat{\mu}_g = \overline{X}_g,$$
$$\hat{\sigma}^2_{\text{TECH};g} = \text{MS}_g^{\text{TECH}},$$
$$\hat{\sigma}^2_{\text{BIOL};g} = \frac{\text{MS}_g^{\text{BIOL}} - \text{MS}_g^{\text{TECH}}}{n}.$$

The mean has expected value and variance given by

$$E(\overline{X}_g) = \mu_g,$$
$$\text{var}(\overline{X}_g) = \frac{\sigma^2_{\text{BIOL},g}}{a} + \frac{\sigma^2_{\text{TECH},g}}{an}.$$

The variance of $\overline{X}_g$ can be estimated by plugging in the estimates of $\sigma^2_{\text{BIOL};g}$ and $\sigma^2_{\text{TECH};g}$

$$\widehat{\text{var}}(\overline{X}_g) = \frac{\text{MS}_g^{\text{BIOL}} - \text{MS}_g^{\text{TECH}}}{an} + \frac{\text{MS}_g^{\text{TECH}}}{an} + \frac{\text{MS}_g^{\text{BIOL}}}{an}$$
$$= \frac{1}{a}\frac{\Sigma_{j=1}^{a}(\overline{X}_{gj} - \overline{X}_g)^2}{a-1} = \frac{1}{a}\widehat{\text{var}}(\overline{X}_{gi}).$$

In other words, the variance of $\overline{X}_g$ is estimated by dividing by a the variance across the biological replicates of the means obtained by averaging across the technical replicates.

The overall mean $\overline{X}_g$ could be affected by outliers among the biological replicates as well as outliers among the technical replicates. Therefore, a resistant version should offer protection against both types of outliers. To begin with, observe that $\overline{X}_g$ is a mean of means; that is, it is the mean across the biological replicates of the a means across the technical replicates

$$\overline{X}_g = \frac{\Sigma_{j=1}^{a}\Sigma_{i=1}^{n}X_{gij}}{an} = \frac{\Sigma_{j=1}^{a}\overline{X}_{gj}}{a},$$

or, in simple terms,

$$\overline{X}_g = \text{mean}_j \ \text{mean}_i(X_{gij}).$$

Resistant and robust estimators of μ_g can be obtained by replacing the means with resistant analogs.

Working along these lines, Amaratunga and Cabrera (2001a, 2001b) analyzed data from a cDNA chip with three biological by three technical replicates for each of two groups. Using other terminology the experiment can be described as three samples per each of two groups and three probes per sample that are technical replicates.

They proposed a three-step process consisting of (i) background subtraction; (ii) standardization by quantiles (now called *quantile normalization*), and (iii) *median-of-medians* (MOM) estimates (proceed with the statistical analysis at the gene level. Step (iii) proposed to use a highly resistant estimator for μ_g called the *median-of-medians* which also can be calculated by a one-step median polish:

$$M_g = \text{median}_j \ \text{median}_i(X_{gij}).$$

However, no simple resistant estimators of σ^2_{BIOL} or σ^2_{TECH} analogous to MAD are readily available. A standard error for M_g can be estimated using a resampling procedure.

Example. Because the control group in Mouse5 has both biological replicates as well as technical replicates, MOM were calculated to summarize the data across the replicates for the genes in the control group. Medians were calculated for the genes in each treatment group. Figure 6.1 shows the treatment group average plotted against the control group average for the first four treatments. The filled circles represent genes that showed a threefold or greater increase or decrease in expression compared to the control group.

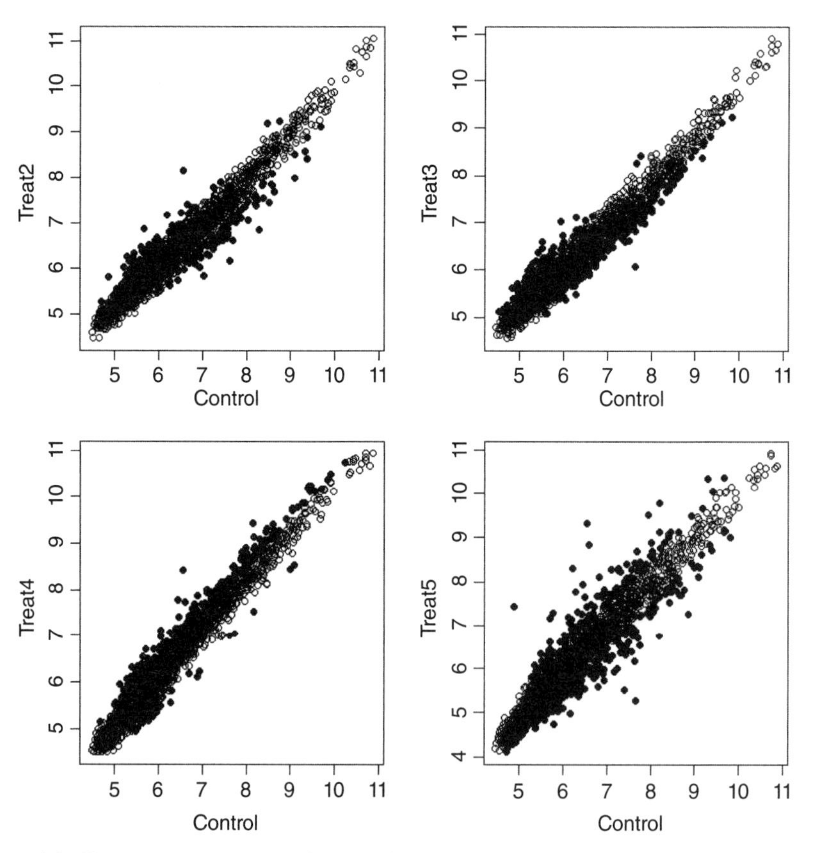

Figure 6.1 Treatment group average plotted against the control group average for the first four treatments.

A robust estimate of μ_g can be obtained by replacing the means with robust analogs:

$$\overline{X}_g = \text{biweightmean}_j \text{biweightmean}_i (X_{gij}).$$

In other words, we first calculate the biweight mean across the technical replicates for each biological replicate. Then the overall biweight mean is the biweight mean across the a biological replicates.

Recall now that the variance of $\overline{X}_g$ is estimated by dividing the variance across the biological replicates of the means obtained by averaging across the technical replicates by a. Analogously, the variance of $\overline{X}_g$ is estimated by dividing the variance across the biological replicates of the means obtained by averaging across the technical replicates by a. In equation form,

$$\widetilde{\text{var}}(\overline{X}_g) = \frac{1}{a}\widetilde{\text{var}}(\overline{X}_{gi}).$$

This, then, produces a robust estimate of the variance of $\overline{X}_g$ as an estimate of μ_g.

6.5 MULTIPLE OLIGONUCLEOTIDE ARRAYS

The expression level of a gene, summarized across multiple oligonucleotide arrays, can be calculated using the methods described below.

A model-based alternative estimation approach was proposed by Li and Wong (2001b) for one probe set in multiple oligonucleotide arrays. For the jth probe pair in this probe set, let PM_{ij} and MM_{ij} denote the (untransformed) expression level measurements for the perfect match probe and mismatch probe, respectively, in the ith microarray.

Let θ_i denote the true expression level of the probe set in the ith array. The model postulates that (i) the observed measurements for MM_{ij} and PM_{ij} are linear functions of θ_i and (ii) for a truly expressed gene, the strength of the PM_{ij} versus θ_i relationship is greater than the strength of the MM_{ij} versus θ_i relationship. Algebraically, the *Li–Wong model* can be written as

$$MM_{ij} = \nu_j + \theta_i \alpha_j + \varepsilon_{ij},$$

$$PM_{ij} = \nu_j + \theta_i(\alpha_j + \phi_j) + \varepsilon_{ij}.$$

The parameters, ν_j, α_j, and ϕ_j, are all assumed to be nonnegative and (ii) above implies that ϕ_j should be strictly positive for a truly expressed gene.

Subtracting the equation for MM from the equation for PM indicates that the PM–MM differences can be modeled by the simpler *reduced Li–Wong model:*

$$Y_{ij} = PM_{ij} - MM_{ij} = \theta_i \phi_j + \varepsilon_{ij}.$$

In words, the perfect match to mismatch difference is, except for random error, the product of a model-based expression index θ_i and a probe sensitivity index ϕ_j. Although some information is lost while using this simpler model, it is easier to use and is often adequate for most practical purposes. The model is overparametrized and some constraint, usually the constraint that $\Sigma\phi_j^2 = J$, is imposed in order to make the model identifiable. The model is fitted by estimating the parameters of this model that minimize the ordinary least squares criterion. They can be obtained by iterative application of a standard least squares routine alternating between estimation of θ_i and ϕ_j until convergence.

Statisticians will recognize the PM−MM difference model as an exponentiated form of the two-way ANOVA linear model with a probe pair effect, an array effect, no intercept term, and no interaction term:

$$\log(Y_{ij}) = \log(\theta_i) + \log(\phi_j) + \varepsilon_{ij}$$

While writing the model in its raw form allows negative values of Y_{ij} to be accommodated, there are certain clear advantages in writing the model the ANOVA way. One is that, if the arrays correspond to different types of samples (e.g., some are from normal tissue and the rest are from diseased tissue), more complex models that include such experimental factors and their interactions can be postulated as in Chapter 8, whereas the Li–Wong model cannot be simply extended beyond the one-way treatment design. For designs in which both models can be fitted, Chu et al. (2004) compared the two-model fits and found that they produced comparable results. On the other hand, the linear model inherently has certain operational advantages because of its linearity; for example, it is easier to fit and the distributional properties of its error term are nicer.

Whichever model is used, there are certainly several benefits to taking a model-based approach over just averaging. By modeling, overly influential observations, such as outliers, can be automatically flagged and the effect of various experimental factors can be statistically assessed.

Efron et al. (2001) discuss a different approach for summarizing data in a 23-factorial experiment involving eight oligonucleotide arrays.

6.6 ESTIMATING FOLD CHANGE IN TWO-CHANNEL EXPERIMENTS

We now consider two-channel microarray experiments. For the gth gene on the ith microarray ($i = 1, \ldots, n$), let X_{1gi} and X_{2gi} refer to the log-transformed and normalized intensity measurements referent to the samples labeled with Channels 1 and 2, respectively. Let $X_{cgi} \sim (\mu_{cg}, \sigma_{cg}^2)$, $c = 1, 2, i = 1, \ldots, n$. One of the principal objectives of two-channel microarray experiments is to estimate the true differential expression for the gth gene, $\rho_g = \mu_{1g} - \mu_{2g}$, and to pick out those that appear to be the most differentially expressed.

The natural estimate of the differential expression is given by

$$\hat{\rho} = \frac{\Sigma_{i=1}^n \overline{X}_{1g} - \overline{X}_{2g}}{n}.$$

This is called the *log fold change* as it is the estimated differential expression on a logarithmic scale, and when transformed back to the original scale,

$$\hat{\phi}_g = e^{\hat{\rho}_g},$$

gives the *fold change*.

The fold change (or log fold change) is a very reasonable, easily understood and readily interpretable estimate of the true differential expression. Consequently, it is also, by far, the most widely used. Nevertheless, it is wise to be cautious when interpreting fold changes across a multitude of genes because a given fold change may have a different interpretation for a gene whose expression level is low in both channels as compared to a gene whose expression level is high in both channels.

The standard error of $\hat{\rho}_g$ is

$$\text{se}(\hat{\rho}_g) = \frac{s_g}{\sqrt{n}},$$

where s_g is the standard deviation of $\{Y_{gi} = X_{1gi}X_{2gi}\}$. The standard error of $\hat{\phi}_g$ is, approximately,

$$\text{se}(\hat{\phi}_g) = \frac{\hat{\phi}_g s_g}{\sqrt{n}}.$$

6.7 BAYES ESTIMATION OF FOLD CHANGE

Newton et al. (2001) attempt to overcome the problem of different interpretations being necessary for genes with different expression levels by using the Bayesian hierarchical modeling approach to estimate the true differential expression. The models are based on the Gamma distribution. This is because Gamma distributions have several features pertinent to this situation: their support is $(0, \infty)$, they are skewed, their coefficient of variation can be controlled, they are easy to work with, and it can be argued that they may be meaningful biologically.

Suppose that X_{gi} and Y_{gi} are the intensity measurements from the sample labeled with Channels 1 and 2, respectively. Assume that they have been suitably transformed and normalized and then transformed back to the original scale. Let $X_{gi} \sim (\mu_{X_g}, \sigma^2 X_g)$ and $Y_{gi} \sim (\mu_{Y_g}, \sigma^2 Y_g)$.

The intensities X_{gi} and Y_{gi} can be modeled as independent Gamma random variables: $X_{gi} \sim \text{Gamma}(a, \theta_X)$, $Y_{gi} \sim \text{Gamma}(a, \theta_Y)$. Because their means are $\mu_X = E(X_{gi})a/\theta_X$ and $\mu_Y = E(Y_{gi}) = a/\theta_Y$, the ratio of their means is $\rho = \mu_X/\mu_Y = \theta_Y/\theta_X$. Their variances are $var(X_{gi}) = a/\theta_X^2$ and $var(Y_{gi}) = a/\theta_Y^2$ so that both X_{gi} and Y_{gi} have the same coefficient of variation, $1/\sqrt{a}$, irrespective of whether or not they have the same variance, which is reasonable to expect after normalization. The hierarchical aspect of the model is that the parameters (θ_x, θ_Y) themselves are modeled as $(\theta_x, \theta_Y) \sim \text{Gamma}(a_0, \nu)$.

The posterior distribution of true differential expression can be derived using the Bayes theorem:

$$p(\rho|X, Y, a, a_0, \nu) \propto \rho^{-(a+a_0+1)}\left\{\frac{1}{\rho} + \frac{X+\nu}{Y+\nu}\right\}^{-2(a+a_0)}.$$

The statistic

$$\hat{\rho}_g^{\text{EB}} = \frac{X_g + \nu}{Y_g + \nu},$$

which lies somewhere in between the mean and the mode of this distribution, is used as the empirical Bayes estimator of the true differential expression. Those familiar with the concept of regularization (see Section 10.3) will recognize that $\hat{\rho}_g^{\text{EB}}$ has the form of a shrinkage estimator. For a gene whose expression level is high in both channels $\hat{\rho}_g^{\text{EB}}$ will be quite close to $\hat{\rho}_g$, whereas for a gene whose expression level is low in both channels $\hat{\rho}_g^{\text{EB}}$ will be shrunk toward 1; the amount of shrinkage is governed by ν. Thus, the empirical Bayes estimator is able to reflect the decreased variation in differential expression with increasing intensity.

Unfortunately, there is no closed form expression for ν. The unknown parameters, (a, a_0, ν), in the model, are estimated by marginal maximum likelihood, details of which are provided by Newton et al. (2001). Besides this, another slight drawback to $\hat{\rho}_g^{\text{EB}}$ is that it does not inherit the natural fold change interpretation of $\hat{\rho}_g$.

Not surprisingly, the ordering of the most significantly expressed genes using the empirical Bayes estimates will generally be quite different from that using the regular estimates.

6.8 ESTIMATING FOLD CHANGE AFFYMETRIX DATA

Similar to two-channel experiments, the natural estimate of the differential expression in Affymetrix experiments (with two conditions) is given by

$$\hat{\rho} = \overline{X}_{1g} - \overline{X}_{2g},$$

and the fold change is exp $(\hat{\rho}_g)$. Here, $\overline{X}_{1g}$ and $\overline{X}_{2g}$ are the sample means under the two conditions.

Example. We illustrate the concept of fold change using the Golub data. The data consists of gene expression data (3051 genes and 38 tumor mRNA samples) from the leukemia microarray study reported by Golub et al. (1999). There are two the tumor classes, 27 ALL cases and 11 AML cases. Figure 6.2a shows the gene-specific estimates for ρ_g. We notice, as expected, that $\|\hat{\rho}\| > 2$ for only few genes, indicating that in most of the gene, the expression levels are not different between the ALL and AML groups. Parameter estimates for

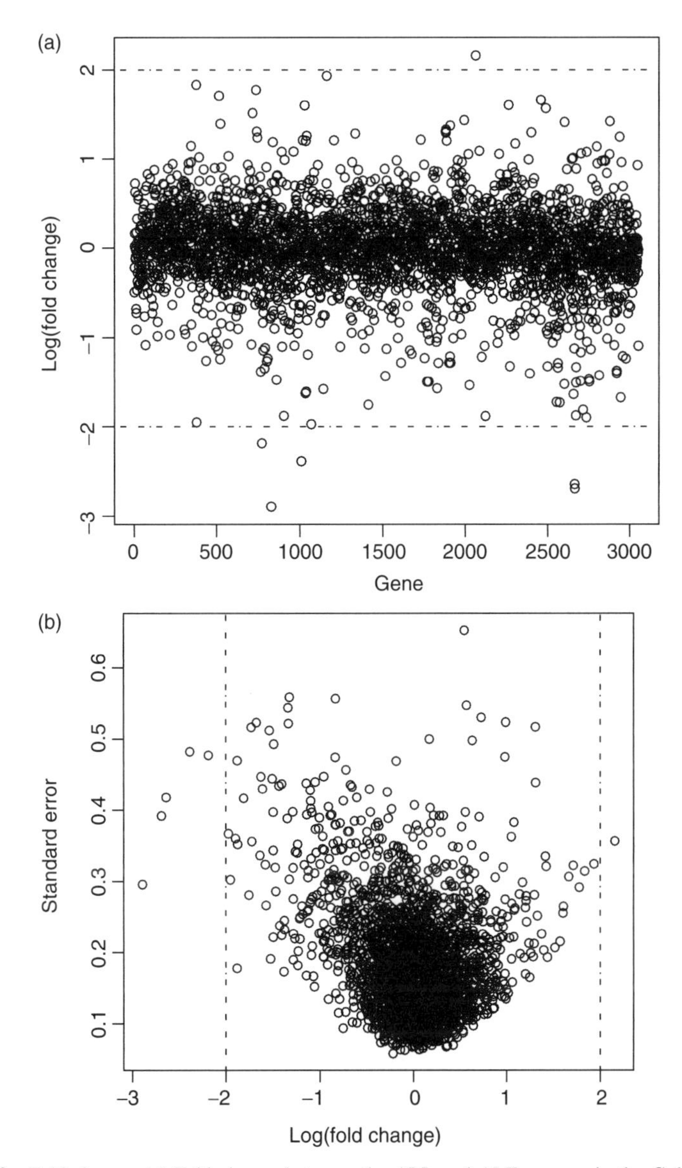

Figure 6.2 Fold change. (a) Fold change between the ALL and AML groups in the Golub data. (b) Fold change versus the empirical standard error.

se($\hat{\phi}_g$) plotted versus the log(fold change) are shown in Figure 6.2b. Finally, Figure 6.3 shows the expression levels for two genes. The log(fold change) is equal to -0.002 and -2.894 for gene 9 and 829, respectively. Note that the log(fold change) is the difference between the two horizontal lines in the lower panels of Figure 6.3.

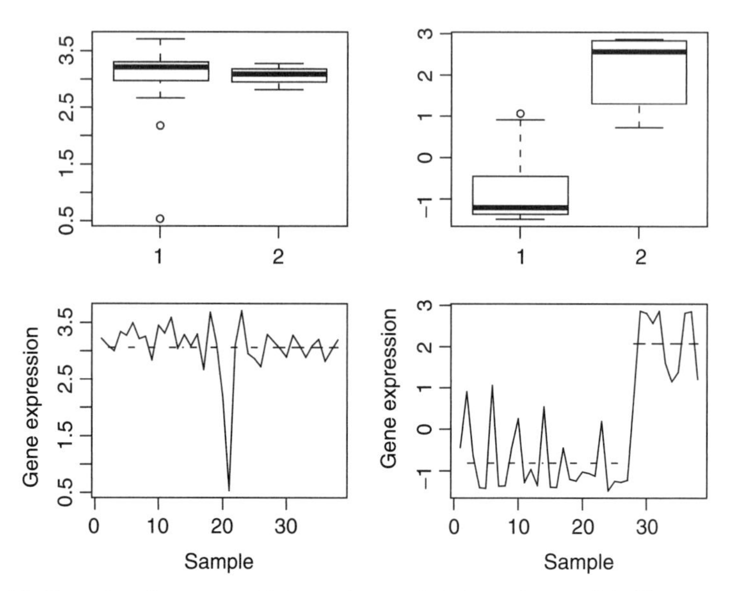

Figure 6.3 Examples of two genes. Right panels: gene 9. Left panels: gene 829. Upper row: boxplot for gene expression. Lower panels: gene expression plot. The first 27 samples belong to the ALL group, while the later 11 to the AML group. Dotted-dashed line represents mean gene expression in the ALL group. Dashed line represents mean gene expression in the AML group.

6.9 RMA SUMMARIZATION OF MULTIPLE OLIGONUCLEOTIDE ARRAYS REVISITED

Example. We use the platinum data to illustrate a *robust multiarray average* (RMA) summarization for multiple oligonucleotide arrays. We focus on the following topics:

- *Probe Intensities and Summarized Data.* Figure 6.4 shows the probe intensities and the summarized intensity per sample for two genes. The summarized intensities per sample (the thick line) are the gene expression levels and could be used as an input for further analysis. Note that the thick line represents the gene's expression level and it was estimated from the model for the log-transformed PM_{ij} discussed in Section 6.5,

$$\log(Y_{ij}) = \log(\theta_i) + \log(\phi_j) + \varepsilon_{ij}.$$

  In the above model, the parameter $\log(\theta_i)$ represents the (log-transformed) gene intensities. Irizarry et al. (2003) proposed to use a three-step procedure consisting of (i) background correction, (ii) quantile normalization, and (iii) the *median polish* method in order to obtain a robust estimate for $\log(\theta_i)$. In Table 6.1, this procedure is compared to the MOM method introduced in Section 6.4.

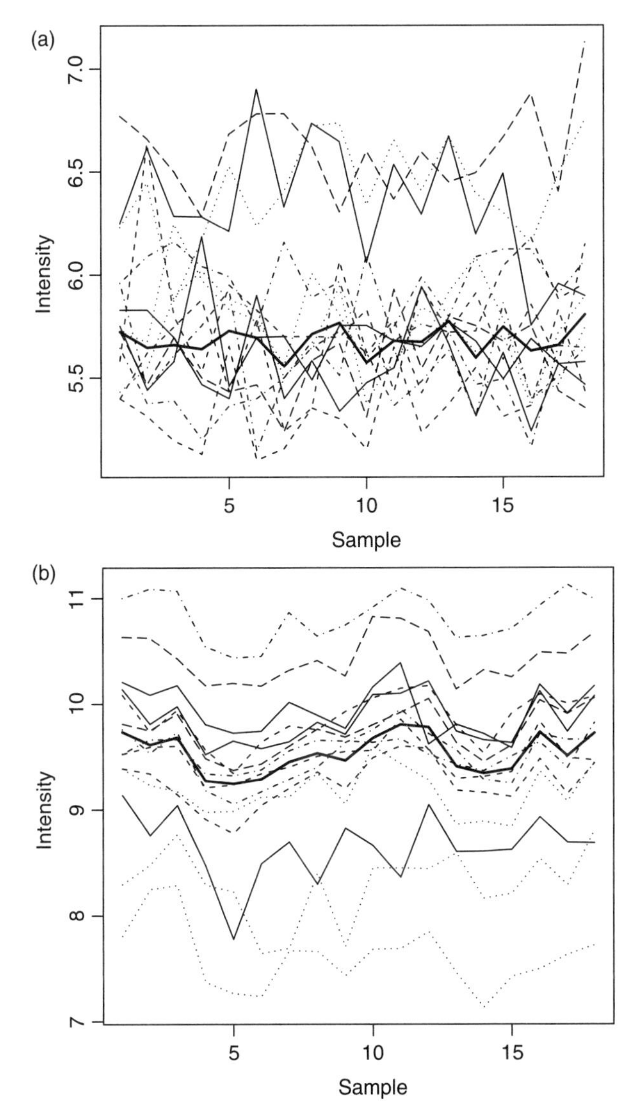

Figure 6.4 Summarization of Affymetrix Platinum data: intensities by sample. Thick line represents the summarized gene intensity per sample. (a) Gene 1636512_s_at. (b) Gene 1631954_at.

Table 6.1 Comparison of RMA and MOM

	RMA (Irizarry et al., 2003)	MOM (Amaratunga and Cabrera, 2001a, 2001b)
1	Background correction	Background subtraction
2	Quantile normalization	Quantile normalization
3	Median Polish	One-step Median Polish
4	Statistical analysis	Statistical analysis

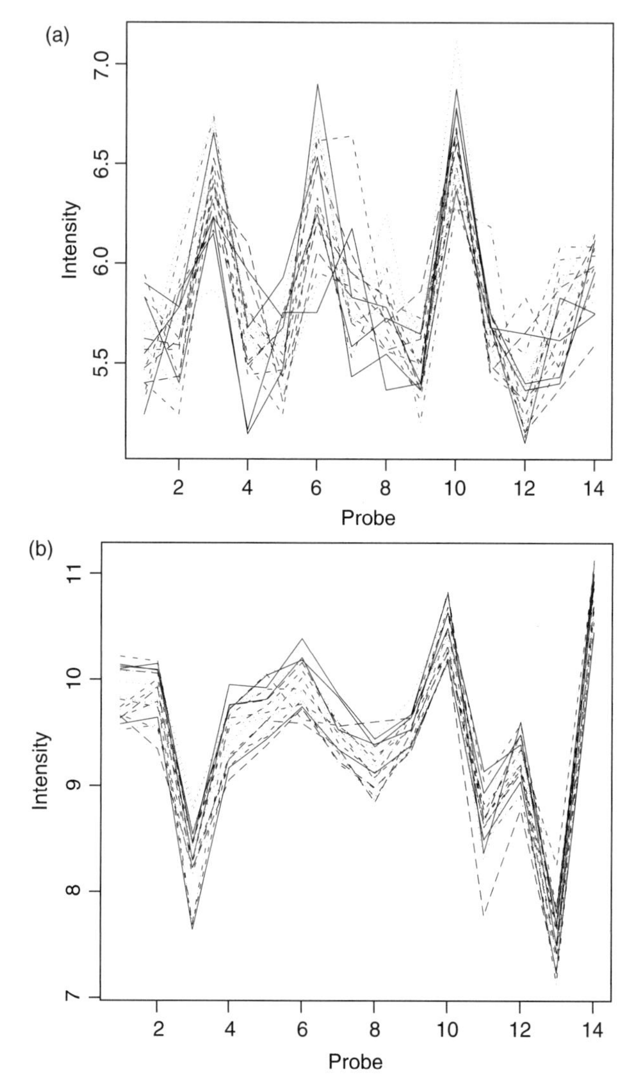

Figure 6.5 Summarization of Affymetrix Platinum data: intensities by probe. (a) Gene 1636512_s_at. (b) Gene 1631954_at.

- *Correlation among Probe Intensities.* Figure 6.5 shows the probe intensities by probe and reveals an important pattern of correlation among the intensities. The correlation among probes of the same gene (probe set) obtained in the same array is expected because all probes measure the same *true and unobserved* gene expression. We notice, however, that the magnitude of the correlation among probe intensities is not the same for the two genes, the correlation gene 1636512_s_at seems to be lower than the correlation among probe intensities in gene 1631954_at. This can be clearly seen in Figure 6.6

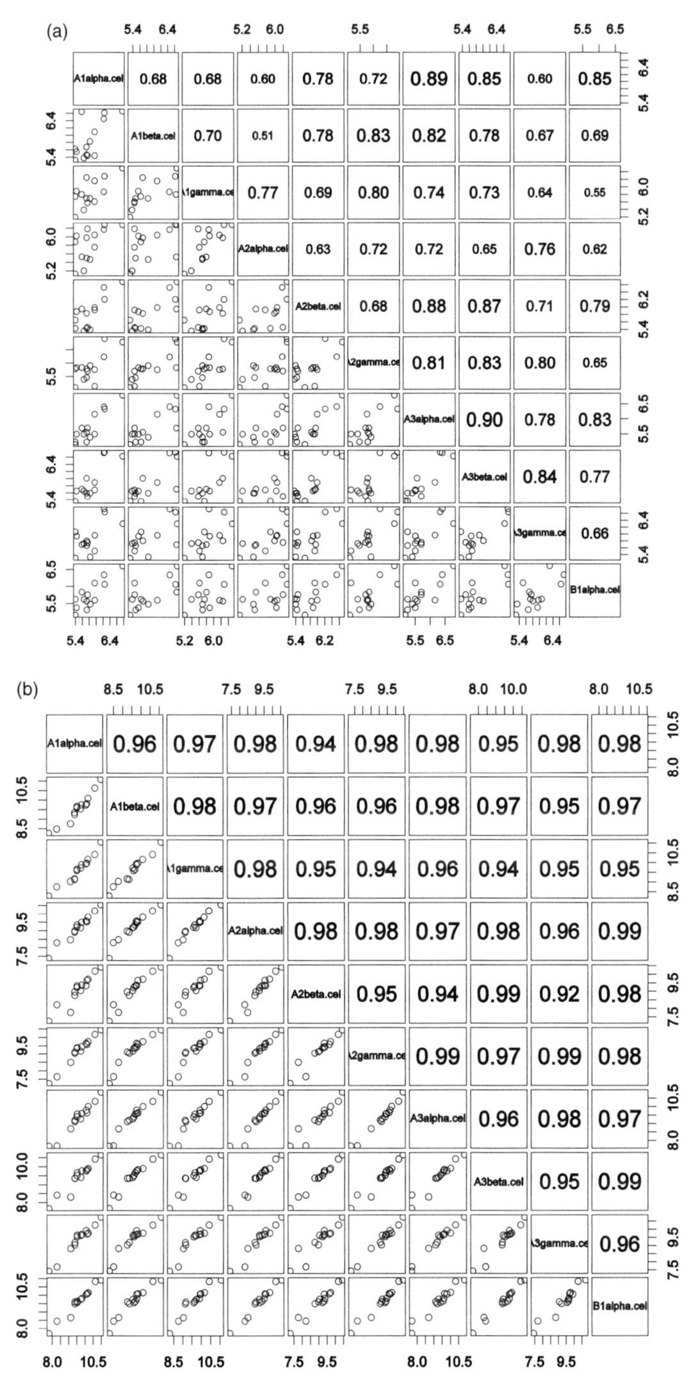

Figure 6.6 Scatterplot matrix for probe intensities. (a) Gene 1636512_s_at. (b) Gene 1631954_at.

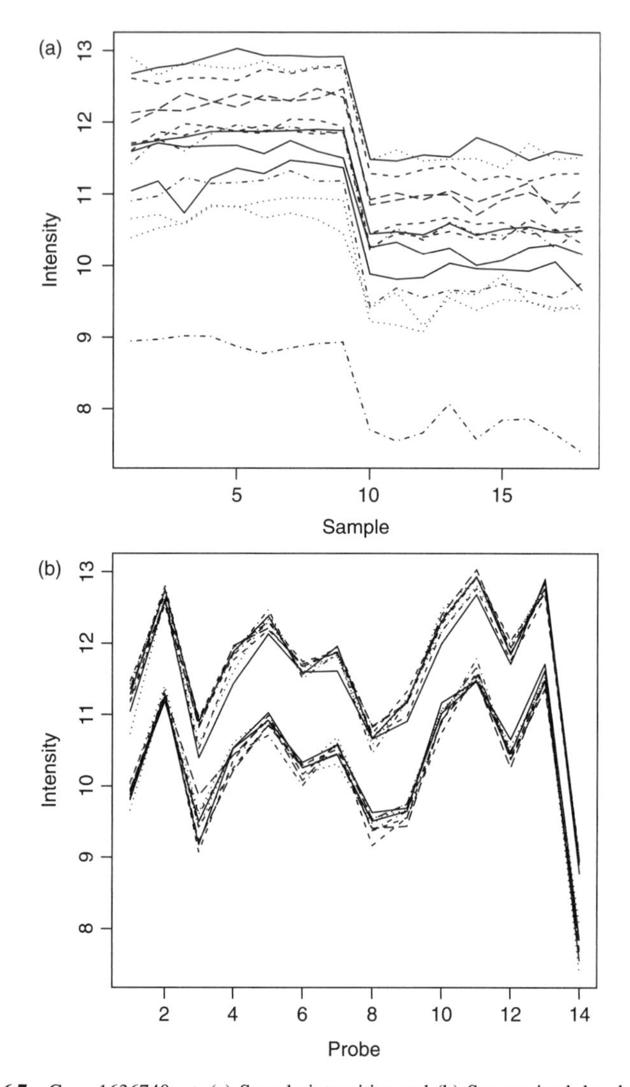

Figure 6.7 Gene 1636740_at. (a) Sample intensities and (b) Summarized data by probe.

that presents the scatterplot matrix for probes intensities for selected probes in the probe set. The correlation among probe intensities is a crucial point for gene filtering which will be discussed in Chapter 7.

- *Condition Effects and (Log) Fold Change.* Figure 6.7 shows the intensities levels of the gene 1636740_at and reveals a clear pattern of condition effect on both probe level and summarized data. Note that the log(fold change), discussed in Section 6.8 is the difference between the mean of the summarized data under the two conditions.

6.10 FACTOR ANALYSIS FOR ROBUST MICROARRAY SUMMARIZATION, FARMS

Factor analysis for robust microarray summarization (FARMS, Hochreiter et al., 2006) is a summarization method that assumes that the log-transformed and normalized PM values can be described by a *factor analysis* model in which the factor represents the true but unobserved gene expression. Hence, the FARMS method implies a multiplicative model for the log (PM) values given by

$$\log(PM_{ij}) = \lambda_j z_i + \varepsilon_{ij},$$

where z_i is the *factor scores* and λ_j are the factor loadings. In this model, the factor scores represent the summarized gene expression levels. Let us consider a probe set with K probes in an experiment with n samples. The probe-set-specific expression matrix of the log-transformed and normalized PM values, $\widetilde{PM}$, is given by

$$\mathbf{Y} = \begin{pmatrix} \widetilde{PM}_{11} & \widetilde{PM}_{12} & \cdots & \widetilde{PM}_{1n} \\ \widetilde{PM}_{21} & \widetilde{PM}_{22} & \cdots & \widetilde{PM}_{2n} \\ \cdot & \cdot & \cdot & \cdot \\ \cdot & \cdot & \cdot & \cdot \\ \cdot & \cdot & \cdot & \cdot \\ \widetilde{PM}_{K1} & \widetilde{PM}_{K2} & \cdots & \widetilde{PM}_{Kn} \end{pmatrix}.$$

The column effects in $\mathbf{Y}$ are the summarized expression level (per sample) and are of primary interest. In RMA, the probe-set-specific expression matrix $\mathbf{Y}$ is summarized using the iterative median polish procedure in which rows, columns, and overall effects are estimated iteratively by the corresponding medians until convergence. Gene expression level for specific sample is the iterative median of the column (or the column effect). In FARMS, $\mathbf{Y}$ is summarized using factor analysis model and the sample-specific gene expression data are the factor scores.

Example. The platinum data set is used for illustration of the FARMS method. Figure 6.8a presents both intensities levels and summarized data by RMA and FARMS for probe set 1627131_at. It shows that the summarized data for this probe set are correlated (see also Fig. 6.8b). Columns effects (sample effects) estimated by RMA and FARMS are shown in Figure 6.9a. Note that both the methods add a constant to the columns effects that represent the overall gene expression (see Figure 6.9b, which presents the gene expression data versus the factor scores.)

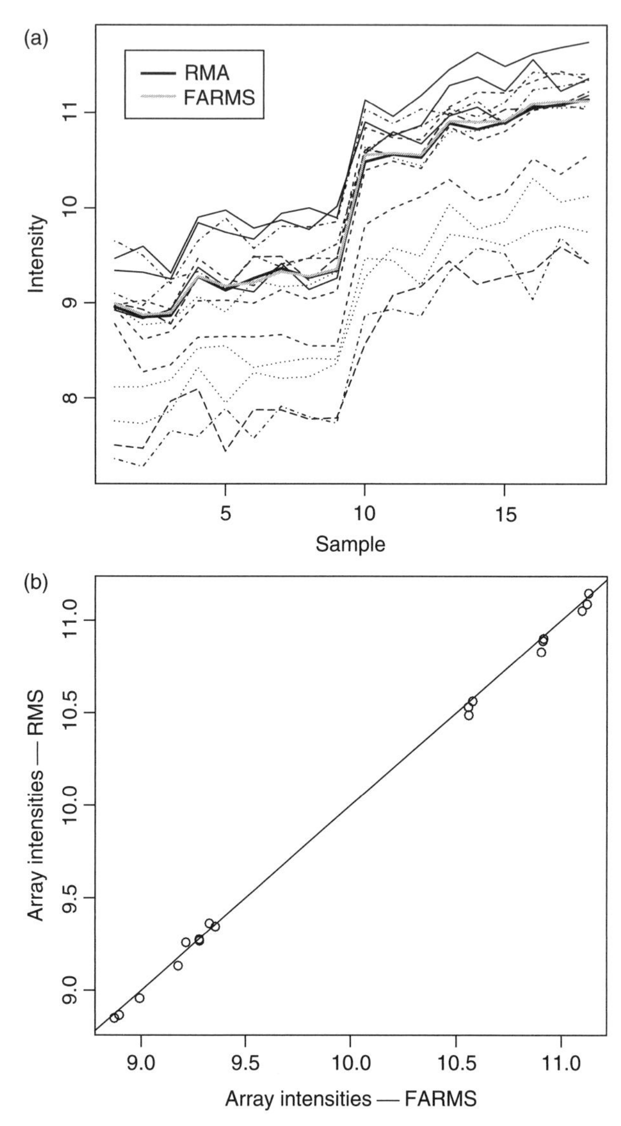

Figure 6.8 Summarization by RMA and FARMS for gene 1627131_at (I). (a) Probe intensities and summarized data by sample. (b) Gene expression data (per sample) summarized by RMA and FARMS.

SOFTWARE NOTES

`DNAMR 2.0`

DNAMR The MOM method for summarization across replicates is available in DNAMR.

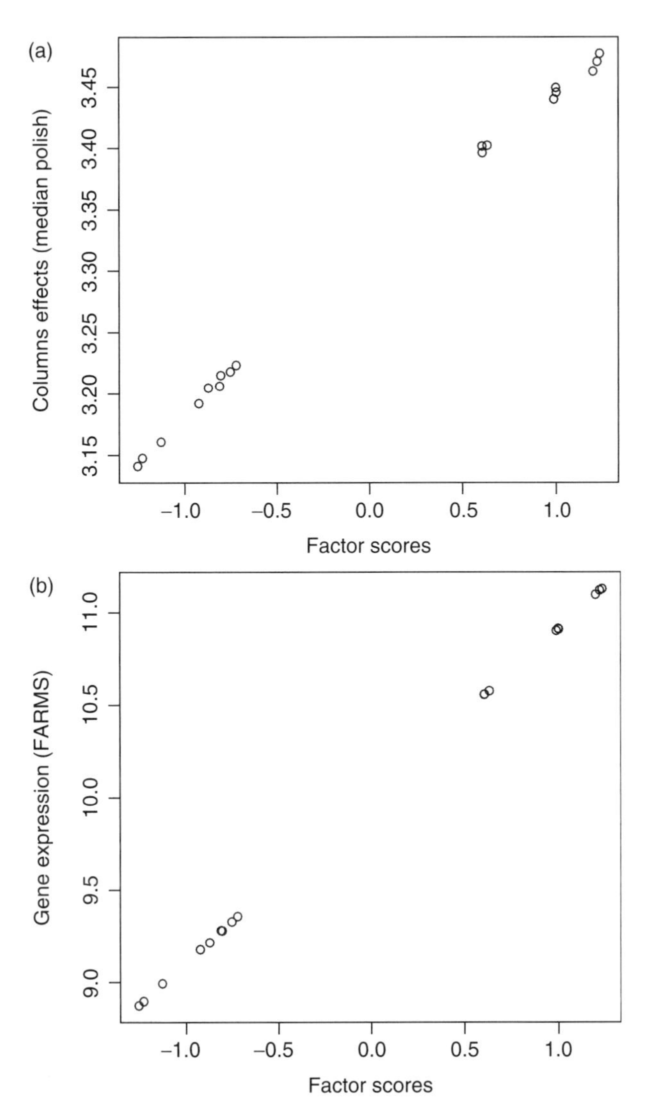

Figure 6.9 Summarization by RMA and FARMS for gene 1627131_at (II). (a) Factor scores versus columns effects obtained by median polish. (b) Factor scores versus summarized gene expression data.

`Affy`

The summarization for oligonucleotide arrays, discussed in Section 6.6, was done using the Bioconductor package `Affy`. In particular, the Li–Wong method, average difference, and the median polish are implemented in the package. Summarization methods implemented in the `Affy` package are discussed in Irizarry et al. (2003) and Li and Wong (2001).

`farms`

FARMS is a model-based technique for summarizing high-density oligonucleotide array data at probe level. The method is implemented in the Bioconductor package `farms`.

EXERCISES

6.1. Explain the need to have both technical replicates and biological replicates in a study.

6.2. Read Efron et al. (2001) and outline the summarization procedure used there.

6.3. For the data in Example E5, calculate the MOM for the control microarrays and the medians for the treatment Group C10. Plot them against one another. Do any genes appear to be differentially expressed in the treatment group compared to the control group?

6.4. For this question use the platinum dataset.

1. Choose a probeset from the platinum dataset and plot the probes intensities (by sample) of the probeset. Do you see a different expression levels across conditions?
2. Use the expression profiles plot from (1) and explain the correlation structure that you see among the probe intensities.
3. Choose several probe sets and summaries the probe levels data using RMA and FARMS. Plot the summarized data obtained from RMA and FARMS and compare the results.

6.5. In this question we use the Golub data for the estimation of the fold change.

1. Estimate the fold change in the Golub data and use boxplot and expression profiles for the 10 genes with the largest (smallest) fold change in the data.
2. For each group of genes, calculate the t-test statistic and plot the fold change versus the test statistics, what are your conclusions?

6.6. Please retrieve the data set `cel_filesday0` from the DNAMR web site which contains the 12 CEL files with from the Sialin day 0 data.

1. Calculate the rma gene expressions and compare the two groups gene by gene using a t test. This should result in a list of p-values, one per gene measuring the differential expression between knock out samples and wild type.
2. Apply the MOM method from the DNAMR package and obtain the corresponding gene p-values.
3. Compare the results of (i) and (ii) by checking the overlap in the sets of 10, 100 and 500 most significant genes.

CHAPTER 7

Two-Group Comparative Experiments

Many microarray experiments are comparative in nature. That is, their objective is to compare the expression levels of a set of genes across two or more conditions and to, in particular, identify genes that are significantly differentially expressed across these conditions. For example, an experiment might be conducted to compare the expression levels of several genes in cancerous liver cells with those in normal liver cells in an attempt to identify the genes that are expressed in cancerous liver cells but not in normal liver cells and vice versa. As another example, an experiment might be conducted to compare the expression levels of several genes in cancerous liver cells in a group of patients treated with a particular test drug with those in a group of untreated patients in an attempt to identify the genes that are expressed in treated cancerous liver cells but not in untreated cancerous liver cells and vice versa.

The simplest way to analyze comparative experiments is to consider each gene in isolation and to compare its expression levels across the groups. At a higher level of complexity, genes can be analyzed in combination, comparing the expression levels of clusters of genes across the groups. The clusters may be prespecified or identified as part of a clustering exercise. Besides finding individual differentially expressing genes, any collection of genes that is found to be differentially expressed across the groups could be used to deduce the regulatory pathways involved in the situation under investigation.

We begin by considering the simplest and most common case: a comparative experiment in which two groups are being compared to one another. In the first few sections of this chapter, we discuss methods for analyzing each gene on its own. The concepts introduced in this initial discussion are important in their own right and will also lay the foundation for more complex and refined analyses, which are discussed in the later sections of this chapter.

Exploration and Analysis of DNA Microarray and Other High-Dimensional Data, Second Edition.
Dhammika Amaratunga, Javier Cabrera, Ziv Shkedy.

Example. In an example that will recur throughout the chapter, we consider a comparison between the gene expression profiles of two groups of four mice. The first group of mice was treated with a vehicle control, while the other group was treated with a test compound. After several hours, a mRNA sample was extracted from the liver of each animal and placed on a microarray containing 4077 genes. Intensity measurements were taken; these were then log transformed and normalized. A scatterplot matrix showing pairwise scatterplots of the gene expression profiles of the eight mice is shown in Figure 7.1.

We use the following notation in this chapter. Suppose that we are comparing the expression levels of a set of G genes in two groups of microarrays, which we shall refer to as Group 1 and Group 2; there are n_1 microarrays in Group 1 and n_2 microarrays in Group 2; the total sample size is $N = n_1 + n_2$. Let x_{gij} denote the intensity measurement for the gth gene in the ith microarray in the jth group, where $i = 1, \ldots, n_j$, $j = 1, 2$; and $g = 1, \ldots, G$. When emphasis on the gene is unnecessary, we will omit the first subscript and denote the intensity measurements x_{ij}. It is assumed that the data have already been suitably transformed and normalized. In addition, let $\overline{x}_j$, $\tilde{x}_j$, s_j, and $\tilde{s}_j$ denote the mean, median, standard deviation, and median absolute deviation from the median (MAD) of the jth group, respectively.

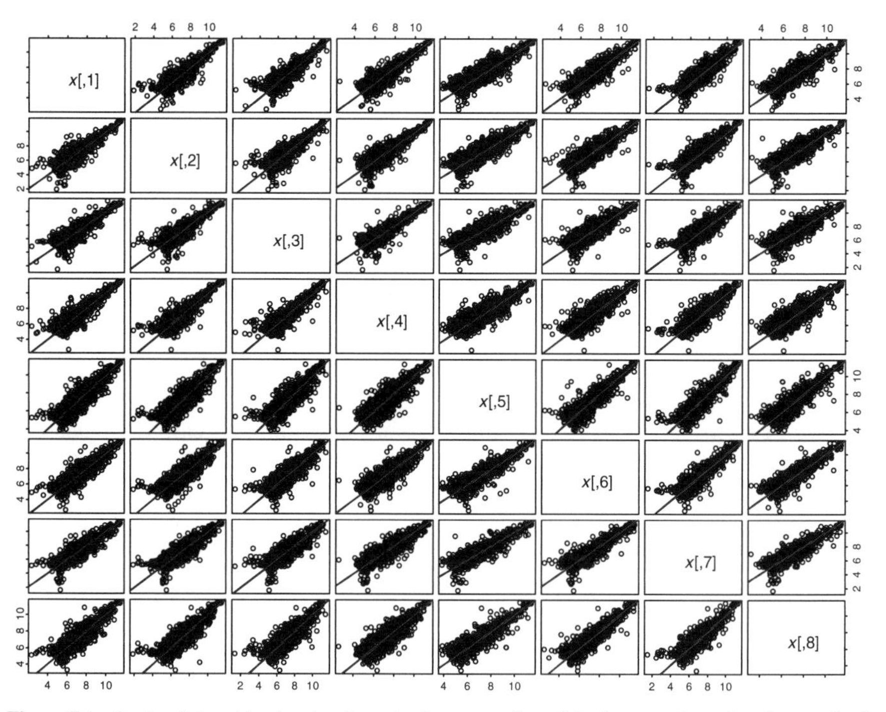

Figure 7.1 Scatterplot matrix showing the pairwise scatterplots of the log-transformed and normalized spot intensities for the eight mice.

7.1 BASICS OF STATISTICAL HYPOTHESIS TESTING

We digress now to review briefly the fundamentals of statistical hypothesis testing. We expect readers with statistics backgrounds to skip this section.

In statistical hypothesis testing, the conjecture that there is no difference between groups is called the *null hypothesis*. With microarray data, there are G null hypotheses being tested, the gth null hypothesis, for $g = 1, \ldots, G$, being that the gth gene is not differentially expressed across the groups. For example, for a two groups experiment, the null hypothesis of no group difference is given by

$$H_0 : \mu_{g_1} = \mu_{g_2},$$

where μ_{g_1} and μ_{g_2} are the mean gene expression in group 1 and 2, respectively.

The result of a hypothesis test is its *decision*. There are two possible decisions: *reject* the null hypothesis and claim that there is a difference between the groups (which can be thought of as a positive finding) or *do not reject* the null hypothesis and declare that there is insufficient evidence to detect a difference between the groups (which can be thought of as a *negative finding*).

If the decision of the test is to reject the null hypothesis, it may be correctly rejecting a null hypothesis that is false (called a *true positive*) or it may be incorrectly rejecting a null hypothesis that is true (called a *false positive* or *a Type I error*), we do not know which. On the other hand, if the decision of the test is not to reject the null hypothesis, it may be correctly not rejecting a null hypothesis that is true (called a *true negative*) or it may be incorrectly not rejecting a null hypothesis that is false (called a *false negative* or a *Type II error*), we do not know which. Table 7.1 is a simple tabular representation of these four possibilities.

In practice, we do not know whether the null hypothesis is true or false. Thus, we really have no way of knowing whether the test might have provided the right decision or reached a false positive or a false negative decision. However, what is fascinating is that it is possible to set up the test to reduce the chances of making such errors. This is what distinguishes a "good" test from a "bad" test.

The key to a good test is a good *test statistic*. The test statistic is generally a sample statistic that reflects how far the observed data are from the situation described by the null hypothesis. Many test statistics, T, have the form r/s. Here, r is the estimate of the size of the biological effect being tested; the further the data are from the null hypothesis (i.e., the more likely that the null hypothesis is false), the larger the value of r. The denominator, s, is the standard error that measures

Table 7.1 Possible Decision in Hypotheses Testing

	Null Hypothesis True	Null Hypothesis False
Null hypothesis not rejected	True negative	False negative (Type II error)
Null hypothesis rejected	False positive (Type I error)	True positive

the variability of r. Thus, T measures how large the biological effect r is relative to its variability s. It is no accident that T has the form of a *signal-to-noise* ratio with r as the "signal" and s as the "noise."

The probability distribution of the test statistic under the null hypothesis is called its *null distribution*. On the basis of the null distribution, we can calculate the p-value, the probability of observing a value as extreme as that observed if the null hypothesis was true. Clearly, the smaller the p-value, the greater the weight of evidence against the null hypothesis. A typical decision rule for a test states that the null hypothesis is rejected if and only if the p-value is less than a specified value called the *significance level* (or just the level) of the test.

The probability of the test reaching a false positive decision is called the *false positive rate* (FPR or the *Type I error probability*) and the probability of the test reaching a false negative decision is called the *false negative rate* (or the *Type II error probability*). Also, the "true positive rate" is called the *specificity* and the "true negative rate" is called the *sensitivity* or *power*. Naturally, we would like both the FPR and the false negative rate to be zero, but this is impossible. On top of that, decreasing one tends to increase the other; in other words, increasing the specificity lowers the sensitivity and vice versa. Thus, we have to arrive at some compromise between the two.

The most popular such compromise is the *Neyman–Pearson approach* to statistical hypothesis testing. In this approach, the FPR is controlled at a specified small value, called the *size of the test*, and then the test is set up to have as small a false negative rate (or, equivalently, as high a true negative rate) as possible—in other words, "fix the size, maximize the power." Generally, the size of the test is bounded above by the significance level.

Of course, life is not so simple. In order to select or develop a good test for a particular situation, it is necessary to make some *assumptions* about that situation. Different assumptions for the same situation will generally lead to quite different tests, and, what is more unsettling is perhaps even quite different test results. Thus, it is important to consider one's assumptions carefully and to keep in mind that, if the assumptions being made are not correct, the size and power properties expected from the test to display might not be achieved. This is why it is always a good idea to run some *diagnostics* to check whether the assumptions underlying the test seem to hold. If they do not appear to hold, it is wise to rethink the testing procedure.

7.2 FOLD CHANGES

Early analyses of microarray data declared a gene differentially expressed if its fold increase or fold decrease exceeded a specified cutoff. For example, in their seminal paper on using microarrays to study gene expression in *Arabidopsis thaliana*, Schena et al. (1995) declared a gene differentially expressed if its expression level showed a fivefold difference between the two mRNA samples.

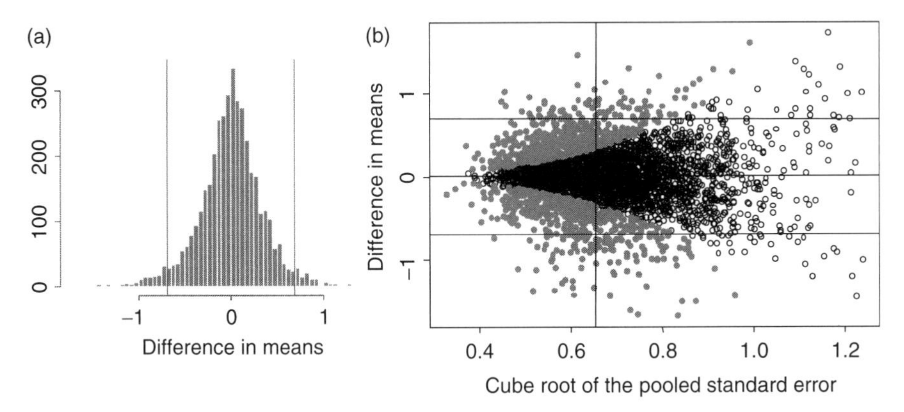

Figure 7.2 (a) Histogram of the difference in means; the two vertical lines refer to twofold changes. (b) Scatterplot of the difference in means versus the cube root of the pooled standard error with those genes found significant by the two-sample t-test shown as filled circles; the central vertical and horizontal lines pass through the medians of the axes, while the other two horizontal lines refer to twofold changes.

On a logarithmic scale, the decision rule that declares that changes of h-fold or greater are significant translates into declaring that a gene should be declared differentially expressed if $|\overline{x}_1 - \overline{x}_2| > \log(h)$.

Example. For the example data set, Figure 7.2a shows a histogram of the values, which range from -1.66 (i.e., a 5.26-fold downregulation compared to control) to 1.72 (i.e., a 5.58-fold upregulation compared to control) with a near zero median of 0.01 with 119 genes showing a twofold or greater upregulation compared to control and 144 genes showing a twofold or greater downregulation compared to control.

The reliance on fold change alone to designate significance has, rightly, been criticized. Keep in mind that the means are merely estimates of the true but unknown mean expression levels and hence are subject to variability. Genes with high variability have a reasonable probability of having a large fold change and looking deceptively interesting. The problem with the fold change approach is that it utterly fails to take this uncertainty into account. It is entirely possible, after all, that a gene might exhibit a 10-fold change and yet not be significant because it has high variability, whereas another gene might exhibit a two fold change and be highly significant, both statistically and biologically, because its expression-level measurements had low variability and were therefore more precise.

The variability of the estimates can be estimated and should be used to adjust the threshold (an early paper on microarrays, Chen et al. 1997), developed some distribution theory in this regard). This is the idea behind the t-test discussed in Section 7.3 and extensions of the t-test that are discussed later. Applying the same arbitrarily chosen threshold to all the genes in the study is just not appropriate.

7.3 THE TWO-SAMPLE t-TEST

The most basic statistical test for comparing two groups is the two-sample t-test. The two-sample t-test statistic, for a two-sided hypotheses testing, is given by

$$T_e = \frac{|\bar{x}_1 - \bar{x}_2|}{s_p\sqrt{\dfrac{1}{n_1} + \dfrac{1}{n_2}}},$$

where

$$s_p^2 = \frac{(n_1 - 1)s_1^2 + (n_2 - 1)s_2^2}{n_1 + n_2 - 2},$$

is the pooled estimate of variance.

If the data are drawn from a normal distribution (the normal distribution is sometimes called the *Gaussian distribution*) and are homoscedastic (i.e., have equal variances), $x_{ij} \sim \mathrm{N}(\mu_j, \sigma_j^2)$, the null distribution of T_e is a t-distribution with degrees of freedom $\nu = n_1 + n_2 - 2$. If the observed value of T_e is $T_{e;\mathrm{obs}}$ then the p-value is given by the probability $p_e = \mathrm{Prob}(|T_e| > T_{e;\mathrm{obs}})$. A gene is declared significantly differentially expressed at level of significance if $p_e < \alpha$.

Example. Of the 4077 genes in the example, 998 are significantly differentially expressed at the 5% level according to the above test; 523 are upregulated compared to control, while 475 are downregulated compared to control. Figure 7.2b shows a scatterplot of the difference in means versus the cube root of the pooled standard error, with the genes found significantly differentially expressed by the t-test plotted as filled circles and the others as clear circles. Figure 7.3a and b shows scatterplots of the p-values versus the differences in means and the cube roots of the pooled standard errors, respectively. These plots indicate that the t-test has a tendency of ignoring those genes that have large differences in means (i.e., large fold changes on the raw scale) if they also should happen to have high variances. This is reasonable, but its inclination to focus on genes with small variances may be too strong when the variances are estimated from small samples from which variance estimates cannot be well estimated. This behavior of the t-test is addressed in Sections 7.10 and 7.11.

Observe that the t-test statistic has the form of a signal-to-noise ratio as mentioned in Section 7.1. The "signal" is the numerator that reflects the difference we are trying to discover; the "noise" is the denominator that reflects the variability of the system.

The two-sample t-test can be modified to test whether the average intensity of the first group is greater or less than that of the second group by some specified

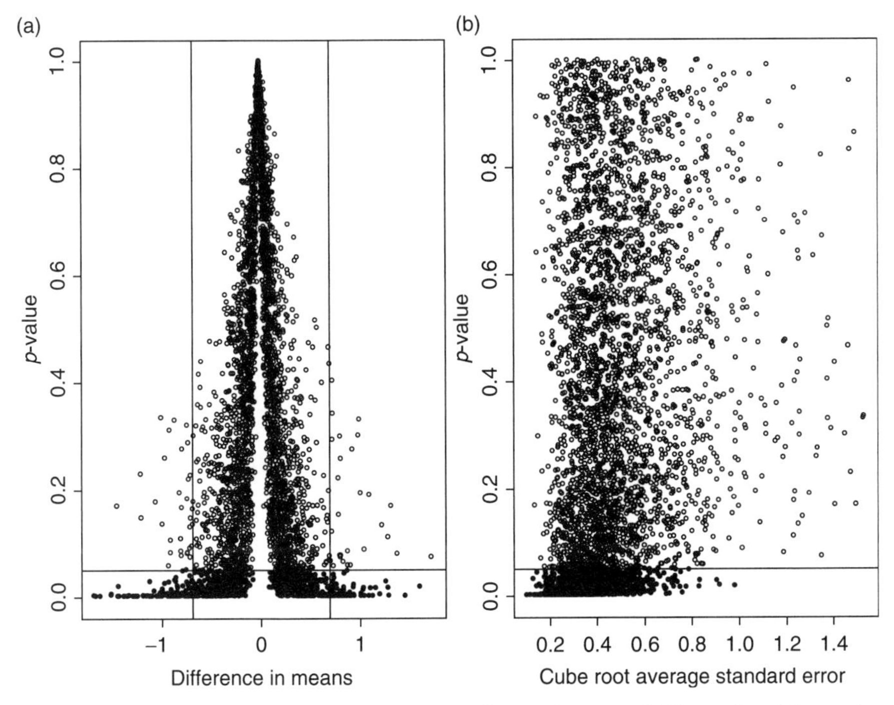

Figure 7.3 (a) Scatterplot of the p-value versus the difference in means. (b) Scatterplot of the p-value versus the cube root of the pooled standard error. Genes found significant by the two-sample t-test are shown as filled circles. The two vertical lines in (a) refer to twofold changes and the horizontal lines in (a) and (b) refer to a p-value cutoff of 5%.

value, δ (e.g., $\Delta = \log(2)$ for a two fold difference). The test statistic for this is

$$T_\Delta = \frac{|\overline{x}_1 - \overline{x}_2| - \Delta}{s_p\sqrt{\dfrac{1}{n_1} + \dfrac{1}{n_2}}}.$$

The null distribution of T_Δ is, again, a t-distribution with degrees of freedom $\nu = n_1 + n_2 - 2$. As very small group differences are usually of no interest and can come up significant because of having unbelievably small variances as outlined above, it is better to use this form of the t-test to focus in on more meaningful differences.

Example. Of the 4077 genes in the example, 223 are upregulated by more than twofold compared to control, while 175 are downregulated by more than twofold compared to control.

The assumptions of normality and homoscedasticity are critical to the t-test functioning properly. For instance, if the underlying distribution has longer tails than a normal distribution, the denominator of the t-test statistic will be inflated and the t-test will generally find it harder to reject the null hypothesis. Therefore, in this case, the t-test will tend to have a lower FPR than expected (because of which it is sometimes claimed that the t-test is robust) but a much higher false negative rate (i.e., lower power) than expected.

When the assumption of normality is tenable but that of homoscedasticity is not, the t-test will tend to have a higher FPR than expected. In an attempt to alleviate this problem, an unequal-variance form of the t-test, called *Welch's test*, has been proposed. The test statistic for Welch's test is given by

$$T_u = \frac{|\overline{x}_1 - \overline{x}_2| - \Delta}{\sqrt{\dfrac{s_1^2}{n_1} + \dfrac{s_2^2}{n_2}}},$$

with $\Delta = 0$ when trying to detect any differences. The null distribution of T_u is, approximately, a t-distribution with degrees of freedom

$$\nu = \frac{\left(\dfrac{s_1^2}{n_1} + \dfrac{s_2^2}{n_2}\right)^2}{\dfrac{1}{n_1 - 1}\left(\dfrac{s_1^2}{n_1}\right)^2 + \dfrac{1}{n_2 - 1}\left(\dfrac{s_2^2}{n_2}\right)^2}.$$

If the observed value of T_u is $T_{u;\text{obs}}$ then the p-value is given by the probability $p_u = \text{Prob}(|T_u| > T_{u;\text{obs}})$. A gene is declared significantly differentially expressed at level of significance α if $p_u < \alpha$.

A test based on T_u can be shown to have, more or less, the correct test size even if $\sigma_1^2 \neq \sigma_2^2$. There is a drawback, however: having fewer degrees of freedom than T_e, T_u also tends to be less powerful. The loss of power may be substantial enough, particularly when n_1 and n_2 are very small, to consider using T_e, even when a moderate amount of heteroscedasticity is present.

Example. For the example, Welch's test finds that 872 genes are significantly differentially expressed, all of which were also found to be significantly differentially expressed by the t-test, demonstrating that the latter flags more differences as being significant; 455 are upregulated compared to control and 417 are downregulated compared to control.

7.4 DIAGNOSTIC CHECKS

The residuals, $r_{ij} = x_{ij} - \overline{x}_j$, form the basis for checking the validity of the assumption that the data follow a normal distribution. Here, the residuals are centered at the median rather than at the mean, because, with the median being relatively unaffected by outliers, it provides a more resistant estimator of the center of the distribution than the mean. When the residuals are sorted and plotted against the quantiles of a normal distribution, the resulting plot, called a *normal probability plot*, should be roughly linear if the underlying distribution was a normal distribution. With microarrays, it is usual to perceive some tapering away at the ends, indicating some degree of longtailedness in the data.

If the variances appear to differ across the groups, the *standardized residuals*, $r_{ij}^* = (x_{ij} - \bar{x}_j)/\tilde{s}_j$, may be used instead. Again a resistant measure of scale, $\tilde{s}_j$, is used instead of the traditional measure of scale, s_j. Large absolute values of r_{ij}^* indicate outliers.

With microarray data, it is in fact useful to gather all the residuals across all the genes $\{r_{ij}^*\}$ for making the normal probability plot.

Example. A normal probability plot of the standardized residuals for the example is shown in Figure 7.4. The plot indicates that the central portion of the distribution of the residuals resembles a normal distribution, but the tails of the residual distribution are considerably longer than those of the normal distribution.

This graphical check is often enough, but there are several formal statistical tests for assessing the normality of the underlying distribution as well. One of the most effective is the Shapiro–Wilk test. Other tests include the Kolmogorov–Smirnov test and its modifications, such as the Anderson–Darling test. With a very large

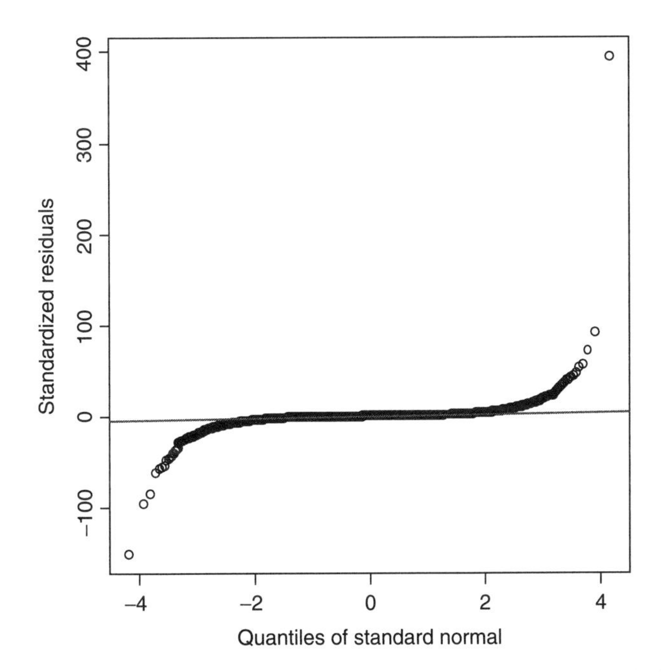

Figure 7.4 Normal probability plot of the standardized residuals. The straight line is the identity line.

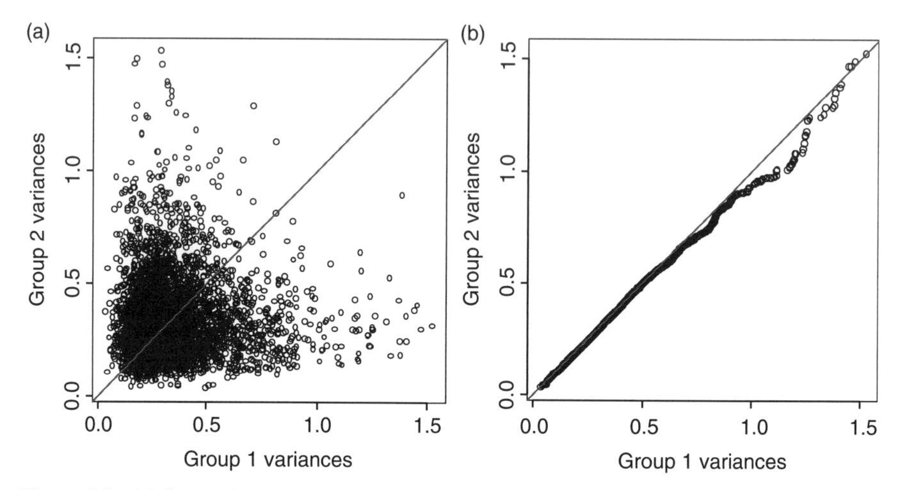

Figure 7.5 (a) Scatterplot (on a cube root scale) and (b) normal probability plot of the variance estimates for Group 1 versus the variance estimates for Group 2. In each plot, the straight line is the identity line.

number of observations, however, these tests will indicate nonnormality even with trivial departures from perfect normality. Therefore, we shall not use them here.

Formal tests for unequal variances across groups, such as Bartlett's test and Levene's test, require larger sample sizes than are generally available in microarray studies. Hence they are not described here. However, it is possible to get some idea as to how close the variances in the two groups are by plotting $\{s_{gi1}^{2/3}\}$ versus $\{s_{gi2}^{2/3}\}$., Here we use the cube root transformation, which brings the distribution of variances closer to a normal distribution (Wilson and Hilferty, 1931).

Example. Figure 7.5a shows a scatterplot of $\{s_{gi1}^{2/3}\}$ versus $\{s_{gi2}^{2/3}\}$. This plot shows that, on an individual gene basis, the variances in the two groups can differ quite markedly. However, the normal probability plot of $\{s_{gi1}^{2/3}\}$ versus $\{s_{gi2}^{2/3}\}$, shown in Figure 7.5b, indicates that the distributions of the variances are the same across the two groups.

7.5 ROBUST *t*-TESTS

If the *t*-test is applied when the data are normally distributed except for a few outliers, these outliers will tend to degrade the power of the test. What happens is that the outliers will inflate the denominator of the test statistic more than its numerator, so that the test statistic is less likely to be large and its propensity of being large when the null hypothesis is false will be dampened. Consequently, the FPR of the test will be low (called *robustness of validity*), which is fine, but the false negative rate of the test will be high (called *lack of robustness of efficiency*).

The t-test can be rendered *robust* (i.e., it can be made to be less influenced by outliers) by replacing the means and variances in the test statistic with robust versions of these sample statistics. One robust form of the t-test is obtained by replacing the means by biweight means (or their one-step counterparts) and the variances by A-estimators or τ-estimators (these estimators are described in Section 6.2).

Example. The robust t-test, with a tuning constant set so that it is very resistant to outliers, finds that 228 genes are upregulated compared to control and 224 genes are downregulated compared to control. The reason for the relatively small number of significant genes is the loss of power due to the high resistance. Raising the tuning constant will give results closer to the t-test. Figure 7.6 illustrates the resistance of the robust t-test. It shows the data for three genes that are declared not significant by the t-test but significant by the robust t-test at the 5% level of significance and one gene that is the reverse. It can be seen that the first three of all have a single extreme outlier that prevents them from turning up significant. This is why it is so important with microarray data to use methods that are not heavily influenced by outliers.

7.6 THE MANN–WHITNEY–WILCOXON RANK SUM TEST

When it is clear that the underlying distribution is far from normal, it may still be reasonable to assume that the distributions for the two groups are identical except for a location effect, so that $x_{i1} \sim F(\mu)$, $x_{i2} \sim F(\mu + \theta)$, where $F()$ denotes a distribution centered at μ. The Mann–Whitney–Wilcoxon test can be used to test the hypothesis that location parameter $\theta = 0$.

Once the observations have been ranked from 1 to N in increasing order, the test statistic for the Mann–Whitney–Wilcoxon test is the *rank sum statistic*, R, the sum of the ranks corresponding to the observations in Group 1. This statistic measures the degree of overlap between the two groups, the smaller the overlap, the further the value of R is from its null value of $n_1(N+1)/2$, indicating a group difference.

The null distribution of R has been tabulated (see, e.g., Hollander and Wolfe, 1999) for small values of n_1 and n_2 using an argument similar to that of permutation tests. For larger values of n_1 and n_2, the fact that

$$\frac{R - \dfrac{n_1(N+1)}{2}}{\sqrt{\dfrac{n_1 n_2 (N+1)}{12}}}$$

has, approximately, a standard normal distribution under the null hypothesis can be used to obtain p-values. If the observed value of R is R_{obs} then the p-value is given by the probability $p_R = \text{Prob}(|R| > R_{\text{obs}})$. A gene is declared significantly differentially expressed at level of significance α if $p_R < \alpha$.

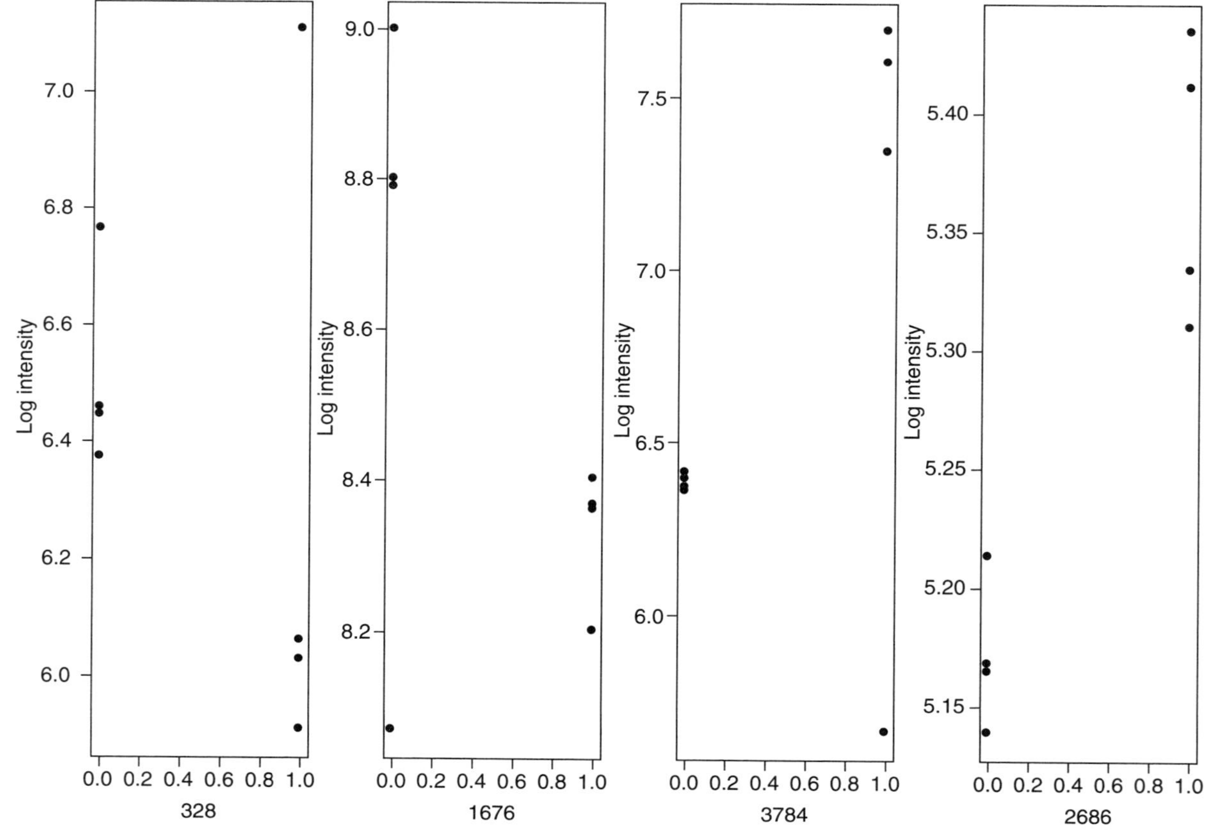

Figure 7.6 Log intensities for the control group and the treatment group for four genes, the first three of which are significant by the robust t-test but not significant by the t-test, the fourth of which is not significant by the robust t-test but significant by the t-test.

Rank-based tests, such as the Mann–Whitney–Wilcoxon test, are referred to as *nonparametric tests* or *distribution-free tests*, as they do not depend on strong distributional assumptions holding to be valid and can be used in a wide range of situations. However, they are less powerful than their parametric counterparts; in other words, their p-values tend to be higher, making it harder to detect real differences as being statistically significant. If the sample sizes are large, the difference in power is minor. On the other hand, with small sample sizes, as in typical microarray experiments, nonparametric tests have very little power to detect differences.

Example. In the example, the Mann–Whitney–Wilcoxon rank sum test finds that 1117 genes are significantly differentially expressed at the 5% level (the actual level is 5.7%, but, as with randomization test, we will not quibble over the extra 0.7%), 952 of which were also found to be significantly differentially expressed by the t-test; 588 are upregulated compared to control, while 529 are downregulated compared to control. The genes that were found to be significantly differentially expressed by the rank sum test but not the t-test had large variance differences across the two groups, demonstrating the loss of power of the t-test when this happens.

Chen et al. (1997), one of the earliest microarray papers to apply a formal statistical test, used the Mann–Whitney–Wilcoxon rank sum test for the segmentation step in image processing. Chambers et al. (1999) apply the Mann–Whitney–Wilcoxon rank sum test to analyze microarray data from a study of human cytomegalovirus infection.

For microarray data, Zhang et al. (2002) propose a different nonparametric scheme. They suggest sorting and scoring the intensities on each array from 1 (for the lowest intensities) to, say, 10 (for the highest intensities) based on the clustering algorithm and then comparing the scores across the groups of arrays. Their rationale is that as much as half the data on an array could be referring to nonexpressing genes and any differences among them is due to experimental variability, so that changes in scores across arrays would be a better than changes in raw values as indicators of differential expression.

7.7 MULTIPLICITY ADJUSTMENT: THE FAMILYWISE ERROR RATE

Analyzing microarray data involves performing a very large number of statistical tests, as a test is being run on each and every gene. One drawback of doing so many tests is that the more the number of statistical tests performed, the higher the overall FPR and the higher the expected number of false positives. Therefore, the microarray researcher must beware of attaching too much importance to all the findings labeled "significant," without making a suitable allowance for multiple testing.

In the case of G statistical tests, each performed at level α, if the tests are independent, the probability of making at least one false positive is $1 - (1 - \alpha)^G$, which is very close to unity for large G, and the expected number of false positives is $\alpha \times G$, which is very large for very large G. Thus, the number of false positives can be so high as to overwhelm and totally obscure any actual effects.

It is possible to alleviate this problem by adjusting the individual p-values of the tests for multiplicity. Indeed, a number of ways of doing so exist in the statistics literature. One major drawback, though, is that such procedures could lower the sensitivity as drastically as they raise the specificity. Indeed, in microarray experiments, G is so large and the number of replicates is so small that the power of the multiplicity adjusted tests is likely to be very small. In other words, aggressively adjusting for multiplicity could seriously impede the ability of the tests to find truly differentially expressing genes.

7.7.1 A Pragmatic Approach to the Issue of Multiplicity

This dilemma can be resolved by taking a pragmatic view as to how the overall objective of the study demands that the p-values be adjusted for multiplicity Nadon and Shoemaker, (2002), for one, make a similar suggestion. For instance, a researcher in a screening study may be willing to accept a fairly large number of false positives in order to improve his or her chances of identifying some truly differentiating genes. In another instance, a researcher's resources may be so limited that he or she would be able to follow up on only a handful of genes that appeared to be the most interesting. In such cases, stochastic multiplicity considerations are useful to the extent that they protect the researchers from assiduously following up on random patterns. However, there is no reason to slavishly adhere to classical cutoffs similar to the one that demands that a p-value should be less than 5% after multiplicity adjustment to declare significance.

In such cases, as long as there is some evidence that the experiment is picking up differences (i.e., the experiment is not a failure, as can be assessed by a quality check of the arrays as briefly outlined in Section 5.8), a reasonable approach is to rank the genes from 1 to G according to some criterion, such as the t-statistic, and to select the H genes with the best ranks for further study. The second researcher would want H to be quite small and would be more selective about how the H are chosen, whereas the first researcher would take a larger H. Multiplicity considerations may help in choosing H. The gene ranking could be based on one or more factors, but it is always preferable to rank a statistic that takes experimental variability into account, such as the t-test statistic, or, equivalently, the p-value associated with the t-test statistic, rather than one that does not, like the fold change.

A modification of this approach is to rank the G genes, select a moderate sized H of them, and then run these H through a cluster analysis (Chapter 9), with the intention of picking either one gene or a very small subset of genes from each tight cluster as the "most interesting" genes. The rationale for doing this is that, because genes mostly express along genetic pathways, an assemblage of coexpressing genes that express differentially across the treatment groups are more interesting than a single gene with a unique expression profile that is differentially expressed across the treatment groups. Annotation information, if available, should also be useful in so picking a subset of interesting genes (Bouton and Pevsner, 2000, 2002). In practice, the most satisfactory gene selection procedure is likely to be some blend of all these considerations.

In later studies, particularly confirmatory studies or studies that are to be submitted for external publication, the researcher would want to protect against an excessively high number of false positives. In such cases, a formal multiplicity adjustment should be applied.

7.7.2 Simple Multiplicity Adjustments

We now outline several ways of adjusting the p-values for the increased FPR resulting from multiple testing. Consider a situation in which G statistical tests have been performed. Let $p_1, \ldots, p_G$ be the G observed p-values. Suppose that, according to the rejection rule, R of the G tests led to rejection of the individual hypotheses they were testing and, unbeknownst to us, V of those were actually false positives.

If we make no adjustments for multiple testing, we are controlling the *per-comparison error rate* (PCER): PCER $= E(V)/G$. This tends to be too permissive in practice, as described above. Most conventional multiplicity adjustments attempt to control the *familywise error rate* (FWER), the probability, $\Pr(V > 0)$, of committing at least one false positive among all the hypotheses tested.

Classical p-value adjustments are single-step procedures in that the same adjustment is applied to each p-value regardless of their ordering.

- *Bonferroni*. The Bonferroni p-value for the kth test is simply $\tilde{p}_k = G p_k$. If it exceeds 1, it is set to 1. The Bonferroni adjustment is highly conservative, in that it produces large adjusted p-values that make it difficult to reject many null hypotheses and, consequently, the adjusted tests have low power.
- *Sidak*. The Sidak p-value (Sidak, 1967) for the kth test is $\tilde{p}_k = 1 - (1 - p_k)^G$. The Sidak p-values are slightly less conservative than the Bonferroni p-values.

Example. The Bonferroni p-values for the example data set can be obtained by multiplying each individual p-value by 4077, the number of genes. When this is done with the t-test p-values, only 12 remain significant, 5 are upregulated, and 7 are downregulated compared to control. In this case, the Sidak method is only slightly more liberal: it finds one additional upregulated gene.

7.7.3 Sequential Multiplicity Adjustments

While such adjustments certainly offer full protection against too many false positives being committed, they are so strong that they result in too many false negatives being committed. An alternative approach is sequential p-value adjustment, a technique pioneered by Holm (1979) and extended by a number of others. These methods take the order of the observed p-values into account with smaller p-values being adjusted more than the larger p-values. For instance, with step-down sequential testing, successively smaller adjustments are made at each step of the procedure. These methods retain control of the FWER and are generally more powerful than single-step p-values adjustments as they do not inflate the p-values as much as the single-step procedures.

Suppose that the unadjusted p-values have been ordered so that $p_1 \leq p_2 \leq, \ldots, \leq p_G$. Sequential methods can be either *step-down* or *step-up*. We now outline a few of the proposed methods.

- *Holm–Bonferroni.* The Holm–Bonferroni step-down p-values are determined as follows:

$$\tilde{p}_1^{\text{HB}} = G p_1,$$
$$\tilde{p}_k^{\text{HB}} = \max\left\{\tilde{p}_{k-1}^{\text{HB}}, (k-1)p_k\right\}.$$

  As always, if any adjusted p-value exceeds 1, it is set to 1.

- *Holm–Sidak.* The Holm–Sidak step-down p-values are determined similarly as

$$\tilde{p}_1^{\text{HS}} = 1 - (1 - p_1)^G,$$
$$\tilde{p}_k^{\text{HS}} = \max\left\{\tilde{p}_{k-1}^{\text{BH}}, (K-1)p_k\right\}.$$

- *Hochberg.* Assuming that the p-values of G are independent and uniformly distributed under their respective null hypotheses, Hochberg (1988) demonstrated that Holm's step-down adjustments control the FWER even when calculated in a step-up manner. The Hochberg step-up p-values are determined in reverse order to the step-down Holm-Bonferroni:

$$\tilde{p}_G^H = p_G,$$
$$\tilde{p}_{G-g}^{\text{H}} = \max\left\{\tilde{p}_{G-g+1}^{\text{BH}}, k p_{G-g}\right\}.$$

  The advantage of doing the adjustments step-up instead of step-down is that the adjustments are uniformly smaller for the former than for the latter. Therefore, the step-up technique is more powerful and the number of false negatives is reduced. However, this improved power comes at the cost of having to make the assumption of independence.

- *Westfall–Young.* The Westfall and Young (1993) step-down p-values (1993) are determined as follows:

$$\tilde{p}_g = \max_{k=1,\ldots,g}\left\{\text{Prob}\left(\max_{l=k,\ldots,G} P_i \leq p_k | H_0\right)\right\}.$$

These adjusted p-values usually have to be estimated by simulation and this is, as a result, a computationally much more intensive method than the others. On the other hand, it has the advantage that (i) unlike the other methods, it takes into account the possibility that the tests may not be independent of one another, a valuable consideration for microarray data as genes rarely act in isolation, and (ii) it is less conservative than the other methods.

Example. Applying the Holm–Bonferroni method to the example finds the same significant genes as the Bonferroni method.

A very different approach to the multiplicity problem in microarray experiments has been taken by Allison et al. (2002). They assess the true positive rate using the fact that if all the null hypotheses were true (i.e., none of the genes are differentially expressed) and the gene expression levels were independent across all genes, then the distribution of p-values would be uniform on the interval [0,1], regardless of the statistical test used or the sample size. On the other hand, if some subset of the genes are differentially expressed, the p-values will tend to cluster at low values. This effect can be mirrored by modeling the set of p-values as a random sample from a mixture of beta distributions. Applying Bayes' rule, the posterior probability that a gene is differentially expressed can then be calculated for each gene.

7.8 MULTIPLICITY ADJUSTMENT: THE FALSE DISCOVERY RATE

7.8.1 Benjamini and Hochberg Procedure

All the FWER-controlling adjustments described in Section in 7.7 are very large. This is because controlling the FWER is a stringent criterion that inherently forces large adjustments. When G is large, as in microarray experiments, FWER-controlling adjustments are likely to be too strong and result in far too many false negatives. This is clearly undesirable, particularly when making a large number of inferences and the overall conclusion is not necessarily erroneous as soon as one of them is incorrect and all that one is concerned about is preventing an inordinately large number of false positives from clouding the results.

In such situations, Benjamini and Hochberg (1995) (see also Yuketieli and Benjamini, 1999) proposed controlling the *false discovery rate* (FDR) instead. The FDR is defined as the expected proportion of false positives among the positive findings.

$$\text{FDR} = E\left[\left.\frac{V}{R}\right| R > 0\right]\Pr(R > 0).$$

If all the null hypotheses were true, the FDR would equal the FWER and controlling the FDR would be equivalent to controlling the FWER. If not every null hypothesis was true, the FDR maintains some control over the number of false positives in an adaptive manner, in the sense that, the more the number of the hypotheses that are truly false, the smaller the FDR. Hence, procedures that control the FDR tend to be more powerful than procedures that control the FWER at the same level. Benjamini and Hochberg (1995) suggested the following step-up procedure to adjust the ordered p-values so as to control the FDR:

- *Benjamini–Hochberg.* The Benjamini–Hochberg-adjusted p-values are

$$\tilde{p}_k^{\text{BH}} = p_k,$$

$$\tilde{p}_{K-k}^{\text{BH}} = \min\left(\tilde{p}_{K-k+1}^{\text{BH}}, \left(\frac{K}{K-k}\right) p_{K-k}\right).$$

These p-values are less conservative than Hochberg's step-up adjustments and are guaranteed to control the FDR when the original p-values are independent and uniformly distributed under their respective null hypotheses.

Example. We illustrate the use of different multiplicity adjustment methods for two microarray experiments. The first study, the Golub study, discussed in Chapters 1 and 5, consists of 38 samples and 3051 genes. For this study, the primary interest of the comparison is between the ALL (27 samples) and ALM (11 samples). The gene expression data for the second example was obtained from a behavioral experiment, in which 24 male experimentally naive Long-Evans rats were randomized into two treatment groups (12 rats in each group). The first group was treated with placebo and the second with antipsychotic compound. Each array measured the expression levels of 5644 genes for each rat. For more details about the study, we refer to Lin et al. (2012). The primary interest is to compare the two treatment groups. For both studies, inference was based on two sample t-test. Table 7.2 shows the number of rejected null hypotheses for error rate of 5%. As expected, within each study, the number of genes declared differentially expressed was higher when the Binjamini–Hochberg (BH) procedure was used to control the FDR as compared to the Bonferroni or Holm procedures, which were used to control the FWER and therefore are more conservative than the BH-FDR. Figures 7.6A and 7.6A plot the fold change versus the $-\log$ ($p-$value) (panel a, the so-called volcano plot). We notice that the range of the fold change in the Golub study is higher than that in the behavioral study. Panel b in Figures 7.6A and 7.6A show the histogram of the unadjusted p-values (raw p-values) in both studies. Notice that the distributions of the raw p-values in the two studies reveal different patterns. In the behavioral study, with a low number of discoveries (i.e., a low number of rejected null hypotheses), the distribution is close to a uniform

Table 7.2 Number of Discoveries for $\alpha = 0.05$

Adjustment Method	Golub Study	Behavioral Study
None	1078	231
Bonferroni	103	10
Holm	103	10
FDR	695	13

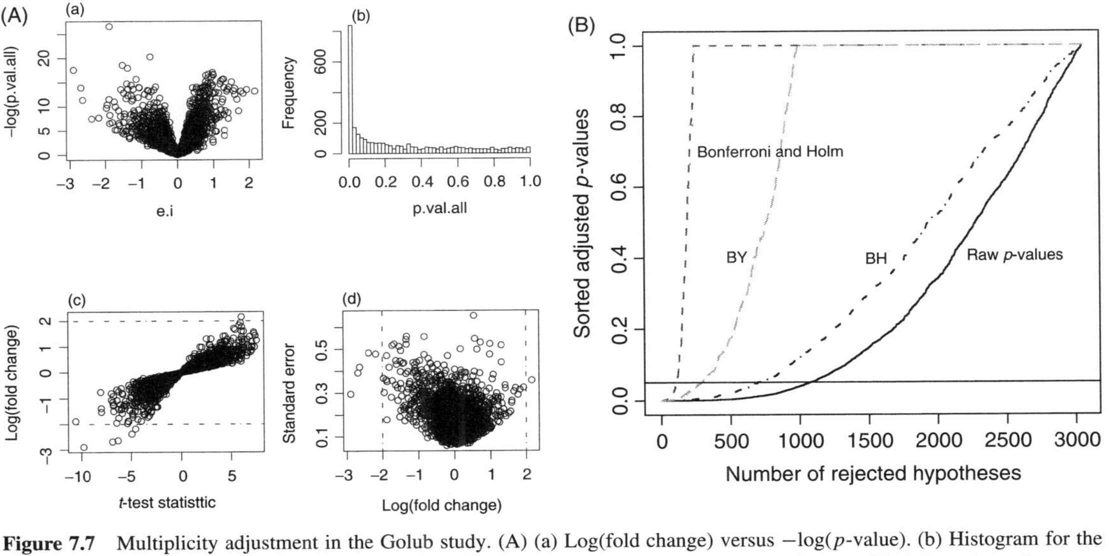

Figure 7.7 Multiplicity adjustment in the Golub study. (A) (a) Log(fold change) versus −log(p-value). (b) Histogram for the raw p-value. (c) Test statistic versus log(fold change). (d) Log(fold change) versus standard error. (B) Adjusted p-values.

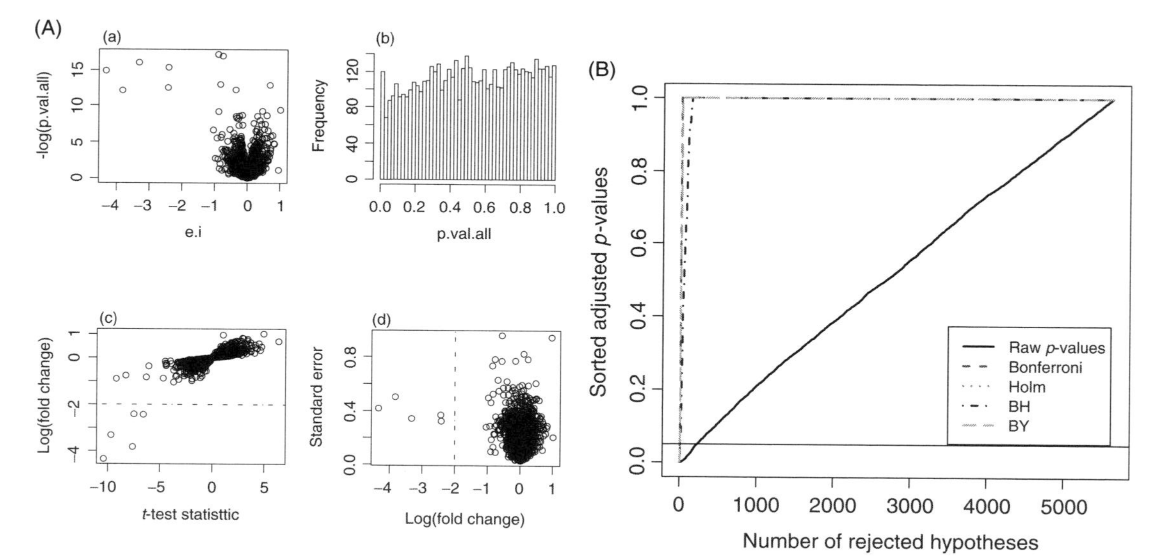

Figure 7.8 Multiplicity adjustment in the behavioral study. (A) (a) Log(fold change) versus −log(p-value). (b) Histogram for the raw p-value. (c) Test statistic versus log(fold change). (d) Log(fold change) versus standard error. (B) Adjusted p-values.

distribution, while the distribution of the raw p-values is skewed to the right with mode between 0 and 0.05, indicating a large number of discoveries. These patterns can be seen in Figures 7.6B and 7.6B that show the raw and the adjusted p-values in both studies. The horizontal line corresponds to an error rate of 0.05. Hence, null hypotheses for which the adjusted p-values are below the horizontal line are rejected.

7.8.2 The Positive False Discovery Rate

Storey and Tıbshirani (2001) proposed a modified version of the FDR, called the *positive false discovery rate* (*pFDR*):

$$\text{pFDR} = E\left[\left.\frac{V}{R}\right| R > 0\right].$$

The pFDR emphasizes the fact that an adjustment is only necessary when there are positive findings.

Given a decision rule, the pFDR can be estimated via a permutation procedure. Suppose that the decision rule is to reject any test statistics, T, that exceed a specified value t_+, and that, of the G test statistics, h_{obs} exceeded t_+. In B^* permutations, suppose that an average number h^* of test statistics exceeded t_+, so that, when there are no true positives, the number of (false) positives observed is h^*. Then, the natural estimate of the pFDR is

$$\text{pFDR} = \frac{h^*}{h_{\text{obs}}}.$$

If the number, G_+, of genes that are truly differentially expressed is not small, then this estimate of pFDR will be too high. The way to improve it is to multiply this crude estimate by an estimate of $\pi_+ = G_+/G$. A somewhat ad hoc estimate of π_+ can be obtained by considering the genes with the smallest values of T (i.e., those such that $T < t_-$, where t_- is some prespecified value) as being truly not differentially expressed, as they are the least likely to be differentially expressed. Suppose that k_{obs} test statistics had $T < t_-$. and that in the B^* permutations, on an average, k^* test statistics had $T < t_-$. Then an estimate of π_+ is k_{obs}/k^* and an improved estimate of pFDR is given by

$$\text{pFDR} = \pi^*\left(\frac{h^*}{h_{\text{obs}}}\right).$$

Example. When analyzing the data in the example with the two-sample t-test, any gene whose $4t$-test statistic exceeded $t_+ = 2.447$ (the 97.5th quantile of a t-distribution with 6 degrees of freedom) in absolute value was flagged as being significant at the 5% level. Recall that 998 such genes were flagged. In the 34 possible permutations of the data, an average of 138.15 genes are flagged, leading to a simple pFDR estimate of $138.15/998 = 13.8\%$. A total of 1259 genes have t-test statistics below $t_{\_} = 0.718$ (the 75th quantile of a t-distribution with 6 degrees of freedom) in absolute value, whereas in the 34 possible permutations of the data, an average of 1958.71 genes have t-test statistics below $t_{\_}$ in absolute value, so that $\hat{\pi}_{+} = 1259/1958.71 = 0.643$, so that the improved estimate of pFDR is $\text{pFDR} = (0.643)(0.138) = 0.089$; that is, about 9%.

Unlike the procedures described in Section 7.8, the pFDR does not actually provide a p-value adjustment. Recalling that the p-value is the smallest Type I error rate at which the null hypothesis is rejected, an analog to the p-value associated with a particular test statistic with the pFDR approach is the q-value (Storey, 2001), which is analogously defined as being the smallest pFDR at which that test statistic is declared significant. Roughly, it could also be thought of as the probability that a statistic as or more extreme is truly null.

Further details of this way of assessing the effect of multiple testing are provided by Storey and Tibshirani (2001). Theoretical aspects of this procedure have been developed by Storey (2001, 2002), Efron et al. (2001) and Efron, Storey and Tibshirani (2001) by embedding it in an empirical Bayes framework.

7.9 RESAMPLING-BASED MULTIPLE TESTING PROCEDURES

In a microarray setting, resampling methods to adjust for multiplicity are often used (Kerr and Churchill, 2001; Reiner et al., 2003; Tusher et al., 2001). The main motivation is to avoid inference based on asymptotic distribution of the test statistics, which, within the microarray setting, can be problematic because of either typically small sample sizes or departure from the assumption about the distribution of the response. Also, in some cases, the asymptotic distribution of the test statistics is unknown (Tusher et al., 2001).

Randomization tests are resampling-based procedures for assessing how reasonable the null hypothesis is in the face of the observed data. As in any hypothesis testing situation, a randomization test proceeds by selecting a test statistic, T, which measures how far the observed data are from the situation described by the null hypothesis.

For the two-group situation, the most natural candidate for a test statistic is the t-test statistic. The observed value of the test statistic, T_{obs}, is compared to the distribution of values of T that are obtained by randomly reassigning the data to the two groups, keeping the sample sizes the same. In other words, the procedure is to repeat the following for every possible permutation of the data:

- Permute the data.
- Assign the first n_1 observations to the first group and the remaining n_2 observations to the second group.

- Calculate the test statistic. Consider a microarray with G genes, and let

$$T_1, \ldots, T_i, \ldots, T_G,$$

be the test statistics of primary interest (e.g., the t-test statistic). By permuting the labels of arrays randomly, the (permutation) test statistics of B genes are recalculated. Let T be the permutation matrix, that is,

$$\mathbf{T} = \begin{pmatrix} T_{11} & T_{12} & \ldots & T_{1B} \\ T_{21} & T_{22} & \ldots & T_{2B} \\ \cdot & \cdot & \cdot & \cdot \\ \cdot & \cdot & \cdot & \cdot \\ \cdot & \cdot & \cdot & \cdot \\ T_{G1} & T_{G2} & \ldots & T_{\text{GB}} \end{pmatrix},$$

where B is the total number of permutations and each element t_{gb} of matrix $\mathbf{T}$ is the test statistic for the gth gene in the bth permutation.

- Count the number of the permutations whose t_{gb} value exceeds the observed test statistic, $t_{g;\text{obs}}$, and divide this count by the total number of permutations to get the proportion, p_{Perm}, of times the value of the t-statistic on the permuted data exceeded the value of the t-statistic on the data we actually obtained. This proportion, p_{Perm}, is an estimate of the probability of such an extreme result under the null. In other words, it functions as a p-value. Hence, the raw p-values are calculated as

$$p_{perm} = \frac{\#(b : |t_{gb}| \geq |t_{g;\text{obs}}|)}{B}.$$

Note that if the number of observations is relatively small then the distribution of the permutation-based p-values is granular. Alternatively, less discrete p-values can be obtained from the marginal distribution of permutation-based test statistics for all the genes in the array,

$$p_{perm} = \frac{\sum_{b=1}^{B} \sum_{g=1}^{G} (|t_{gb}| \geq |t_{g,\text{obs}}|)}{B \times G}.$$

The raw p-values obtained by using either methods can be used as an input in the procedures for multiple testing adjustment discussed in Section 7.7 and 7.8.

Example 1. In the example, there are two groups of four, making for 35 possible permutations. We use the difference in means, $T_d = \overline{x}_2 - \overline{x}_1$, as test statistic and will regard T_d as significant if the observed value $|T_{d;\text{obs}}|$ of $|T_d|$ exceeds $|T_d|$ in at most one permutation, which constitutes a two-sided test of level $2/35 = 5.7\%$, which we will call 5% without quibbling over the extra 0.7%. This test finds that 1384 genes are significantly differentially expressed; 651 are upregulated compared to control, while 733 are downregulated compared to control.

Example 2. Figure 7.9A shows the histogram for the marginal distribution of the permutation test statistics of two-sample t-test for the Golub data for two genes. The vertical line is the observed test statistic and the permutation p-value for one sided test is the proportion of permutation test statistics greater than the observed test statistics. Figure 7.9B shows the scatterplot matrix for the raw p-values. We notice that indeed raw p-values calculated for each row in the permutation matrix separately by $p_g = \#(b : |t_{gb}| \geq |t_{g;\text{obs}}|)/B$ are more discrete compare to the raw p-values calculate when all permutation test statistics are taken into account, that is, $p_g = \sum_{b=1}^{B} \sum_{g=1}^{G} (|t_{gb}| \geq |t_{g,\text{obs}}|)/B \times G$.

7.10 SMALL-VARIANCE-ADJUSTED t-TESTS AND SAM

Let us now revisit the t-test. With small samples, the t-test statistic tends to be highly correlated with the standard error term that appears in its denominator. As a result, the test has a propensity for picking up significant findings at a higher rate from among those genes with low variance than from among those with high variance (as observed in Fig. 7.2). This property of the t-test is especially troubling because it is difficult to estimate standard errors well when the sample size is low and small standard errors could occur purely by chance. Because the sample sizes used in microarray experiments are typically very small, the small sample effect of the t-test tends to manifest itself in such experiments as a high FPR for genes whose variability is low and a high false negative rate for genes whose variability is high. This effect is somewhat related to the problem of competition bias in model selection, where when several models compete to be selected, those that appear the best with the data at hand get selected. This is clearly an undesirable state of affairs and proposals to avoid this problem have begun to appear in the microarray data analysis literature.

Example. Figure 7.10 shows scatterplots of the two-sample t-test statistics versus the pooled standard errors for the two groups (Fig. 7.10a) and the absolute value of the two-sample t-test statistics versus the pooled standard errors for the two groups (Fig. 7.10b). The scatterplot on the left has a rotated volcano shape indicating that genes with small variances have large t-test statistics and vice versa. Figure 7.11 shows the proportion of significant t-statistics as a function of the pooled standard errors for values of 0.05, 0.01, and 0.001. The graphs demonstrate that the problem of obtaining too many significant t-statistics for small values of the pooled standard error.

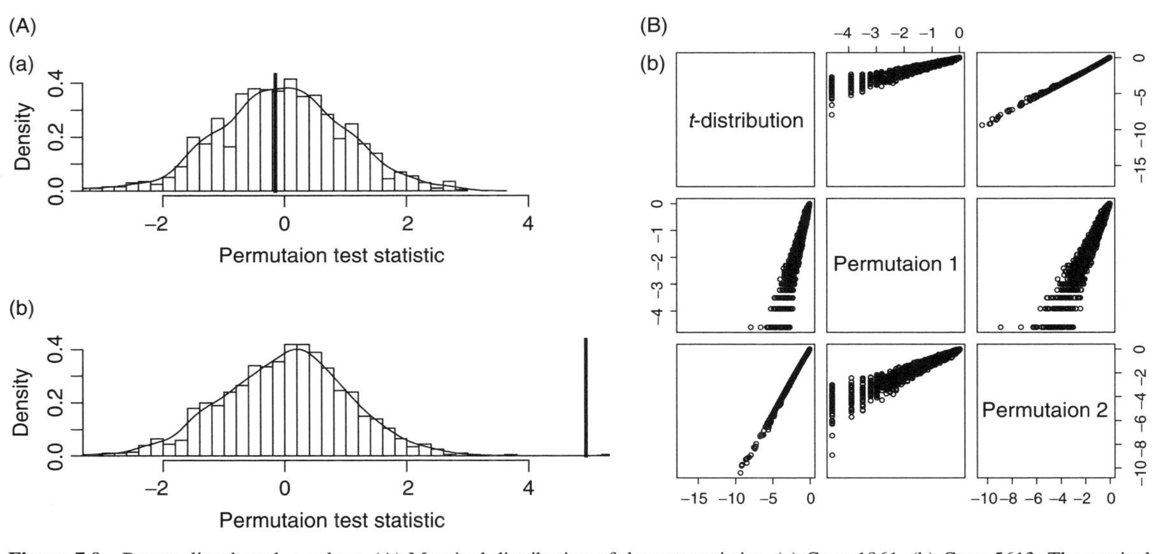

Figure 7.9 Resampling-based p-values. (A) Marginal distribution of the test statistics. (a) Gene 1961. (b) Gene 5613. The vertical lines represent the observed test statistic. (B) Permutation versus asymptotic raw p-values.

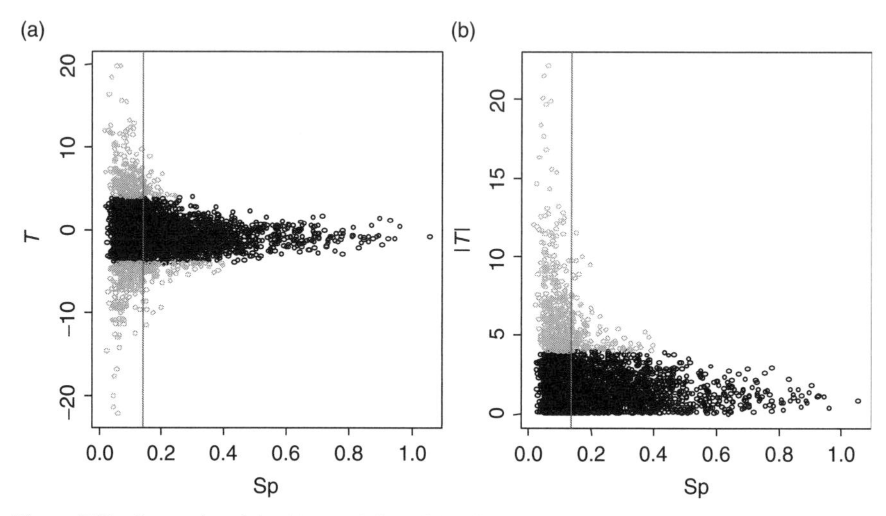

Figure 7.10 Scatterplot of the (a) t-statistic and (b) absolute value of the t-statistic versus the pooled standard error. In each graph, the gray dots refer to genes declared significant by the two-sample t-test, the vertical line is the median pooled standard error.

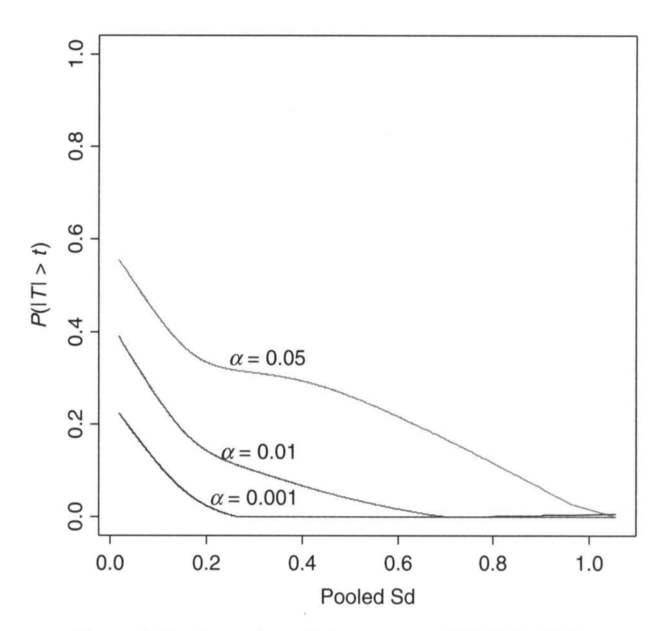

Figure 7.11 Proportion of $|t| > t_{\alpha/2}$, $\alpha = 0.05, 0.01, 0.001$.

7.10.1 Modifying the t-Statistic

One solution to the problem was suggested by Tusher et al. (2001) (see also Efron and Tibshirani, 2002). They add a carefully chosen constant, the so-called "fudge factor," to the denominator of the t-statistic. Recall that the t-test statistic, T_g, for the gth gene, has the form $T_g = r_g/s_g$, where $r_g = |x_g - y_g|$ and $s_g = s_{gp}\sqrt{1/n_1 + 1/n_2}$ (see Section 7.3). The adjusted t-statistic is

$$T_g(c) = \frac{r_g}{s_g + c},$$

where c is the fudge factor. This test statistic is often called the *SAM t-statistic*, where SAM stands for "significance analysis of microarrays."

$T_{g(0)}$ is, of course, the ordinary t-statistic, T_g. $T_{g(c)}$ with a very large value of c is equivalent to the t-statistic without its denominator, that is, to r_g. The plan is to choose an intermediate positive value of c for which, given c, the dependence of $T_{g(c)}$ on s_g is as small as possible. The simplest way to do this in practice is to study the relationship of $T_{g(c)}$ versus s_g for a number of different values of c, with the intention of retaining as the fudge factor, c, the one for which the dependence of $T_{g(c)}$ on s_g is least.

Tusher et al. (2001) (see also the documentation accompanying the software package, SAM) implement this is as follows. Let s^α be the αth percentile of the $\{s_g\}$ values and let $T_g(s^\alpha) = r_g/(s_g + s^\alpha)$. Compute the percentiles, $q_1 < q_2 <, \ldots, < q_{100}$, of the s_g values. For $\alpha \in \{0, 5, 10, \ldots, 100\}$, compute the MAD (median absolute deviation from the median), $v_j(\alpha)$, of the $T_g(s^\alpha)$ values within the interval $[q_j, q_{j+1}]$, for $j = 1, 2, \ldots, n$. Then compute $cv(\alpha)$, the coefficient of variation of the $v_j(\alpha)$ values. Choose as $\hat{\alpha}$ the value of α that minimizes $cv(\alpha)$. Fix as $\hat{c}$ the value $\hat{s}$.

An alternative proposal for estimating the fudge factor (Broberg, 2002) involves studying the false negative rate versus the FPR, a relationship called the *receiver operating characteristic* (ROC) curve, for various values of c, and choosing as the fudge factor the value of c that corresponds to the point on the ROC curve that is nearest the origin.

7.10.2 Assessing Significance with the SAM t Statistic

Once the SAM t-statistics, $T_g(\hat{c})$, are calculated, the critical value of $T_g(\hat{c})$ that separates significance from nonsignificance must be set. For the ordinary t-statistic, this is done by looking up the quantiles of a t-distribution. However, the null distribution of the SAM t-statistic, $T_g(\hat{c})$, is not a t-distribution, so this is no longer correct. In fact, the null distribution is intractable. Therefore, Tusher et al. (2001) assess the significance of the observed $T_g(\hat{c})$ values via a permutation procedure.

Suppose that a suitable $\hat{c}$ has been identified and that the $T_g(\hat{c})$ values have been calculated and sorted into increasing order: $T_{(1)}(\hat{c}) \le T_{(2)}(\hat{c}) \le, \ldots, \le T_{(G)}(\hat{c})$.

The permutation procedure proceeds by permuting the columns of the data matrix, $\boldsymbol{X}$, and assigning the first n_1 columns to Group 1 and the remaining n_2 columns to Group 2. A total of B such permutations will be done. For the bth permutation, compute the test statistics, $T_g^{*b}(\hat{c})$, and the corresponding order statistics: $T_{(1)}^{*b}(\hat{c}) \leq T_{(2)}^{*b}(\hat{c}) \leq, \ldots, \leq T_{(G)}^{*b}(\hat{c})$.

Hence, the SAM procedure requires to sort each one of the columns in the permutation matrix discussed above such that the first row of the sorted matrix in the minimum test statistics across permutations and the last row is the maximum, that is,

$$\boldsymbol{T} = \begin{pmatrix} T_1^{*1}(\hat{c}) & T_1^{*2}(\hat{c}) & \ldots & T_1^{*B}(\hat{c}) \\ T_2^{*1}(\hat{c}) & T_2^{*2}(\hat{c}) & \ldots & T_2^{*B}(\hat{c}) \\ \cdot & \cdot & \cdot & \cdot \\ \cdot & \cdot & \cdot & \cdot \\ \cdot & \cdot & \cdot & \cdot \\ T_G^{*1}(\hat{c}) & T_G^{*2}(\hat{c}) & \ldots & T_G^{*B}(\hat{c}) \end{pmatrix} \Rightarrow T^{\text{SAM}} = \begin{pmatrix} T_{(1)}^{*1} & T_{(1)}^{*2} & \ldots & T_{(1)}^{*B} \\ T_{(2)}^{*1} & T_{(2)}^{*2} & \ldots & T_{(2)}^{*B} \\ \cdot & \cdot & \cdot & \cdot \\ \cdot & \cdot & \cdot & \cdot \\ \cdot & \cdot & \cdot & \cdot \\ T_{(G)}^{*1} & T_{(G)}^{*2} & \ldots & T_{(G)}^{*B} \end{pmatrix}.$$

Let $\boldsymbol{T}^{\text{SAM}}$ be the sorted permutation matrix and let $T_{(1)}(\hat{c}) \leq \cdots \leq T_{(G)}(\hat{c})$ be the sorted observed statistics. The expected value of the observed statistic is the mean of the rows of $\mathbf{T}^{\text{SAM}}$,

$$\mathbf{T}^{\text{SAM}} = \begin{pmatrix} T_{(1)}^{*1} & T_{(1)}^{*2} & \ldots & T_{(1)}^{*B} \\ \hline T_{(2)}^{*1} & T_{(2)}^{*2} & \ldots & T_{(2)}^{*B} \\ \hline \cdot & \cdot & \cdot & \cdot \\ \hline \cdot & \cdot & \cdot & \cdot \\ \hline \cdot & \cdot & \cdot & \cdot \\ \hline T_{(G)}^{*1} & T_{(G)}^{*2} & \ldots & T_{(G)}^{*B} \end{pmatrix} \Rightarrow \begin{pmatrix} \frac{1}{B}\sum_{b=1}^{B} T_{(1)}^{*b} \\ \frac{1}{B}\sum_{b=1}^{B} T_{(2)}^{*b} \\ \cdot \\ \cdot \\ \cdot \\ \frac{1}{B}\sum_{b=1}^{B} T_{(G)}^{*b} \end{pmatrix} = \begin{pmatrix} \overline{T}_{(1)}(\hat{c}) \\ \overline{T}_{(2)}(\hat{c}) \\ \cdot \\ \cdot \\ \cdot \\ \overline{T}_{(G)}(\hat{c}) \end{pmatrix}.$$

Any gene g that is such that its $T_g(\hat{c})$ value substantially exceeds its $\overline{T}_{(g)}(\hat{c})$ value is possibly differentially expressed.

This can be examined further by plotting the $T_{(g)}(\hat{c})$ values versus the $\overline{T}_{(g)}(\hat{c})$ values. The central part of this plot lies along the identity line, where $T_g(\hat{c}) = \overline{T}_{(g)}(\hat{c})$, indicating genes that are not differentially expressed. The ends tail away from this line; the further a gene is located from the identity line, the more likely it is that the gene is significantly differentially expressed.

The procedure to declare significance is as follows. For a fixed threshold, Δ, starting at the origin and moving up to the right, find the first i_1 genes such that $T_g(\hat{c}) - \overline{T}_{(g)}(\hat{c}) > \Delta$ and call all genes past i_1 "significant positive." Similarly, starting at origin and moving down to the left, find the first i_2 genes such that

$T_g(\hat{c}) - \overline{T}_{(g)}(\hat{c}) < -\Delta$ and call all genes past i_2 "significant negative." For a given value of Δ, call the smallest value of $T_g(\hat{c})$ among the significant positive genes the "upper cut-point," $\mathrm{cut}_{\mathrm{up}}(\Delta)$, and the largest value of $T_g(\hat{c})$ among the significant negative genes the "lower cut-point," $\mathrm{cut}_{\mathrm{lo}}(\Delta)$.

This process can be carried out for a series of Δ values. For each value of Δ, count the total number of significant genes and determine the average number of genes falsely identified as differentially expressed. For the latter, compute the median, k_m, and the 90th percentile, $k_{0.9}$, of the proportions of values among each of the B sets of $T^{*b}_{(g)}(\hat{c})$ values that fall in between the cut points, $\mathrm{cut}_{\mathrm{lo}}(\Delta)$ or $\mathrm{cut}_{\mathrm{up}}(\Delta)$. The proportion of genes that is truly not differentially expressed (i.e., π_+ in Section 7.9.1) is taken to be twice the proportion of values, $T_g(\hat{c})$, that falls in between the quartiles of all the values of all the $T^{*b}_{(g)}(\hat{c})$ values. The values of k_m and $k_{0.9}$ are multiplied by this proportion and used to calculate the pFDR, as k_m (or $k_{0.9}$) divided by the number of significant genes. By evaluating pFDR for several values of Δ, a suitable strategy can be devised to decide which genes are significantly differentially expressed.

Example. Figure 7.12a shows a scatterplot of the sorted SAM t-statistics versus their expected values for the example - the oblique lines correspond to $\Delta = 2$. Figure 7.12b shows the proportion of significant genes produced by SAM versus the pooled standard error. Table 7.3 gives a list of typical values of Δ, the number of false discoveries, the number of genes declared significant, the pFDR for both 50% and 90% and the FPR for both 50% and 90%.

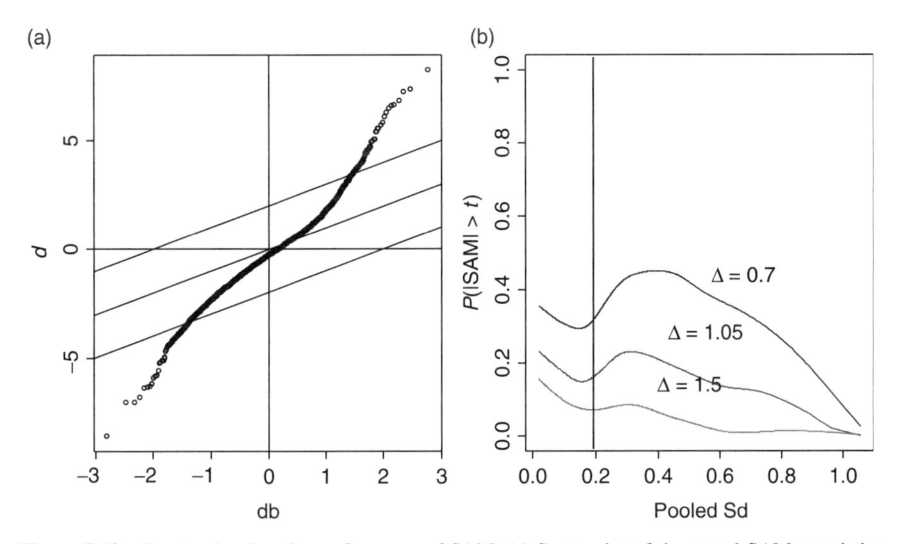

Figure 7.12 Graphs showing the performance of SAM. (a) Scatterplot of the sorted SAM t-statistics versus their expected values—the oblique lines correspond to $\Delta = 2$. (b) Proportion of significant genes produced by SAM versus pooled standard error.

Table 7.3 The Δ Table: Summary of a SAM Analysis

Δ	FP50%	FP90%	Called	FDR50%	FDR90%	FPR(50%)	FPR(90%)
0.1	1847	1951	3514	0.526	0.555	0.453	0.479
0.2	1351	1515	2996	0.451	0.506	0.331	0.372
0.3	949	1130	2550	0.372	0.443	0.233	0.277
0.4	645	812	2182	0.296	0.372	0.158	0.199
0.5	400	538	1787	0.224	0.301	0.098	0.132
0.6	249	366	1567	0.159	0.233	0.061	0.090
0.7	143	228	1306	0.109	0.175	0.035	0.056
0.8	76	135	1112	0.068	0.121	0.019	0.033
0.9	39	80	931	0.042	0.086	0.010	0.020
1.0	20	45	746	0.027	0.061	0.005	0.011
1.1	10	28	628	0.017	0.045	0.002	0.007
1.2	6	16	537	0.011	0.030	0.001	0.004
1.3	4	8	446	0.008	0.019	0.001	0.002
1.4	2	5	389	0.005	0.014	0.000	0.001
1.5	1	3	311	0.004	0.010	0.000	0.001
1.6	1	2	269	0.002	0.009	0.000	0.000
1.7	0	2	226	0.000	0.008	0.000	0.000
1.8	0	71	186	0.000	0.003	0.000	0.000
1.9	0	71	154	0.000	0.004	0.000	0.000
2.0	0	71	139	0.000	0.004	0.000	0.000

7.10.3 Strategies for Using SAM

As the pFDR does not actually provide a p-value adjustment and pFDR is not monotone in Δ, it is sometimes unclear as to how to decide which genes are significantly differentially expressed, that is, essentially, how to set Δ. Some strategies for selecting a suitable value for Δ are as follows:

1. Settle on the highest pFDR the researcher is willing to tolerate (say, 5% or 1%). Select the smallest value of Δ that corresponds to that pFDR. In our example, in Table 7.3, if we choose pFDR (90%) = 1% this corresponds to $\Delta = 1.2$.
2. It is sometimes difficult to prespecify a value for pFDR or Δ. In this event, it may be more convenient to stay with the more familiar 'classical' strategy of choosing a Δ that corresponds to a fixed proportion of false positives, say 0.01. From Table 7.3, this method would produce $\Delta = 1.1$.
3. Begin with strategy (2) to pick a Δ, then check the pFDR for that Δ, and, if the pFDR is too high, increase Δ as long as (i) there is a sizeable reduction in the pFDR and (ii) the number of genes declared significant does not decrease substantially. For Table 7.3, we may argue that $\Delta = 1.1$ corresponds to a pFDR of 4.5%, which is sufficiently low.

4. Begin with an initial number of genes the researcher would like to follow up on. Calculate the pFDR and FPR for that number. If they are satisfactorily small, stop. Otherwise, adjust the number of genes until both pFDR and FPR are at comfortable levels.

We may still pick up genes exhibiting fold changes that are so small as to be biologically irrelevant. In the event that we want to omit them and pick up only those genes that exhibit at least an h-fold change, then, in addition to being significant positive or significant negative, a gene must also satisfy $|x - y| > \log(h)$ in order to be declared significantly differentially expressed.

7.10.4 An Empirical Bayes Framework

The theoretical underpinnings of the SAM approach were investigated by Efron et al. (2001) by casting it in an empirical Bayes framework. This framework is as follows. Suppose that p_E is the probability that a gene is differentially expressed and that $f_E(z)$ and $f_0(z)$ denote the probability density functions of $Z = T(c)$ for genes that are differentially expressed and not differentially expressed respectively. Then,

$$f(z) = (1 - p_E)f_0(z) + p_E f_E(z)$$

is the probability density function for the mixture distribution of Z.

Applying Bayes' rule to this model gives the posterior probability that a gene is differentially expressed:

$$p_E(z) = 1 - \left[(1 - p_E)\frac{f_0(z)}{f(z)}\right].$$

The density $f(z)$ can be estimated from the observed $\{Zg\}$ values. The null density $f_0(z)$ is estimated by permuting the columns of X as with the SAM procedure. Efron et al. (2001) describe how to use logistic regression to estimate $f_0(z)/f(z)$. The probability p_E is set equal to its maximum value: $1 - \min)Z[f(Z)/f_0(Z)]$. On the basis of these estimates, the posterior probability $p_1(z)$ that a gene is differentially expressed can be determined for each gene.

7.10.5 Understanding the SAM Adjustment

In order to understand what SAM does, we present a careful analysis of the original microarray data question and explain the behavior of SAM.

Microarray data typically exhibits a strong dependence relationship between mean and variance of gene effect, that is, between μ_g and σ_g (see Figure 7.13). This dependence is reflected in the values of $\overline{x}_g$ and s_g in the raw data. This is one reason why a transformation such as log or square root, followed by a normalization step, are applied to the original data as described in Chapter 5. The hope is that, by doing these transformations, some or all of the following problems will be resolved for the overwhelming majority of the genes.

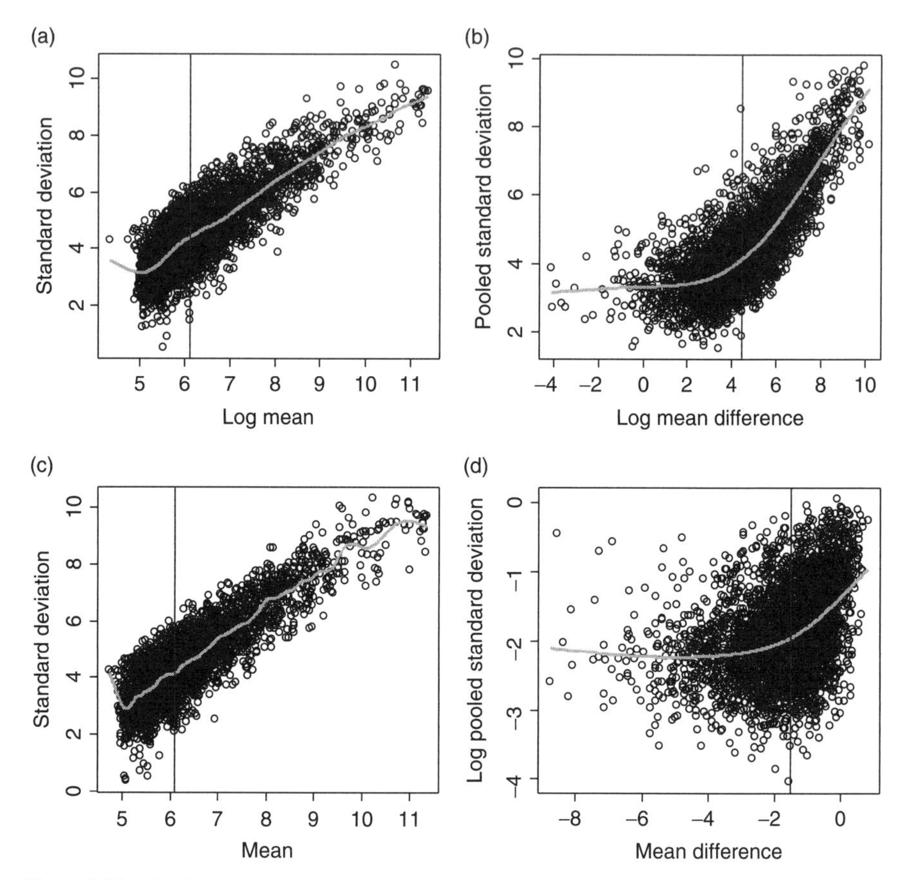

Figure 7.13 The four graphs show the strong dependence between location and scale for the logged data. But when considering the pool standard error and mean differences of the logged data, the dependence is much smaller. (a) Raw control; (b) raw scale; (c) raw treatment; and (d) log scale.

1. Dependence between μ_g and σ_g.
2. Even if μ_g and σ_g are independent, σ_g are not homogeneous, because they vary from gene to gene.
3. σ_g varies from group to group.

One cannot expect to change or eliminate all these problems with a simple transformation. It may be possible to eliminate (1) or even (2) alone but, in practice, we may expect combinations of the three or all the three problems to exist in one data set.

Example. For the example, Figure 7.13 shows that the dependence has been reduced somewhat after log transformation and normalization.

This background is useful because it lets us study different scenarios that may arise in practical situations and enables us to understand what SAM will do in each of these cases. Here are the scenarios.

- *Case 1.* Assume that σ_g is constant for all the groups and all the genes and σ_g is independent of μ_g for all groups.
  In this case, $T_g(c)$ and s_g are dependent for all values of c, but the correlation goes to zero as c goes to infinity. SAM will choose a value of α close to 100%. SAM with a large constant is equivalent to using the t-statistic without the denominator, and finding the critical value for the t-statistic that corresponds to significance.
- *Case 2.* Assume that (i) σ_g is the same for both groups and is distributed as F_σ and (ii) σ_g is independent of μ_g for both groups.
  In this case, $T_g(c)$ and s_g are negatively correlated for small c, but the correlation becomes positive as c goes to infinity. SAM will choose a fudge factor, c, that makes the correlation more or less zero. Simulation results suggest that, when the distribution of σ_g is very skewed to the right, such as a chi-squared distribution with 1 or 2 degrees of freedom, the resulting fudge factor, c, corresponds to very small values of α near 0%. However, when the distribution of σ_g is not heavily skewed, SAM will choose values of α close to 100%. This does not imply that there is no dependence between $T_g(c)$ and s_g, because, for almost all distributions F_σ, there exists no constant, c, that makes the distribution of $T_g(c)$ independent of s_p. However, SAM may produce a reasonable reduction of the dependence.
- *Case 3.* Assume that σ_g is the same for all groups and σ_g is dependent of μ_g for all groups and their joint distribution is $F_{\mu,\sigma}$.
  In this case, it appears also unlikely that a constant c would totally eliminate the dependence of the distribution of $T_g(c)$ from s_g. However, again, SAM should produce a reasonable reduction of the dependence.
- *Case 4.* In addition to Case 3, assume a correlation structure among the genes. The column permutations in SAM preserves the correlation structure, but the same comments as above apply.

Example. Figures 7.1 and 7.13 indicate that σ_g and μ_g are very positively correlated. On the other hand, this correlation structure is reduced when we subtract the gene means, so it may be just a result of the high variation among gene mean effects. Nevertheless, it is worth noting that this effect should be checked before using the methods for Cases 2 or 3 and some modifications may be necessary to account for it.

7.11 CONDITIONAL t

Amaratunga and Cabrera (2009) propose a novel method of addressing the dependence of T_g from s_g by determining, from the distribution of T_g conditioned on

s_g, the critical value of T_g that separates significance from nonsignificance. This method is called the *conditional t* (CT) method.

The CT method provides a solution to the problem of small sample standard deviations by estimating the conditional distribution of T_g given s_g and calculating the critical values $t_\alpha(s)$ that help us to decide which genes are up- or downregulated and which are not according to whether or not $T_g > t_\alpha(s_g)$.

The justification of the CT method starts with Case 1, which assumes that $\sigma_g = \sigma$ is constant for all $1 \leq g \leq G$ and therefore it is estimable with a very small error by $\hat{\sigma} = \sum_{g=1}^{G} s_g/G \cong \sigma$. Under the null hypothesis (H_0) that the differential expression is zero, the conditional distribution of the t-statistic $T_g|s_g$ is Normal$(0, \sigma^2/s_g^2)$ and the optimal rejection region is $n\{|Z_g| > z_{\alpha/2}n\} = n\{|T_g| > \sigma/s_g \quad z_{\alpha/2}n\}$, which has a wedge shape.

In reality, it is unlikely that σ_g is constant but it is distributed by some unknown distribution F_σ as in Case 2, but the correct wedge-shaped rejection region could be approximated by doing a simulation and estimating the distribution of $T_g|s_g$ by nonparametric quantile regression.

The procedure to calculate the critical values, $t_\alpha(s)$, will depend on which of the above four cases is assumed. We start with the basic method that will be used for handling Case 2. Case 1 is difficult to separate from Case 2 in practice because we never know when the variances are constant or variable. Procedures for Case 3 and Case 4 are extensions of the procedure for Case 2. *CT for Case 2.* The simplest development of the method is in the situation in which σg is a realization from the distribution F_σ, where F_σ is the same for all the groups and all the genes and σ_g is independent of μ_g. The procedure comprises two steps:

1. Estimate F_σ.
2. Estimate the conditional distribution of $T_g|s_g$, and, as a consequence, estimate the values $t_\alpha(s_g)$ for a few α's.

These steps are now described in more detail.

1. Estimate F_σ. We know that the empirical distribution of s_g, namely, $\hat{F}_\sigma$, is a biased estimator of the distribution $F_\sigma$in the sense that the low quantiles of the empirical are biased downwards, whereas the high quantiles are biased upwards. This bias is especially large for very small sample sizes as is typical of many microarray experiments. The reason for the large bias is that the distribution of $s_p^2|\sigma^2$ is approximately $\sigma^2\chi^2/(n-1)$. It follows that, for small n, the marginal distribution of s_p^2 has heavier tails than those of $F\sigma$. This bias can be corrected by using a simulation method initially proposed in Amaratunga and Cabrera (2001b). This method by itself is a version of the target estimation procedure of Cabrera and Fernholz (1999). The idea is to estimate the function $g : [0:1] \to [0,1]$ defined by $g(F_\sigma(x) = \hat{F}(x)$. Because g is strictly monotonic, it can be inverted in order to obtain an estimate of $F_\sigma(x)$. The steps to estimate $F_\sigma(x)$ are as follows:

(a) Generate a null distribution for the data by subtracting the sample means and dividing by the standard deviations.

(b) Assume that $\hat{F}_s(x)$ is the true distribution of σ. Then resample from the null distribution of x and multiply each sample by a σ generated from $\hat{F}_s(x)$. Repeat this 10,000 times and, this way, get 10,000 pairs of samples for 10,000.

(c) From each pair of samples, calculate a value for the pooled sample standard deviation, namely, s_g^*, for $g = 1, \ldots, 10,000$. Let $\hat{F}_{s*}(x)$ be the empirical distribution of the s_g^*'s. Then the estimator of g is obtained by mapping the empirical distribution $\hat{F}_s$ into $\hat{F}_{s*}$. More precisely,

$$\hat{g}(y = \hat{F}_s(x)) = \hat{F}_{s*}(\hat{F}_s^{-1}(y)) \text{ and } \hat{g}^{-1}(y) = \hat{F}_s(\hat{F}_{s*}^{-1}(y)).$$

Hence, the estimator of F_σ is

$$\hat{F}_\sigma(x) = \hat{F}(x)(\hat{F}^{-1}(\hat{F}_s(x))).$$

$\hat{F}_\sigma(x)$ will be used in the second part of the method to generate the standard deviations of the gene populations.

An alternative iteration for (c) is based on the multivariate version of the target method (Cabrera and Fernholz, 2004). The idea is to modify the target method by adding a sorting steps that guarantees that the steps of the iteration yield distribution functions. Suppose that $\hat{\boldsymbol{F}}_\sigma$ is a vector with the observed quantiles of the empirical distribution of the s_g's. Then the following iteration produces the target estimator of $\boldsymbol{F}_\sigma$

$$\tilde{\boldsymbol{F}}_\sigma^{(i+1)} = \text{SORT}\left\{\tilde{\boldsymbol{F}}_\sigma^i - \frac{1}{i}(g(\tilde{\boldsymbol{F}}_\sigma^i) - \hat{\boldsymbol{F}}_\sigma)\right\},$$

where $\tilde{\boldsymbol{F}}_\sigma^1 = \hat{\boldsymbol{F}}_\sigma$ and $g(F) = E_F(\hat{\boldsymbol{F}}_\sigma)$. The sequence $\tilde{F}_\sigma^{(i+1)}$ will converge to the target estimator $\tilde{\boldsymbol{F}}_\sigma$ of $\boldsymbol{F}_\sigma$. This estimator shrinks the distribution $\hat{\boldsymbol{F}}_\sigma$ toward the center, which is also what Empirical Bayes (Limma) does, whereas SAM will shift the estimator towards the right. In addition, the target estimator is nonparametric, so it does not make any normality assumptions that are made by Empirical Bayes.

2. The second part of the method involves generating the conditional distribution of $t|s_d$, and the first steps are the same as Steps (a) and (b) of the above algorithm.

(a) Generate a null distribution for the data by subtracting the sample means and dividing by the standard deviations.

(b) Resample from the null distribution of x and multiply each sample by a σ generated from $\hat{F}_\sigma(x)$. Repeat this 10,000 times and, in this way, obtain 10,000 pairs of samples. From each pair of samples, calculate a value for the pooled sample standard deviation and the two-sample t-statistic, namely, s_g and t_g for $g = 1, \ldots, 10{,}000$.

(c) We estimate $t_\alpha(s_g)$ using a quantile regression estimate for t_g versus s_g and estimate the regression quantile curve for the $1-\alpha$ quantile. A crude but effective way to estimate the quantile curve is to split the 10,000 points into 100 groups of 100 points sorted by s_g and calculate the $1-\alpha$ quantile for each group and call it $t_{(j)}$ and calculate the group medians for s_g and call it $s_{(j)}$ $j = 1, \ldots, 100$. Then estimate $t_\alpha(s_g)$ by fitting a smoother such as lowess or a smoothing spline to $t_{(j)}$ versus $s_{(j)}$. To estimate the quantile function, it is recommended to take the log of $t_{(j)}$ and $s_{(j)}$ first and then to estimate the quantile function.

CT for Case 3. Now assume that σ and μ are not independent. The main difficulty is that, instead of estimating the distribution of σ alone, we must now obtain and estimate the joint distribution of μ and σ. Conceptually, this is not a problem, but computationally it requires using two-dimensional smoothers and inverting two-dimensional functions.

The first part of the procedure is more complicated than for Case 2 because we need to invert a function $h : R^2 \to R^2$. We can assume that h is continuous and differentiable and g has to be one-to-one in order to have a well-defined inverse h^{-1}.

The second part of the procedure in Case 2 can be replicated for Case 3, with the exception that σ_g and μ_g are sampled from their joint distribution. As in Case 2, we estimate the cutoff, $t_\alpha(s_p)$, from the joint distribution of t_α and s_p by conditioning on s_p. Moreover, it is also possible to estimate the cutoff conditioning also on the overall sample mean, $t_\alpha(s_g, \overline{x}_g)$.

It is easy to see that the overall error rate of the CT procedure is α. Let s and t be the random variables representing the pooled variance estimate and the t-statistic for a randomly selected gene. Let $f(t, s)$ be the joint probability density function of t and s. This is a mixing distribution since s has a distribution that depends of the gene. The CT procedure consists of rejecting a null hypothesis if $t > h(s)$ and conditioning on s the probability of Type I error is α. The following calculation shows that the overall unconditional probability of Type I error is also α:

$$\int_0^\infty \int_{h(s)}^\infty f(ts)\, dt\, ds = \int_0^\infty \left(\int_{-\infty}^\infty f(t,s)dt \right) \frac{\int_{h(s)}^\infty f(t,s)dt}{\int_{-\infty}^\infty f(t,s)ds}$$

$$\int_0^\infty \int_{-\infty}^\infty f(t,s)dt\alpha ds = \alpha \int_0^\infty \int_{-\infty}^\infty f(t,s)dt\alpha ds = \alpha$$

Example. Figures 7.14 and 7.15 show a comparison between the pooled standard errors of the genes and three distributions: χ distributions with 0.5, 2, and 6 degrees of freedom. If the assumption of equal variances was true (and the genes were all independent of one another), we would expect that the pooled standard errors would be approximately proportional to a χ distribution with 6 degrees of freedom. Instead, they appear to be closer to a χ distribution with 0.5 degrees of freedom. Such a large difference strongly suggests that the gene variances are heterogeneous. Therefore, we apply the CT method for Case 2. The

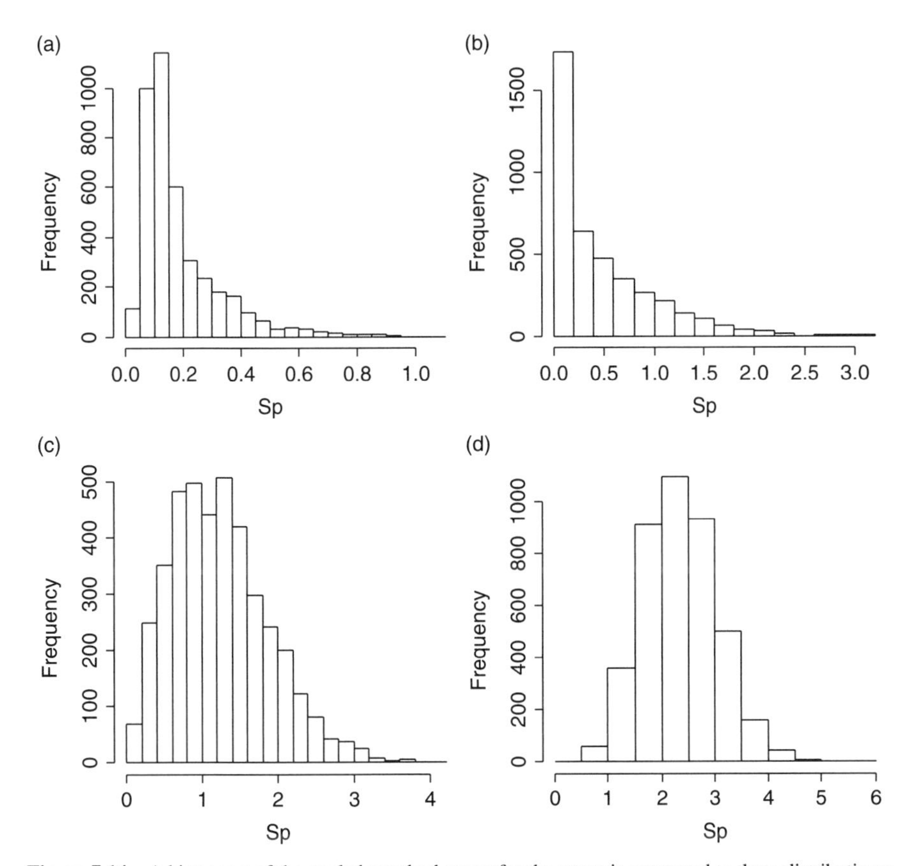

Figure 7.14 A histogram of the pooled standard errors for the genes is compared to three distributions: Case 1, chi-square with 0.5 degrees of freedom. Case 2, Chi-square with 2 degrees of freedom. Case 3, chi-square with 6 degrees of freedom. (a) E7 data; (b) case 1; (c) case 2; (d) case 3.

curves in Figure 7.16 represent the proportion of significant genes reported by the CT procedure using the method for Case 2. It is clear that the CT method greatly reduced the dependence of the significance of the t-statistic on s_g. Even though SAM does an exemplary job of correcting the problem at the low range of s_g, it is not clear that a simple constant correction will produce a homogeneous t across the whole range of s_g values. The CT approach is a more direct means, although perhaps making more assumptions, but it should produce, in general, a more homogeneous result.

7.12 BORROWING STRENGTH ACROSS GENES

Inferences drawn from experiments with little replication can be terribly unreliable and nonreproducible. To a large extent, this is because the fewer the number of

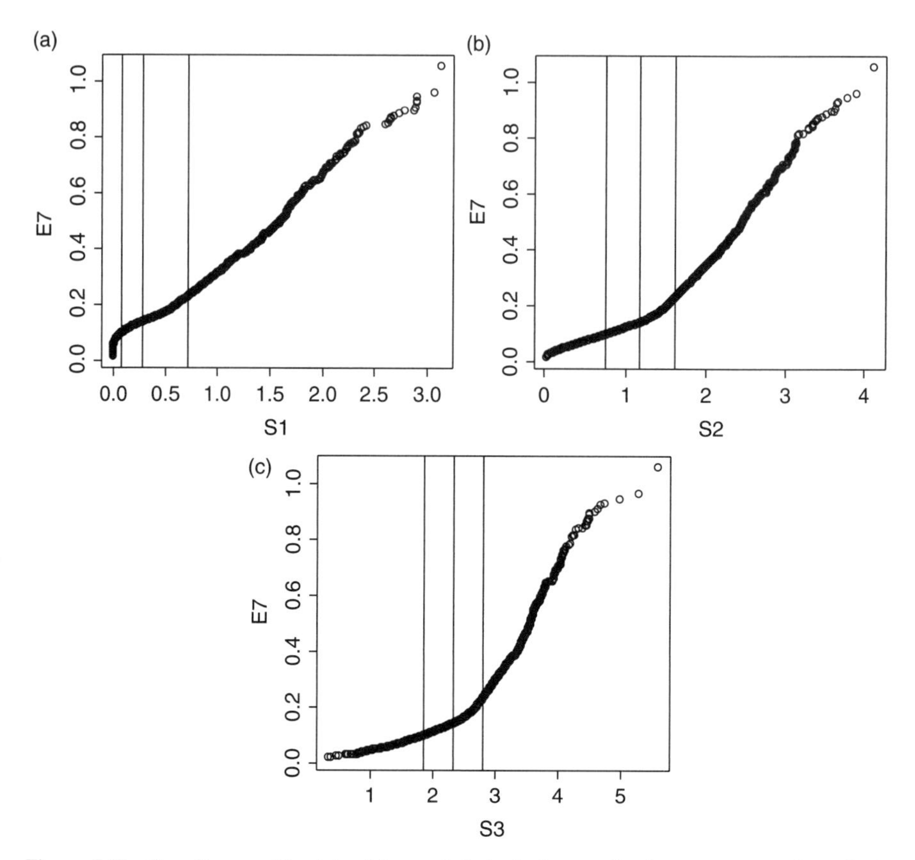

Figure 7.15 Quantile–quantile plots of the pooled standard errors for the genes versus three distributions: (a) Case 1, chi-square with 0.5 degrees of freedom. (b) Case 2, chi-square with 2 degrees of freedom. (c) Case 3, chi-square with 6 degrees of freedom.

samples used in an experiment, the less precise the variance estimates are. Using the signal-to-noise analogy, without a reasonable estimate of "noise," it becomes difficult to separate the "signal" from the "noise."

This is of particular concern with microarray experiments as they are notorious for having few true replicates, particularly biological replicates. Statistical inferences reached purely on an individual gene basis could be driven by weak variance estimates and may not be particularly trustworthy. On the other hand, even though a microarray experiment may have only a few replicates, there is always data on a large number of genes. Thus, an appealing idea for improving inferences from microarray experiments is to "borrow strength across genes."

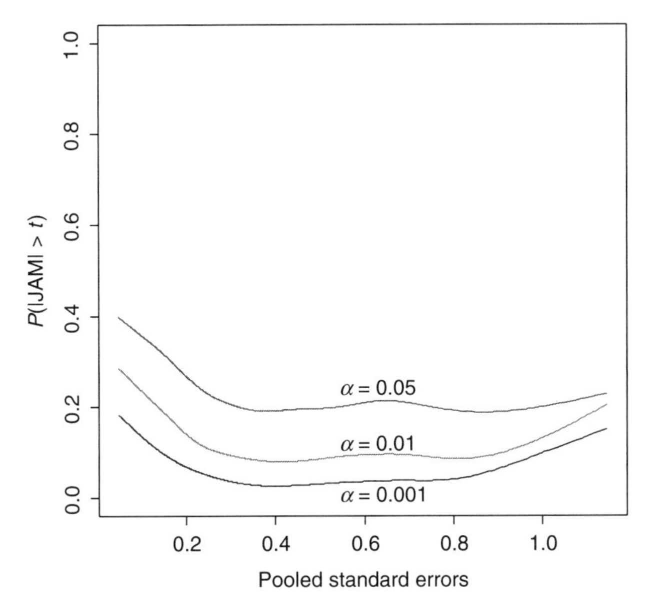

Figure 7.16 Proportion of significant genes produced by the conditional t method for values of $\alpha = 0.05, 0.01, 0.001$ versus the pooled standard errors.

7.12.1 Simple Methods

The simplest approach is to assume that every gene has the same variance and then estimate that variance as the average variance across all the genes:

$$s_{g1}^2 = \frac{\Sigma_{h=1}^{G} s_h^2}{G}.$$

Amaratunga and Cabrera (2001b) describe such a situation, although they use a different approach.

However, rarely is it the case that all genes have the same variance. More often, the variance tends to be high for genes whose expression levels are high and low for genes whose expression levels are low; variances of genes whose expression levels are similar to one another tend to be closer than genes whose expression levels are very different from one another. In this case, it is reasonable to assume that $\sigma_{gt}^2 = f(\mu_{gt})$, where f is a smooth continuous function. In this case, we can fit the model

$$s_g^2 = f(\overline{x}_g) + e_g$$

using a semiparametric smoothing procedure such as lowess or a spline smoother, and take the fitted value as s^2:

$$s_g^2 = \hat{f}(\overline{x}_g).$$

Another approach on the same lines is to use as σ_{g2}^2 the local average of the standard deviation for genes showing similar expression levels as gene g. To do this, first order all the genes within a treatment group according to their average expression levels. Then consider the given gene and the k next higher expressing genes and the k next lower expressing genes. Take the average of the standard deviations of these $2k + 1$ genes as s_{g2}^2.

Using either s_{g1}^2 or s_{g2}^2 may produce an overly smooth estimator of σ_g^2. This can be remedied by estimating σ_g^2 by a composite estimator, which is a weighted combination of the observed variance of the gth gene and the smoothed variance estimate:

$$\hat{\sigma}^2 = \lambda s_g^2 + (1 - \lambda)s_{g1}^2 \text{ or } \hat{\sigma}^2 = \lambda s_g^2 + (1 - \lambda)s_{g2}^2.$$

Doing this results in increased precision for variance estimates and inferences are made more trustworthy. However, the question remains how to choose λ?

7.12.2 A Bayesian Model

Baldi and Long (2001) present a formal development of this idea by casting it in a Bayesian framework. They begin by assuming that the data has a normal distribution, so that for a particular gene in a particular group

$$x_i \sim \mathrm{N}(\mu, \sigma^2),$$

where, in the interest of simplicity, we have omitted the subscript g for gene and j for group. Let $\overline{x}$ and s^2 denote the sample mean and sample variance for the gene in this group.

Following fairly standard Bayesian practice, the variance parameter, the prior distribution of μ and σ^2 is defined in two parts as follows: σ_g^2 , is taken to follow an inverse gamma distribution, while, given σ_g^2, the mean parameter, μ_g, is taken to follow a normal distribution, that is,

$$\mu|\sigma \sim \mathrm{N}\left(\mu, \frac{\sigma^2}{\lambda}\right),$$

$$\sigma^2 \sim \mathrm{IG}(\nu_0, \sigma_0^2).$$

This formulation corresponds to a conjugate prior. A bonus is that the resulting joint prior distribution of (μ, σ^2) forces μ and σ^2 to be dependent, as can be observed in many microarray experiments.

Applying Bayes's theorem, followed by some algebraic manipulations, we can obtain the posterior distribution:

$$(\mu, \sigma|x) \sim \mathrm{N}\left(\mu, \frac{\sigma^2}{\lambda}\right) \mathrm{IG}(\nu_0, \sigma_0^2),$$

with

$$\begin{aligned}
\mu_n &= \frac{\lambda_0}{\lambda_0 + n}\mu_0 + \frac{n}{\lambda_0 + n}\overline{x},\\
\lambda_n &= \lambda_0 + n,\\
\nu_n &= \nu_0 + n,\\
\nu_n\sigma_n^2 &= \nu_0\sigma_0^2 + (n-1)s^2 + \frac{\lambda_0 n}{\lambda_0 + n}(\overline{x} - \mu_0).
\end{aligned}$$

Observe that the parameters of the posterior distribution combine information from the prior and the data. The posterior mean is a weighted average of the prior mean and the sample mean. The posterior degrees of freedom is the prior degrees of freedom plus the sample size. The posterior sum of squares is the prior sum of squares plus the sample sum of squares plus the residual uncertainty due to the discrepancy between the prior mean and the sample mean.

The prior mean is usually set to the sample mean: $\mu_0 = \overline{x}$, so that $\mu_n = \overline{x}$. The mean of the posterior distribution is

$$\begin{aligned}
\mu_P &= \mu_n = \overline{x},\\
\sigma_P^2 &= \frac{\nu_n}{\nu_n - 2}\sigma_n^2 = \frac{\nu_0\sigma_0^2 + (n-1)s^2}{\nu_0 + n - 2}
\end{aligned}$$

provided that $\nu_0 + n > 2$.

Baldi and Long (2001) use a simple rule of thumb to assign a value to ν_0. They assume that a minimum of K points are necessary to adequately estimate a standard deviation (they use $K = 10$, but Tukey has made persuasive arguments that $K = 30$) and choose 0 so that $\nu_0 + n = K$.

These values are then plugged into the t-test statistic. A robust Bayes version has been proposed by Amaratunga and Cabrera (2003c). There have also been Emprical Bayes procedures that have been proposed (see, e.g., Efron, Storey and Tibshirani, 2001). In some sense the conditional t (CT) approach also has connections to these concepts (Amaratunga and Cabrera, 2009).

7.13 TWO-CHANNEL EXPERIMENTS

Consider a two-channel microarray experiment whose objective is to compare two types of samples, A_1 and A_2. Suppose that there are K microarrays and on each microarray, there are two channels, one channel corresponding to A1 and the other channel corresponding to A_2. Let X_{gjk} be the log-transformed and normalized spot intensity level for gth gene and the channel of the jth array that corresponds to sample type A_k; here $g = 1, \ldots, G,\ j = 1, \ldots, n,$ and $k = 1, 2$.

The value $Y_{gj} = X_{gj1} - X_{gj2}$ is the difference in log $_2$ expression level between the two channels in the jth sample for the gth gene (or equivalently the log of the fold change between the two channels); $\overline{Y}_g = \Sigma_{j=1}^{n} Y_{gi}/n$ is the mean and $V_g = \Sigma_{j=1}^{n}(Y_{gi} - \overline{Y}_g)^2/(n-1)$ is the variance of the $\{Y_{gj}\}$ values for the gth gene.

7.13.1 The Paired Sample t Test and SAM

The *paired sample t-test* statistic for testing for differential expression is

$$T_g = \frac{\overline{Y}_g}{\sqrt{V_g/n}}$$

If the data are drawn from a normal distribution, the null distribution of T_g is a t-distribution with degrees of freedom $\nu = n - 1$. If the observed value of T_g is $T_{g;\text{obs}}$ then the p-value is given by the probability $p_g = \text{Prob}(|T_g| > T_g; \text{obs})$. A gene is declared significantly differentially expressed at level of significance α if $p_g < \alpha$.

As described in Section 7.10 for the two-sample t-test, the paired sample t-test can also have the problem that, with small samples, that the t-test statistic tends to be highly correlated with the standard error term appearing in its denominator. This results in a high false positive rate for genes whose variability is low and a high false negative rate for genes whose variability is high. The SAM modification to the t-statistic described in Section 7.10.1 can also be used here. The modified SAM t-statistic is

$$T_g = \frac{\overline{Y}_g}{(\sqrt{V_g/n}) + c}$$

where the fudge factor, c, is estimated as described in Section 7.10.1. The rest of the procedure then proceeds as described there.

7.13.2 Borrowing Strength Via Hierarchical Modeling

Several authors (Lee et al., 2000; Efron et al., 2001; Newton et al., 2001; Pan et al., 2002; Lonnstedt and Speed, 2002) have proposed various ways of borrowing strength across genes via Bayesian hierarchical modeling. These constructions begin by assuming that some unknown proportion, p_E, of the G genes are actually differentially expressed. For those genes, the indicator variable $I_g = 1$, while, for the rest, $I_g = 0$. The question is to determine, based on the data, which genes are the most likely to truly have $I_g = 1$.

A mixture model is developed as follows. Suppose that p_E is the probability that gene g is differentially expressed and that $f_E(y)$ and $f_0(y)$ denote the probability density functions of Y_g for genes that are differentially expressed and not differentially expressed, respectively. Then,

$$f(y) = (1 - p)E)f_0(y) + p_E f_E(y),$$

is the probability density function for the mixture distribution of Y_g.

Lee et al. (2000) assume a normal distribution for Y_g, for each g, the various components of the mixture model can be estimated using, for example, the EM algorithm (Dempster et al., 1977).

Lonnstedt and Speed (2002) similarly assume $Y_{gj} \sim \mathrm{N}(\mu_g, \sigma_g)$. In the prior distribution, genes having no previous evidence of effects are considered exchangeable, making the posterior mean effect for each gene borrow strength from the observed effects of the other genes. Thus, a large observed effect of a gene will be shrunk toward zero in the posterior mean when the gene is exchangeable with other genes that have mostly small observed effects. Candidate genes, for which there is some prior evidence for an effect, will be treated separately.

Following fairly standard Bayesian practice as before (Section 7.3.2), the variance parameter, σ_g^2, is taken to follow an inverse gamma distribution, while, given σ_g^2, the mean parameter, μ_g, is taken to follow a normal distribution

$$\tau_g = \frac{na}{a\sigma_g^2} \sim \Gamma(\nu, 1),$$

$$\mu_g|\tau_g = \begin{cases} 0 & \text{if } I_g = 0 \\ N\left(0, \frac{cna}{2\tau_j}\right) & \text{if } I_g = 1. \end{cases}$$

This formulation implies a correlation between the difference in means and the variance for those genes that are differentially expressed.

Applying Bayes' rule, we can work out the log posterior odds for the gth gene to be differentially expressed as

$$B_g = \log\left[\frac{\mathrm{Prob}(I_g = 1|M_{gi})}{\mathrm{Prob}(I_g = 0|M_{gi})}\right]$$

which works out to

$$B_g = \log\left(\frac{p}{1-p}\right)\frac{1}{\sqrt{1+nc}}\left[\frac{a + s_g^2 + \overline{M}_g^2}{a + s_g^2 + \dfrac{\overline{M}_g^2}{1+nc}}\right]^{\frac{\nu n}{2}}$$

The B_g values provide a ranking of the genes with respect to the posterior probability of each gene being differentially expressed.

Generally, it is impossible to estimate simultaneously all the four parameters p, νa and c. To circumvent this problem, p is fixed at some prespecified value, then ν and a are estimated by the method of moments, while c is estimated from the top proportion of genes.

Another approach to this problem is given by Newton et al. (2001) based on the model given in Section 6.3.

7.14 FILTERING

As we saw in the previous sections, for a gene-by-gene analysis in which the inference is based on a gene-specific test, each gene corresponds to a null hypothesis. In this case, rejection of null hypotheses becomes difficult as the number of genes increases. Therefore, a preselection of biological relevant genes for the analysis is crucial because it could be expected to increase both the number of discoveries and power. In this section, we discuss a preselection procedure called *gene filtering*. We discuss two different approaches; the first is based on the summarized data, while the second is based on the probe-level data before summarization. Figure 7.17a shows the intensity levels of the probes of the gene 1636740_at from the platinum data set discussed in Chapter 6. It shows the main difference between the two approaches. The first approach uses the summarized data (the thick black line) in order to make a decision as to whether to include the gene in the analysis or not, while the latter uses the probe intensity levels for the filtering procedure.

7.14.1 Filtering Based on Summarized Data

Gene filtering based on summarized data is a two-stage procedure in which the preselection step is based on the *gene-specific filtering statistic*, U_g^I, and the inference at the second stage is based on the *gene-specific test statistic*, U_g^{II}. The filtering statistic U_g^I is *nonspecific* or *unsupervised* (Bourgon et al., 2010) because it is calculated for each gene without taking into account the effect under investigation (i.e., the treatment or group). This implies that variability caused by condition effect, such as the one that was observed in Figure 7.17a, is "translated" to a high value of U_g^I. Therefore, genes with high condition effects will be included in the analysis, while genes with "flat" expression profiles will be excluded. Hackstadt and Hess (2009) reported that doing this increased the number of discoveries for several examples of gene expression data and different filtering methods. Bourgon et al. (2010) pointed out that, as long as the null distribution of U_g^{II} is independent of U_g^I, the error rate in the second stage can be controlled.

Example. For the Golub data, Figure 7.18 shows the histogram for three possible nonspecific filtering statistics, the standard error, the inter quartile range $Q_3 - Q_1$, and the MAD. We notice that all filtering statistics reveal the same

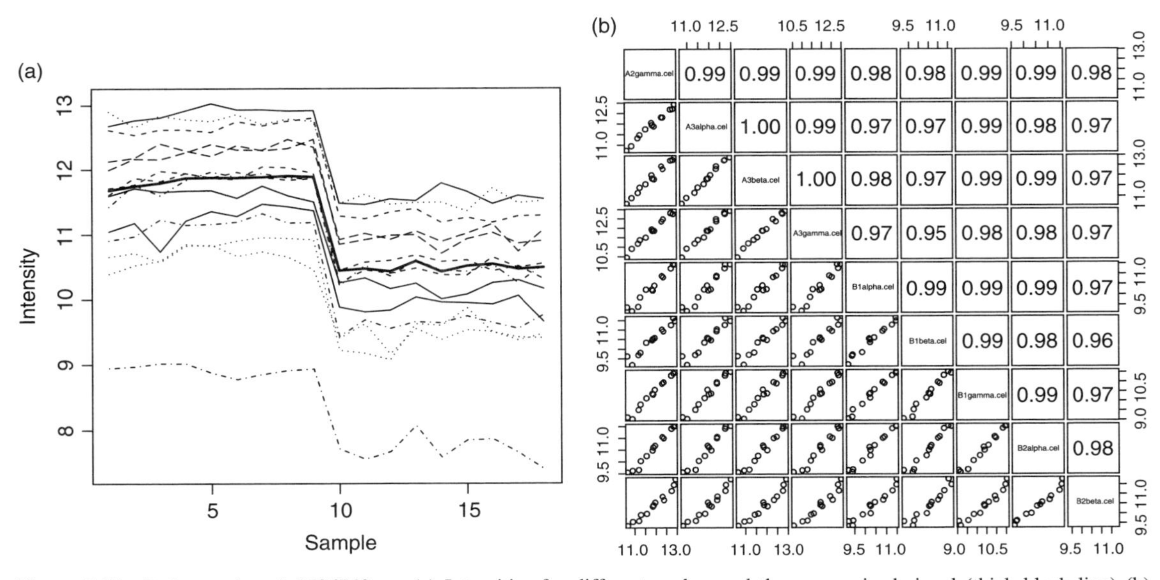

Figure 7.17 Probe set (gene) 1636740_at. (a) Intensities for different probes and the summarized signal (thick black line) (b) Scatterplot of probe intensities for selected probes in the probe set.

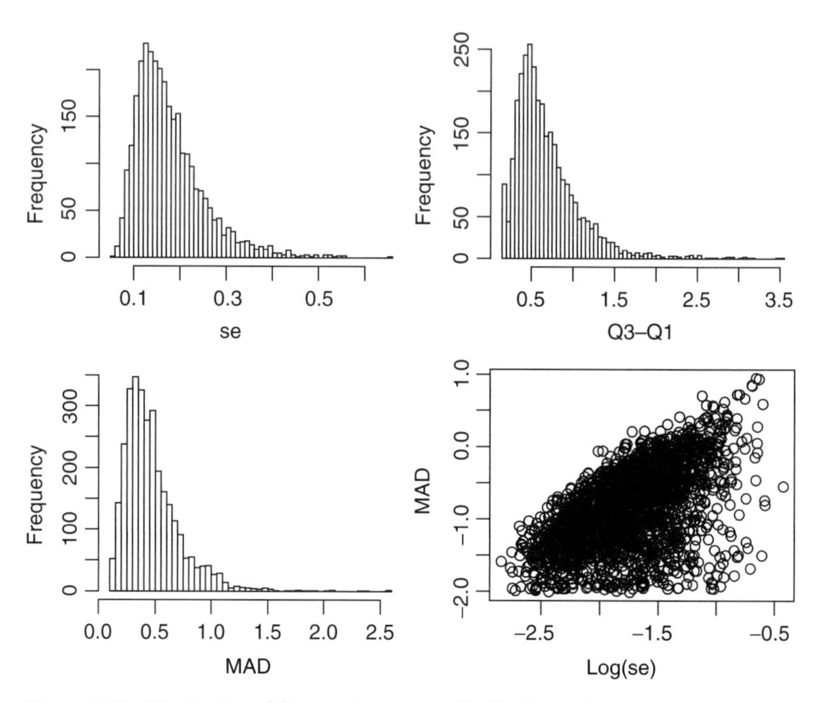

Figure 7.18 Distribution of the possible nonspecific filtering statistics in the Golub data.

pattern; their distribution is skewed to the right, that is for most of the genes the variability is low, while a minority of the genes have high variability. Intuitively, we would like to filter out those genes with low variability and include in the analysis only those genes with high variability. Figure 7.19 shows an example of randomly selected genes for which the standard error belongs to either the lower 5% (Fig. 7.19a) or the upper 5% (Fig. 7.19b) of the distribution. The difference between the two horizontal lines is the fold change, $\overline{x}_{\mathrm{ALL}} - \overline{x}_{\mathrm{AML}}$. Clearly, the fold change of genes with standard error belonging to the upper tail of the distribution is higher than that of the genes with standard error belonging to the lower tail of the distribution.

Without filtering and after FDR adjustment for multiplicity, 695 genes (out of 3051) were declared differentially expressed. As a filtering score, we used the interquartile range $(Q_3 - Q_1)$, a robust measure for the variability in the center of the distribution. Genes for which the interquartile range was below $(Q_3 - Q_1)_{10\%}$ (i.e., in the 10% lower tails of the distribution) were not included in the analysis. This implies that only 2745 were included in the analysis and 306 were filtered out. After filtering, the number of rejected null hypothesis increased to 712. The impact of filtering in terms of the fold change is visualized in Figure 7.20 that presents the volcano plots and the distribution of the fold change in both subset of genes that were filtered in (Fig. 7.20a and b) and filtered out (Fig. 7.20c and d). We can see clearly that the genes that were filtered out have in general lower fold

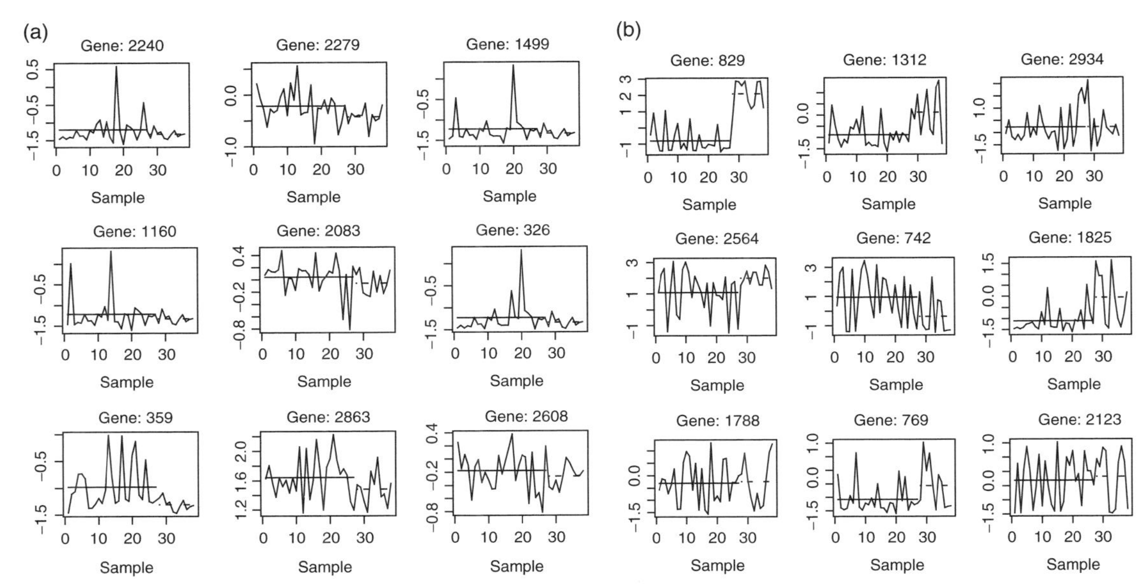

Figure 7.19 Expression levels for a random selection of genes. (a) Genes with se $\leq s_{5\%}$. Genes were selected from the subset of genes for which the standard error is belong to the lower 5% of the distribution. (b) Genes with se $\geq s_{95\%}$. Genes were selected from the subset of genes for which the standard error belongs to the upper 5% of the distribution. The horizontal lines are the mean gene expression levels for the acute lymphoblastic leukemia (ALL) group and the acute myeloid leukemia (AML) group.

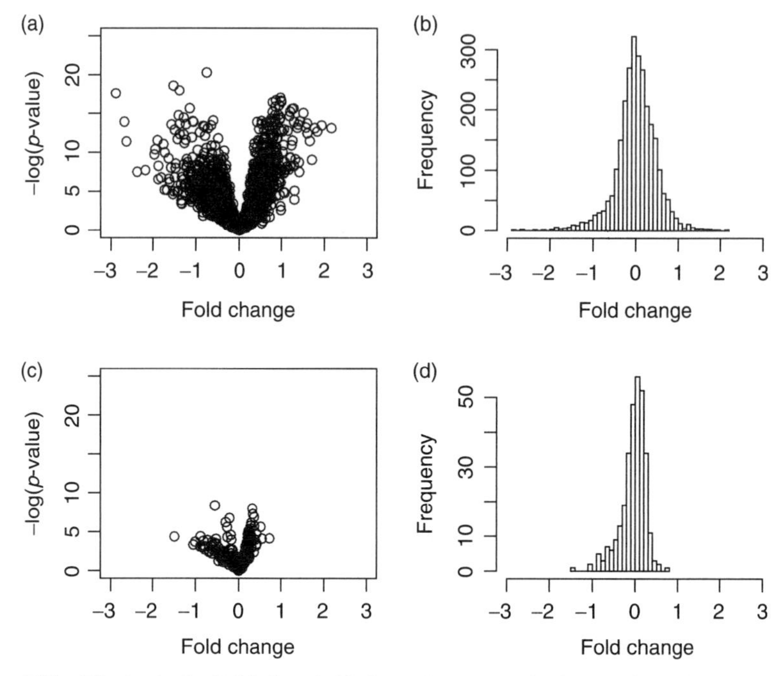

Figure 7.20 Filtering in the Golub data. (a, b) Genes that were retained. (c, d) Genes that were filtered out. (a, c) Fold change versus $-\log(p\text{-values})$. (b, d) Distribution of the fold change.

changes compared to the genes that were selected for the analysis. The distribution of the raw p-values (before adjustment for multiplicity) is shown in Figure 7.21.

Figure 7.22a shows the number of rejected null hypotheses versus the proportion of genes with the highest interquartile range that were selected in the first stage and illustrate the advantage of filtering. If 7.5% of the genes are filtered out, the number of rejected null hypotheses increases from 695 (when all genes are included) to 712. Figure 7.22b illustrates the price that we pay when initial filtering is performed. In case that the cutoff point for U_g^I is too low (i.e., if a large number of genes are filtered out, it is possible that) some of the genes that are filtered out are actually differentially expressed.

7.14.2 Filtering Based on Probe-Level Data

The second filtering approach is based on the probe-level intensities and not on the summarized data as in Section 7.14.1. Let PM_{ij} be the jth probe intensity measured on array i of the perfect match in a given probe set. Talloen et al. (2007), Hochreiter et al. (2006), Calza et al. (2007), and Kasim et al. (2010) pointed out that because all measurements PM_{ij} belong to the same probe set, they should measure the same quantity, the *unobserved and true intensity*, of the jth gene. Hence, for an informative probe set, the intensity measurements should be correlated. Such a pattern can be clearly seen in Figure 7.17b, while Figure 7.23 shows an example

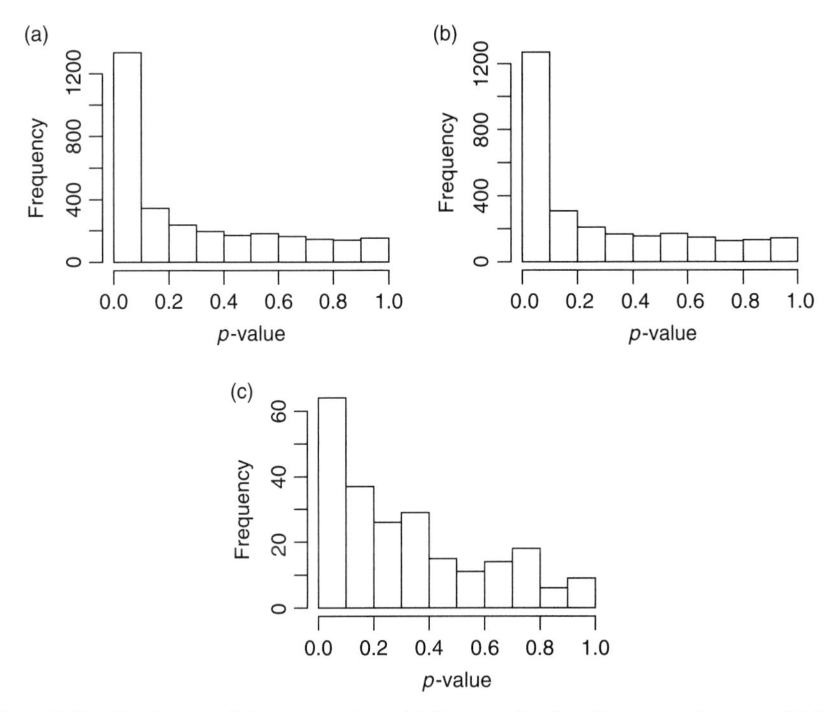

Figure 7.21 Distribution of the raw p-values. (a) Raw p-value for all genes in the array. (b) Raw p-values for genes that were filtered in. (c) Raw p-values for genes that were filtered out.

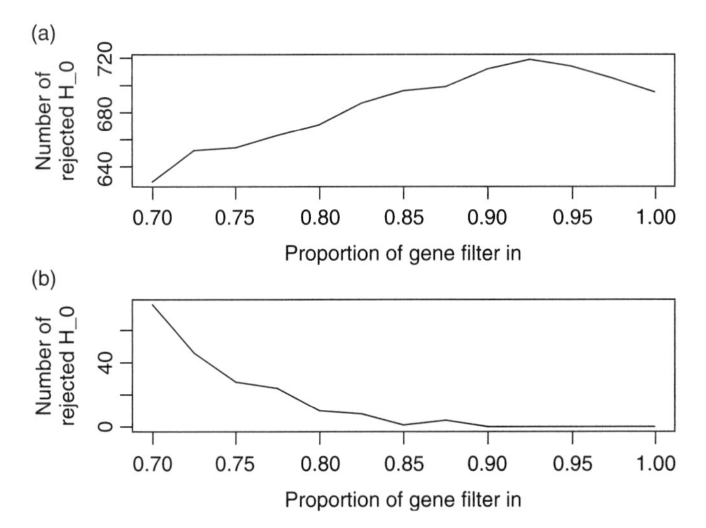

Figure 7.22 Number of rejected null hypotheses versus the proportion of genes that were filtered in. (a) Number of rejected null hypotheses for genes that were filtered in. (b) Number of rejected null hypotheses for genes that were filtered out.

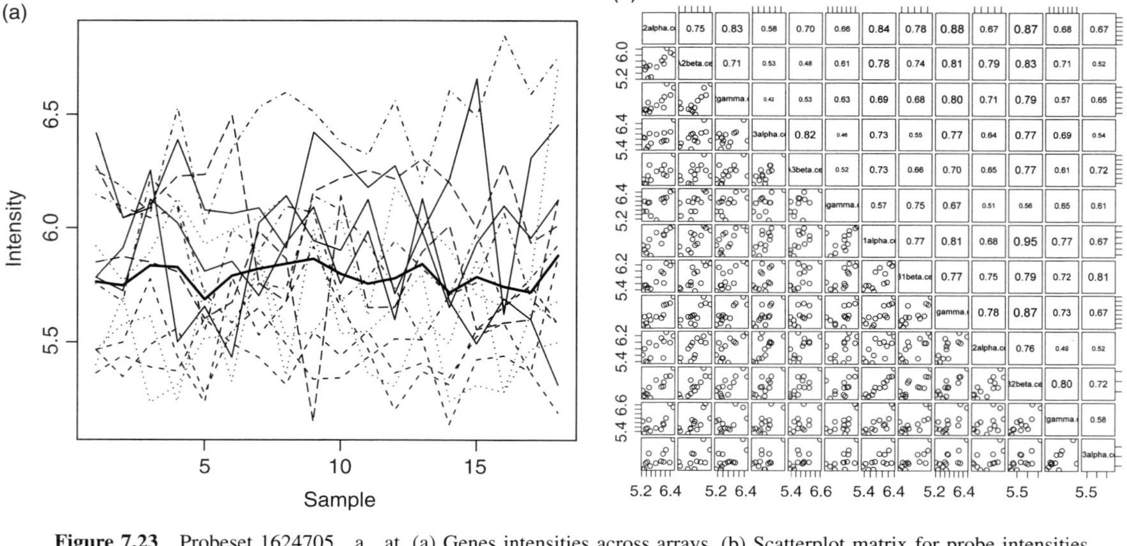

Figure 7.23 Probeset 1624705_ a_ at. (a) Genes intensities across arrays. (b) Scatterplot matrix for probe intensities.

of a probe set for which the probe intensities are not correlated. Hence, the probe sets can be divided into two subsets: (i) informative probe sets, which carry relevant biological signal, and (ii) noninformative probe sets, which do not contain relevant biological information. We expect that probe-level intensities will be correlated for informative probe sets and will not be correlated for noninformative probe sets. A good filtering procedure should filter out noninformative probe sets from the analysis.

The modeling framework for filtering based on probe-level data is based on the assumption that the $\log_2(\mathrm{PM}_{ij})$ consists of two sources of variability: The first is the variability because of *measurement error* and the second is an *array-to-array variability*. In Figure 7.17a, the second sources of variability is associated with the difference between the intensity profiles of different arrays (*between-array variability* or *array-to-array variability*), while the first source of variability is associated with the variability of within each intensity profile (*within-array variability* or *measurement error*). Kasim et al. (2010) formulated a linear mixed model (Verbeke and Molenberghs, 2000) for $\log_2(\mathrm{PM}_{ij})$ and in particular assumed

$$\log_2(\mathrm{PM}_{ij}) = \mu_j + b_i + \varepsilon_{ij}, \quad i = 1, \cdots, n, \quad j = 1, \cdots, K.$$

Here, b_i is an array-specific effect, $b_i \sim \mathrm{N}(0, \sigma_b^2)$, μ_j is probe specific effects, and $\varepsilon_{ij} \sim \mathrm{N}(0, \sigma_\varepsilon^2)$. The parameters of variance components in the model σ_ε^2 and σ_b^2 represent the two sources of variability in the data, the variability within the arrays and the variability between the arrays, respectively. Note that the filtering model of Kasim et al. (2010) is the same as the summarization model of Irizarry et al. (2003), discussed in Chapter 6, with $\log(\theta_j) = \mu_j$ and $\log(\phi_i) = b_i$.

Within the mixed model framework, the probe intensities measured on the same array form a cluster, and it is expected that observations within a cluster are correlated if they all measure the same true expression levels for the probe set. The probe-set-specific intracluster correlation (Verbeke and Molenberghs, 2000), that is, the correlation between probes on the same array, is given by

$$\rho_g = \frac{\sigma_b^2}{\sigma_b^2 + \sigma_\varepsilon^2}, \quad g = 1, \ldots, G.$$

Note that for the case in which σ_b^2 is relatively larger than σ_ε^2, the array-to-array variability is larger than the measurement errors. In that case, the probe set is considered to be informative. On the other hand, $\rho_g \to 0$ when $\sigma_b^2 << \sigma_\varepsilon^2$. In that case, the probe intensities are independent and there is no coherence within the probe set and the probe set is considered to be noninformative. The cutoff point $\rho = 0.5$ represents the case that $\sigma_b^2 = \sigma_\varepsilon^2$. Thus, probe sets with $\rho_g > 0.5$ are considered to be informative.

Example. Kasim et al. (2010) used the spiked-in data set to compare several filtering procedures based on the probe-level data. Figure 7.24 shows examples of informative (Fig. 7.24a) and noninformative (Fig. 7.24b) probe sets. We notice that for the spiked-in probe sets, probe intensities are highly correlated as expected, while for the noninformative probe sets, because the probe sets do not carry any biological signal, the probe intensities are not correlated as expected.

SUPPLEMENTARY READING

Many basic statistical textbooks (e.g., Triola, 2001, 2002) describe the fundamentals of statistical hypothesis testing. Cox and Hinkley (1974) present a more advanced philosophical discussion. Manly (1992) describes the use of randomization methods in biology.

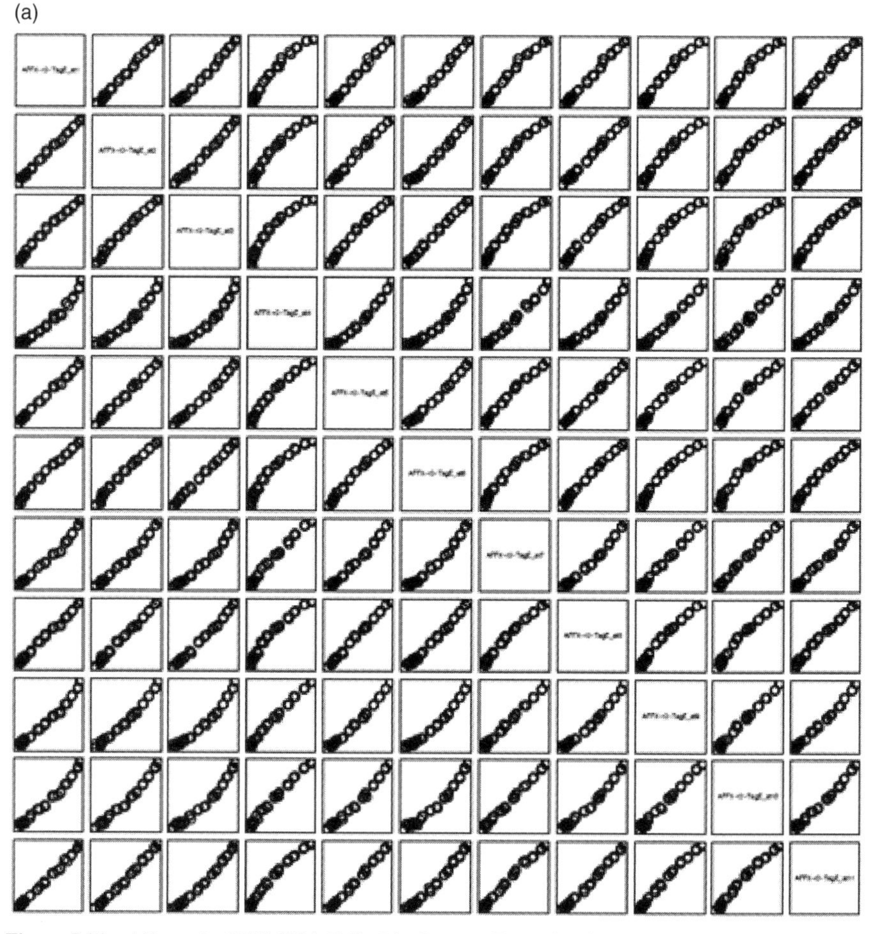

Figure 7.24 Affymetrix HGU-133A Spiked-in data set. Example of probe-level intensities for informative and noninformative probe sets. (a) Informative probe set.

SOFTWARE NOTES

`DNAMR 2.0`

This package implements some of the methods that are included in this chapter which are (i) conditional t (CT) (ii) SAM and corresponding graphs.
`www.rci.rutgers.edu/~cabrera/DNAMR.`

`ct`

R script for CT (conditional t) is available in DNAMR and from the authors.

`multtest`

The bioconductor package `multtest` uses several multiple testing procedures for controlling the FWER, generalized familywise error rate (gFWER), and FDR.

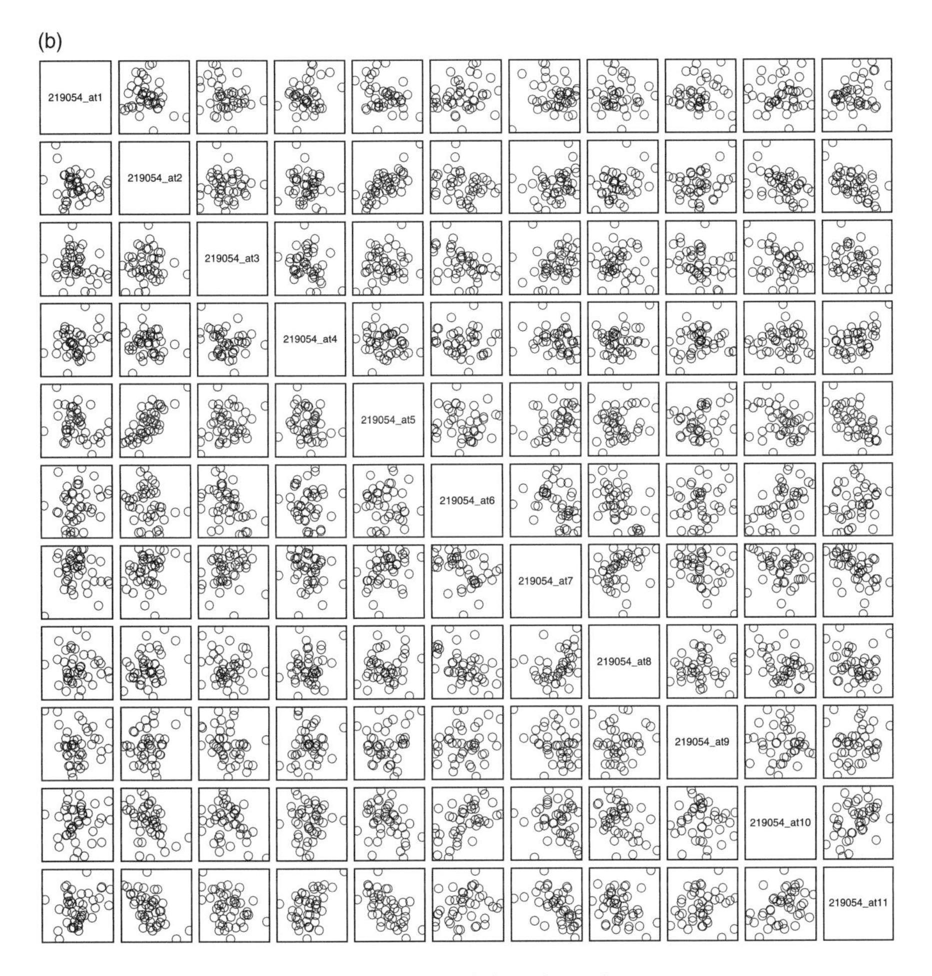

Figure 7.24 (b) Noninformative probe set.

Single-step and step-wise methods, discussed in Section 7.8, are implemented. The results are reported in terms of adjusted p-values and test statistic cutoffs. The methodology implemented in the package is discussed by Dudoit and Van der Laan (2008).

`genefilter`

Filtering based on summarized data, discussed in Section 7.14, was done using the bioconductor package `genefilter`. Methodological issues related to two-stage filtering are discussed in Bourgon, Gentleman, and Huber (2010).

`samr`

The CRAN package `samr` was used to produce the output for the SAM (Tusher et al., 2001) discussed in Section 7.10.

`farms`

Factor Analysis for Robust Microarray Summarization (FARMS) is a model-based technique for summarizing high density oligonucleotide array data at probe level for. The bioconductor package `farms` use the methodology discussed in Talloen et al. (2007) for filtering.

EXERCISES

7.1. Consider the following subset of data related to four genes, G1, G2, G3, and G4. Their expression levels (log transformed and normalized) in four control tissues C1, C2, C3, and C4, and four test tissues, T1, T2, T3, and T4, are shown below.

	C1	C2	C3	C4	T1	T2	T3	T4
G1	9.011	9.064	9.067	9.008	8.944	9.087	8.963	9.074
G2	10.556	10.373	10.657	10.336	10.101	10.073	10.095	11.273
G3	11.967	12.014	11.757	12.101	11.604	11.782	11.503	11.861
G4	10.211	10.282	10.284	10.087	10.104	9.981	10.131	10.473

(a) Are any of these genes significantly differentially expressed in test tissue versus control tissue if the investigator decides to regard twofold or greater fold changes as significant?

(b) Use a two-sample t-test at the 5% level (two-sided) to test whether any of the genes are significantly differentially expressed in test tissue versus control tissue.

(c) Repeat using Welch's test.

(d) Repeat using the Mann–Whitney–Wilcoxon test.

(e) Repeat using the robust t-test.

(f) Repeat using a permutation test with the difference in medians as test statistic.

(g) For each gene, examine the residuals to check whether any observations can be considered outliers. Observe that there are two extreme outliers. Remove them and repeat (a)–(f). Do any conclusions change?

7.2. Golub et al. (1999) (data available online) compared the gene expression profiles of 11 AML patents with that of 27 ALL patients.

(a) What method did the authors of this article use to select 50 genes?

(b) Determine which genes are statistically significantly differentially expressed in AML versus ALL using (i) t-test, (ii) Welch's test, (iii) robust t-test, (iv) SAM test, and (v) Wilcoxon–Mann–Whitney rank sum test, with and without a Bonferroni adjustment for multiplicity. Compare these lists with each other and the list obtained by the authors of the article.

(c) Determine the q-values for each of the unadjusted tests in (b).

7.3. The data set `mice` in the library DNAMR contains eight biological samples representing the expression levels for cell tissue for eight rats. Four of the rats are treated with a drug and the other four are treated with a placebo.

(a) Calculate the mean, variance, and t-test statistics for each gene and construct the following plots for this data: cube root variance versus mean (average across groups), t-test statistics versus mean, and t-test statistics versus cube root variance. Do you observe any volcano effect in your graph? Produce a list of significantly expressed genes.

(b) Use the SAM methodology. Compare the four SAM strategies suggested in Section 7.10.3 and choose an appropriate value for Δ. Produce a list of differentially expressed genes that come out for your choice of Δ and report the pFDR and the expected number of false discoveries.

(c) Using the functions included in the DNAMR library for `R/SPLUS`, determine the significant genes using the CT method. Finally, compare this list with the previous lists from parts (a) and (b) and try to reach a conclusion as to which genes are differentially expressed.

7.4. (a) For the Khan data (mentioned in Section 1.4.3), compare the gene expression profiles of the 23 EWR cells to those of the 20 RMS cells using individual t-tests. Calculate p-values and compare the distribution of these p-values to a uniform distribution (which is the distribution one would expect if none of the genes were differentially expressed) using a histogram and a q-q plot. Comment.

(b) Randomly permute these 43 cells (so that none of the genes should be differentially expressed) and repeat the above. Comment.

(c) In each of the above, calculate q-values.

(d) What effect does the number of differentially expressed genes have on the calculation of q-values?

(e) What effect does a possible lack of uniformity of the distribution of non-differentially-expressed genes have on the calculation of q-values?

7.5. Carry out the following simulation.

(a) Simulate two gene expression matrices X and Y with 10000 rows (genes) and 5 columns (samples), where all the entries are randomly drawn from a N(0,1) distribution. Add the value 1 to the first 100 rows of X.

(b) Compare each row of X to the corresponding row of Y using t-tests. How many of the 100 significantly differentially expressed genes are declared significant?

(c) Repeat (b) using the conditional t approach.

(d) Repeat (b) using limma.

(e) Repeat (a) to (d) 99 more times for a total of 100 simulations. In general, which of t, *Ct* and limma are better able to detect the truly differentially expressing genes? Comment on the usefulness of "borrowing strength across genes".

7.6. The Sialin data contains 4 control samples and 4 Slc17A5 knocked out samples at two time points, day 0 and day 18. Using the CT method implemented in the DNAMR library for R/SPLUS, determine the 100 most significant genes at time 0 and at time 18. Is there any overlap? Are there any genes that are highly significant at both time points?

7.7. In this question we use the Golub Data.

1. Read the paper by Bourgon et al. (2010) "Independent filtering increases detection power for high-throughput experiments."
2. Use Variance and fold change filtering, and use the wilcoxon test statistic to test between the two groups. Use different cut off point for filtering and compare the results between the variance and fold change filtering.
3. Use variance filtering and compare the distribution of the row p-values between the features that were filtered out and filter in.

7.8. In this question we use the Platinum Affymetrix data.

1. Read the letter by Talloen et al (2010): "Filtering data from high-throughput experiments based on measurement reliability".

2. Talloen et al (2010) advocate the use of filtering methods based on probe level data. Use FARMS in order to filter features in the platinum data based on I/NI calls.
3. Use RMA to summarize the platinum data and use variance filtering based on the summarized data. Compare the results (in terms of number of features included in the analysis) between (2) and (3).

7.9. Use the Golub data to compare between SAS and two sample t-test.

1. Use both SAM and t-test to test the null hypothesis of no group effect and compare the results.
2. Plot the modified test statistics of SAM versus the t-test statistics. Where can you see the modification effect of SAM.
3. Plot the row p-values obtained from the two sample t-test to the q values obtained from SAM.
4. Explain what is the influence if the value of Δ on the number of significant tests in SAM.

7.10. Use the behavioral study to investigate the influence of the modification of the test statistics of the SAM method.

1. Calculate the mean difference (the fold change) and plot it versus the standard error (and log(standard error)). Do you see any relationship between the fold change and the standard error?
2. Plot the SAM test statistics with and without modification of the fudge factor versus the standard error of the mean difference and use these plot to explain the main ideas behind the SAM modification.

CHAPTER 8

Model-Based Inference and Experimental Design Considerations

Over the years, a significant number of applied statistics problems have been successfully solved by, applying statistical linear modeling techniques, either directly or indirectly. Therefore, it is not surprising that this workhorse of mainstream applied statistics has been tried and found to be useful for analyzing comparative microarray experiments as well. In addition to being of practical value for analysis, these models also provide a constructive framework upon which to reflect on what experimental designs might be appropriate for a proposed microarray experiment, which is an essential, but often sadly neglected, aspect of any research endeavor.

The literature on this topic has been growing rapidly. Kerr and Churchill (2001a, 2001b) and Kerr et al. (2000, 2002) are "early" references on the application of linear modeling techniques for the analysis of data from multichannel cDNA microarrays. They also advocated the application of sound experimental design principles to microarray experimentation and proposed various innovative designs for multichannel cDNA microarray experiments. Churchill (2002) and Yang and Speed (2002) have done subsequent reviews of this work. Wolfinger et al. (2001) proposed a two-stage approach for fitting linear models, including mixed effect models. Chu et al. (2002) discuss linear models and Smyth (2004) discusses mixed effect models for oligonucleotide array experiments. Lin et al. (2012) discussed in detail methods for modeling dose–response and other order-restricted microarray data.

Here, we review some of the statistical models that have been used for analyzing microarray data. Obviously, the model that one would consider using in a particular circumstance depends totally on the experimental design of the situation, and, because it would be far too space consuming to cover a large range of situations,

Exploration and Analysis of DNA Microarray and Other High-Dimensional Data, Second Edition.
Dhammika Amaratunga, Javier Cabrera, Ziv Shkedy.

we shall focus only on some common ones. Experimental design issues are also addressed.

8.1 THE *F*-TEST

Consider a simple comparative microarray experiment whose objective is to investigate how genes express differentially across a single factor, V. The factor might represent treatments, tissue types, times, or something else. Following Kerr and Churchill (2001a, 2001b), we will use the generic term "varieties" to refer to them. Let Y_{gij} be the suitably transformed and normalized expression-level measurement for the gth gene ($g = 1, \ldots, G$) in the jth microarray ($j = 1, \ldots, J_i$) assigned to variety i, ($i = 1, \ldots, I$). Let $N = \Sigma_{i=1}^{I} J_i$ denote the total sample size.

The simplest approach is to model the data for each gene separately as

$$Y_{gij} = \mu_g + V_{ig} + \varepsilon_{gij},$$

where μ_g represents the average signal for the gth gene, V_{ig} represents the additional signal due to the effect of the ith variety on the gth gene, and ε_{gij} represents an *error* term that subsumes all sources of variability not accounted for by the terms in the model, including random noise. The traditional assumption is that the $\{\varepsilon_{gij}\}$ are independently and identically distributed as a normal distribution with mean 0 and variance σ_g^2, which we shall write as $\varepsilon_{gij} \sim \text{NID}(0, \sigma_g^2)$.

This model is fitted for each gene using ordinary least squares and statistical theory shows that the estimates so obtained have several desirable optimality properties. The primary hypothesis of interest, is whether the gth gene is differentially expressed across the varieties, that is, whether $Vig = 0$ for all i, and can be tested for statistical significance via an F test. This type of approach is called analysis of variance (ANOVA).

The F-test statistic for testing whether the gth gene is differentially expressed across the varieties involves the *mean square among varieties*

$$\text{MS(V)} = \frac{\Sigma_{i=1}^{I}(y_{ij} - \overline{y})^2}{I - 1},$$

and the *mean square error*

$$\text{MS(E)} = \frac{\Sigma_{i=1}^{I}\Sigma_{j=1}^{J_i}(y_{ij} - \overline{y}_i)^2}{N - 1},$$

where $\overline{y}_i = \Sigma_{j=1}^{J_i} y_{ij}/j_i$ is the mean of the ith group and $\overline{y} = \Sigma_{i=1}^{I}\Sigma_{j=1}^{J_i} y_{ij}/N$ is the overall mean (the subscript g has been omitted from all the equations for simplicity). The F-test statistic,

$$F = \frac{\text{MS(V)}}{\text{MS(E)}}$$

is the average squared difference in intensities across the varieties, as measured by MS(V, relative to the variability or "noise" in the observations, as measured by MS(E). Under the null hypothesis of no difference in intensities across the varieties, both MS(V) and MS(E) are estimates of the error variance σ_g^2, so that their ratio, F, is close to unity and is distributed as a F-distribution with $I - 1$ and $N - I$ degrees of freedom. When there are differences among the varieties, MS(V) would generally be substantially larger than MS(E) and F would generally be substantially greater than unity. The larger the value of F, the greater the weight of evidence against the null hypothesis. If the observed value of F is F_{obs} then the p-value is given by the probability $p_F = \text{Prob}(F > F_{\text{obs}})$. A gene is declared significantly differentially expressed at level of significance α if $p_F < \alpha$.

Example. Experiment E8 was conducted to study the gene expression profiles of mice in response to a particular drug. Nine mice were treated with the drug and after 1, 2, and 3 h of treatment, three mice were randomly sacrificed and mRNA from their liver was harvested. In addition, there were three control mice to provide 0-h information. A dozen microarrays (one for each mouse) containing 2004 genes were challenged with the mRNA and intensity data collected. Applying the F-test for each gene separately, 335 were found to be significantly differentially expressed across the four treatments. When a Bonferroni correction was applied, only two genes were found to be significantly differentially expressed across the four time points.

The F-test is an extension of the t-test that can be applied when $I \geq 2$. When $I = 2$, the F-test is equivalent to the usual two-sample t-test based on T_e described in Section 7.3.With very small sample sizes, the F-test statistic, similar to the t-test statistic, tends to be highly correlated with the mean square error term that appears in its denominator, causing it to pick up significant findings at a higher rate from among those genes with low variance than from among those genes with high variance, resulting in a high false positive rate for genes whose variability is low and a high false negative rate for genes whose variability is high.

In the SAM approach of Tusher et al. (2001), the F-test statistic is regularized to adjust for this effect as follows:

$$F = \frac{\text{MS(V)}}{\text{MS(E)} + c},$$

where c is a fudge factor whose value is estimated as for the t-test statistic as described in Section 7.4 to reduce the dependence of $F(c)$ versus c.

8.2 THE BASIC LINEAR MODEL

In a simple comparative microarray experiment whose objective is to investigate how genes express differentially across a single factor, varieties, V, there are three *effects* or *factors*: varieties (V), arrays (A), and genes (G), which could potentially influence the expression-level measurements $\{Y_{gij}\}$, where Y_{gij} is the suitably transformed and normalized expression-level measurement for the gth gene ($g = 1, \ldots, G$) in the jth microarray ($j = 1, \ldots, J_i$) assigned to variety i ($i = 1, \ldots, I$). Therefore, it is reasonable to try to formulate a model that describes the relationship between Y_{gij} and these three effects and their interactions or some subset of them. We can use the platform of this model to estimate the extent of the influence of each effect and to assess how significant it is.

Before we write down a model, it behooves us to think about what effects we ought to include in it and what effects, if any, may be acceptable, or even necessary, to exclude. The obvious candidates for any model are the main effects:

- An array effect, A, would account for overall differences in expression-level measurements among the arrays after the effects of all the other factors in the model have been removed. If the normalization effort was successful, the array effect should be fairly small.
- A gene effect, G, would account for differences among the average expression-level measurements across the multitude of genes. Such an effect transpires owing to many causes such as the facts that some genes have higher natural expression levels than others, some sequences tend to be labeled more efficiently than others because of factors such as sequence length and sequence composition, and some genes tend to hybridize more efficiently than others.
- A variety effect, V, would account for differences in expression-level measurements of some of the varieties are substantially higher or lower overall than others.

Then, there are the various *two-factor interaction effects:*

- A variety–gene interaction effect, VG, would account for how a gene expresses differentially across the varieties. Given a particular gene g, if any one of the $(VG)_{gi}$ terms is larger than the others relative to the underlying variability, it means that that particular variety is inducing a higher level of expression than the other varieties. Clearly, contrasts among the $(VG)_{gi}$, for each g, are the quantities of greatest interest in comparative microarray experiments.
- An array–gene interaction effect, AG, would account for the variability of a spot across the arrays averaged over all the spots. This effect would be observed if the concentration or amount of DNA spotted on the microarrays varied from array to array.
- A variety–array interaction effect, VA, would account for variability across the varieties for arrays. This effect, however, is not estimable as each array contains only a single variety.

The simplest additive linear model that can be fitted to all the genes simultaneously involves the factors V, A, G, and VG :

$$Y_{gij} = \mu + V_i + A_{j(i)} + G_g + (VG)_{gi} + \varepsilon_{gij}.$$

Here, μ represents the average signal across the whole experiment and the errors ε_{gij} are independently and identically distributed as a normal distribution with mean 0 and variance $\sigma_2 : \varepsilon_{gij} \sim \text{NID}(0, \sigma^2)$. The model is fitted using ordinary least squares and hypotheses of interest, such as whether each gene is differentially expressed across the varieties, can be tested for statistical significance via F-tests.

With microarray data, it is possible that none of the assumptions of normality, independence and homoscedasticity holds:

- *Nonnormality.* Empirical evidence seems to indicate that it is reasonable to assume that the error distribution is symmetric and normal-like (i.e., bell shaped) in the middle. The problem is in the tails. For one thing they tend to be quite heavy (see Chapter 7 and, except for very well-behaved experiments, there tend to be a handful of extreme outliers that could damage some estimates severely. In addition, there is a truncation effect at very high gene expression levels as a result of saturation.
- *Lack of Independence.* Genes rarely express in isolation but rather in biological pathways. Therefore, it would be wrong to assume that the expression levels of the genes in the experiment are totally independent of one another. On the other hand, it is impossible to model any aspect of the gene correlation structure in advance and the size of the samples used in typical microarray experiments just does not permit it to be inferred from the data. Therefore, generally, the best one can do is to assume independence and hope that it does not affect the properties of the test too much and there is reason to believe that this might be the case. Follow-up analyses, such as cluster-based methods, can then address the lack of independence should it remain a concern.
- *Heteroscedasticity.* In some microarray experiments, it can be observed that all the genes appear, perhaps after a transformation, to have the same variance, in which case, it is fine to assert that $\varepsilon_{gij} \sim (0, \sigma^2)$. However, in most microarray experiments, it appears to be the case that those genes that exhibit high expression levels also tend to exhibit high variances and vice versa. In such instances, it is more appropriate to write $\varepsilon_{gij} \sim (0, \sigma_g^2)$, which postulates a gene-specific variance. In fact, it may even be appropriate, in some situations, to write $\varepsilon_{gij} \sim (0, \sigma_{gi}^2)$ to cover the eventuality that if gene g is differentially expressed across the different varieties i, that it also has different variances across the varieties. In some instances, it may be better to model the variance to level relationship explicitly by $\sigma_g^2 = f(\mu_g)$ or $\sigma_{gi}^2 = f(\mu_{gi})$, where μ_g denotes the true overall mean expression level of the gth gene and μ_{gi} denotes the true mean expression level of the gth gene in the ith variety.

8.3 FITTING THE MODEL IN TWO STAGES

There is a natural categorization of the effects in a microarray experiment into *gene-specific effects* (effects involving G) and *global effects* (effects not involving G). These two sets of effects are *orthogonal* to one another; that is, they are statistically independent of one another and the effect of one does not mask or interfere the other.

Motivated by this categorization and the computational and statistical disadvantages associated with fitting a linear model in one giant step, Wolfinger et al. (2001) suggested breaking the fitting down into two stages, essentially fitting two submodels, one submodel to the global effects (they call this the *normalization model*) and one submodel to the gene-specific effects (they call this the *gene model*).

The normalization model,

$$Y_{gij} = \mu + V_i + A_{j(i)} + \delta_{gij},$$

is fitted first and serves to adjust the data for the global effects that otherwise could bias the gene-specific inferences. The array effect could be regarded as a random effect. There are no gene-specific effects in the model. The error term $\delta_{gij} \sim (0, \sigma^2)$.

In the second stage, the residuals, R_{gij}, from the normalization model are regarded as gene-expression-level measurements that have been centered and normalized for extraneous effects and used as input to the gene model:

$$R_{gij} = G_g + (VG)_{gi} + \varepsilon_{gij},$$

where the error term $\varepsilon_{gij} \sim (0, \sigma^2)$.

In principle, the two-stage fit and the one-stage fit should produce results that are close, if not identical, to each other, because the effects being fitted in the normalization model are orthogonal to the effects being fitted in the gene model. However, this is not exactly the case as the residuals, R_{gij}, are generally slightly correlated to one another. Nevertheless, this effect should be small, and in practice, there should be little difference between the two sets of results.

There are a few key advantages to the two-stage process:

- It is computationally much less demanding.
- When fitting the gene model, it is possible to accommodate gene-specific heteroscedasticity by letting $\varepsilon_{gij} \sim (0, \sigma^2)$.
- The first fit residuals, R_{gij}, can be used as input to clustering.

8.4 MULTICHANNEL EXPERIMENTS

In multichannel experiments, in addition to the effects mentioned in Section 8.1, there is a global effect due to dye (D). Some dyes tend to produce consistently higher fluorescent signals compared to other dyes. Therefore, when modeling such experiments, a dye main effect that measures the overall effect of dye-to-dye variability on expression-level measurement should be included in the model. Now, let Y_{gijk} denote the suitably transformed and normalized expression-level measurement for the gth gene with the kth dye in the jth microarray representing variety i. Including the dye effect in the model, we can model this situation as

$$Y_{gijk} = \mu + V_i + A_j + D_k + G_g + (VG)_{gi} + \varepsilon_{gij}.$$

To account for spot-to-spot variation, we can add a term AG:

$$Y_{gijk} = \mu + V_i + A_j + D_k + G_g + (VG)_{gi} + (AG)_{gi} + \varepsilon_{gij}.$$

In addition, to account for the possibility that dyes might be interacting with genes, we can add a dye–gene interaction effect DG:

$$Y_{gijk} = \mu + V_i + A_j + D_k + G_g + (VG)_{gi} + (AG)_{gi} + (DG)_{gi} + \varepsilon_{gij}.$$

8.5 EXPERIMENTAL DESIGN CONSIDERATIONS

Most experiments involve studying how a variable of interest is affected by a series of factors. The design of such an experiment refers to the assignment of samples over the levels of the various factors. For microarray experiments, the variable of interest is the expression level of a gene and the experimental design refers to the assignment of samples over the levels of factors such as variety and dye. The number of replicates to use for the various different types of replication is also an experimental design consideration.

8.5.1 Comparing Two Varieties with Two-Channel Microarrays

We will commence our discussion with multichannel microarray experiments, where the scope for improving inference by applying principles of classical experimental design is most apparent.

The following simple example can be used to illustrate some of the key points to keep in mind when designing a microarray experiment. An experimenter is planning to perform a DNA microarray experiment to compare the effects of two varieties A and B and intends to use 2 two-channel cDNA microarrays, A_1 and A_2. We shall call the two channels R and G to represent the two dyes, red and green, that are most often used. There are four obvious designs.

In design D_1, array-specific effects are *confounded* with variety effects in that, if a gene is differentially expressed in A_1 versus A_2, it will be impossible to know whether to attribute it to array or to variety (Table 8.1). Thus, it is better to avoid this design if possible. Of course, with single-channel arrays, this aspect is

Table 8.1 Design D_1

	Array A_1	Array A_2
Channel R	A	B
Channel G	A	B

Table 8.2 Design D_2

	Array A_1	Array A_2
Channel R	A	A
Channel G	B	B

Table 8.3 Design D_3

	Array A_1	Array A_2
Channel R	A	B
Channel G	B	B

unavoidable. Incidentally, in experimental design parlance, arrays are essentially experimental blocks with as there are channels; in two-channel experiments, they are blocks of size two.

In design D_2, dye-specific effects are confounded with variety effects (Table 8.2). As it is known that sizeable dye effects are possible, some care must be taken if using this design.

In design D_3, the dyes assigned to the two varieties in the first array are switched in the second array (Table 8.3). Making this modification makes it possible to separate out both array-specific effects as well as dye-specific effects by fitting the model

$$Y_{gijk} = \mu + V_i + A_j + D_k + G_g + (VG)_{gi} + (AG)_{gi} + (DG)_{gi} + \varepsilon_{gij},$$

or one of the other smaller models mentioned above. In the two-stage modeling approach, the normalization model would be

$$Y_{gij} = \mu + V_i + A_j + D_k + \delta_{gij},$$

with each of the effects having 1 degree of freedom. The gene model would be

$$R_{gij} = G_g + (VG)_{gi} + (AG)_{gj} + (DG)_{gk} + \varepsilon_{gij}.$$

Table 8.4 Design D_3'

	Array A_1	Array A_2	Array A_3	Array A_4
Channel R	A_1	B_1	A_2	B_2
Channel G	B_1	A_1	B_2	A_2

Table 8.5 Design D_4

	Array A_1	Array A_2
Channel R	A	B
Channel G	REF	REF

Table 8.6 Design D_1

	Array A_1	Array A_2	Array A_3
Channel R	REF	REF	REF
Channel G	A	B	C

For obvious reasons, this type of design is called a *dye-swap design* or *dye flip design*. While there is a clear advantage to dye-swap designs, they do require some extra effort on the part of the experimenter because each sample has to be labeled with both dyes.

If there are biological replicates, it is advisable for the dye-swap design to be applied to each pair of biological replicates, giving rise to the *replicated dye-swap design* Here, A_i refers to the ith biological replicate given variety A and B_i refers to the ith biological replicate given variety B.

Design D_4 includes REF, a reference variety (Table 8.5). While it is useful to have such a variety to which hybridization results can be referred, if the primary objective of the experiment is to compare varieties A and B, it is not advisable to use this design. It is more efficient to make a key comparison directly on one array rather than indirectly via an intermediate comparison.

8.5.2 Comparing Multiple Varieties with Two-Channel Microarrays

Now, suppose that an experimenter is planning a microarray experiment to compare the effects of several varieties (for illustration, say three varieties, A, B, and C) and intends to use two-channel microarrays. Suppose that a reference variety, REF, of no intrinsic interest, is also available. Two possible designs are the reference sample design and the loop design. The *reference sample design* is given in Table 8.6. In this design, dye effects are confounded with test variety versus reference variety effects but, because these are not of intrinsic interest, this is not a problem.

Table 8.7 Design D_2

	Array A_1	Array A_2	Array A_3
Channel R	A	B	C
Channel G	B	c	A

Table 8.8 Design D_3

	Array A_1	Array A_2	Array A_3	Array A_4	Array A_5	Array A_6
Channel R	A	B	C	B	C	A
Channel G	B	C	A	A	B	C

Table 8.9 Design D_4

	Array A_1	Array A_2	Array A_3	Array A_4
Channel R	REF	A	B	C
Channel G	A	B	C	REF

The *loop design* was proposed by Kerr and Churchill (2001) as a natural extension of the dye-swap design (Table 8.7).

A dye swap could be included in the loop design to yield a *saturated design* (Table 8.8).

The reference variety could be included in the loop design if necessary:

The loop design has two clear advantages over the reference sample design. One is that the dye effect is estimable in the loop design. The second is that there is essentially double the amount of information in the loop design for the varieties of interest compared to the reference sample design. Loop designs are useful for temporal studies. In this case, A, B, and C would be three successive time points.

However, despite their nice properties, there are some drawbacks to loop designs as well. One is that, similar to dye-swap designs, they require some extra effort on the part of the experimenter because each sample has to be labeled with both dyes. However, doing so is also likely to introduce additional variability. Another risk, particularly with large experiments is this. Microarray technology is still fallible and it is not uncommon to have a problem with an array. If this happens with a loop design and the defective array cannot be salvaged, there may be quite some difficulty in drawing proper conclusions from the study unless there was adequate replication.

Now consider the situation in which one of the varieties, say A, is a control, and the goal of the experiment is to compare the other two varieties, B

Table 8.10 Design D_5

	Array A_1	Array A_2
Channel R	A(control)	B (control)
Channel G	B	C

and C, to A. As a general rule, if a pairwise comparison is considered important, it is always advisable to have an array that represents that comparison in the design. Thus, a sensible design for this situation is the *comparison to control design* (Table 8.10).

The general guidelines outlined above are applicable to complex settings as well. An example is Churchill and Oliver (2001), who apply them to propose an alternative design for a complex microarray experiment described by Jin et al. (2001) and involving three factors: strain, sex, and age. Finally, to establish a library of gene expression data or to compare many samples to one another, one could use two-channel arrays with a common reference sample or, provided the experiment is well under control, single-channel arrays.

8.5.3 Single-Channel Microarray Experiments

The experimental designs used in single-channel microarray experiments should also require careful consideration. For example, consider an experiment in which four treatments, A, B, C, and D, are being compared. Each treatment is to be given to four animals. If the sample from each animal corresponded to one array, there would be 16 arrays in all, which we can refer to as $A_1, A_2, A_3, A_4, B_1, B_2, B_3, B_4, C_1, C_2, C_3, C_4, D_1, D_2, D_3, D_4$. Suppose that the facility is a small one, so that at the most four arrays can be performed in any one day. This means that the experiment has to be run over a period of 4 days. Assume that the experiment was run as given in Table 8.11.

In this case, if there was a day effect (and such an effect has been observed in practice), then the treatment effect is totally confounded with day effect. Instead it is much better to run as given in Table 8.12.

In this design, day effects can be estimated and these estimates can be used to adjust the treatment–gene effects.

Table 8.11 A Four-Treatment Design

Day	Arrays
Day 1	A_1, A_2, A_3, A_4
Day 2	B_1, B_2, B_3, B_4
Day 3	C_1, C_2, C_3, C_4
Day 4	D_1, D_2, D_3, D_4

Table 8.12 A Four-Treatment Design

Day	Arrays
Day 1	A_1, B_1, C_1, D_1
Day 2	A_2, B_2, C_2, D_2
Day 3	A_3, B_3, C_3, D_3
Day 4	A_4, B_4, C_4, D_4

8.6 MISCELLANEOUS ISSUES

In general, it is advisable to adhere, as much as possible, to the fundamental precepts of the theory of design of experiments (*DOE*): randomization, replication, and balance.

- *Randomization.* Arrays should be assigned to varieties at random.
- *Replication.* It was described in Section 6.1. While the examples in this section have been shown with the minimum number of arrays possible for illustrative purposes, it is always advisable to replicate as much as possible.
- *Balance.* Ultimately, the power of experimental design lies in being able to study many factors with few arrays, and doing so in such a way so as to maximize the information content. One of the keys to this is proper statistical balance. An effect is balanced with respect to another if the first effect occurs equally often with the second effect. Balance confers orthogonality on the two effects and prevents an effect of interest being influenced by another effect. For example, by balancing varieties with dyes (i.e., by ensuring that each variety is labeled with each dye an equal number of times), the variety–gene interactions of interest are not biased by dye–gene interactions. This is particularly crucial when genes are not replicated on arrays, as in this case, the dye–gene effect interaction would not be estimable and it would not be possible to adjust the variety–gene interaction for it.

The more carefully planned an experiment is, the better the use that can be made of available resources.

8.7 MODEL-BASED ANALYSIS OF AFFYMETRIX ARRAYS

8.7.1 One-Way ANOVA

In this section, we discussed several model-based approaches for the analysis of Affymetrix microarray data such as one-way ANOVA, SAM for one-way ANOVA, limma, conditional F, joint modeling of gene expression and clinical outcome, and order-restricted analysis including dose–response data and analysis of time course data.

***F*-Test**

In this section, we apply the ANOVA model, discussed in Section 8.1 to Golub data. We consider the following gene-specific linear model,

$$Y_{gij} = \mu_g + V_{gi} + \varepsilon_{gij},\ g = 1, \ldots , 3051,\ j = 1, \ldots , 38, i = 1, 2,$$

where μ_g represents the overall average signal for the gth gene, V_{ig} represents the effect of the additional signal due to tumor class (ALL or AML). Note that because there are only two tumor classes, the V_{ig} is set to be equal to zero for the ALL group, and it represents the additional signal in the AML class. Similar to Section 8.1, we assume that $\varepsilon_{gij} \sim \text{NID}(0, \sigma_g^2)$.

As we mentioned in Section 8.1, we can use the F-test to test the null hypothesis of not tumor class effect,

$$H_0 : V_{g,\text{AML}} = 0, \text{ versus } H_0 : V_{g,\text{AML}} \neq 0.$$

A gene is declared differentially expressed whenever the null hypothesis is rejected. After adjustment for multiple testing using the BH-FDR procedure, 681 genes were found be differentially expressed. Figure 8.1a shows the distribution of the F-test statistic, while Figure 8.1b shows the fold change versus the F-teat statistic. As expected, the F-statistics increases for genes with high/low fold

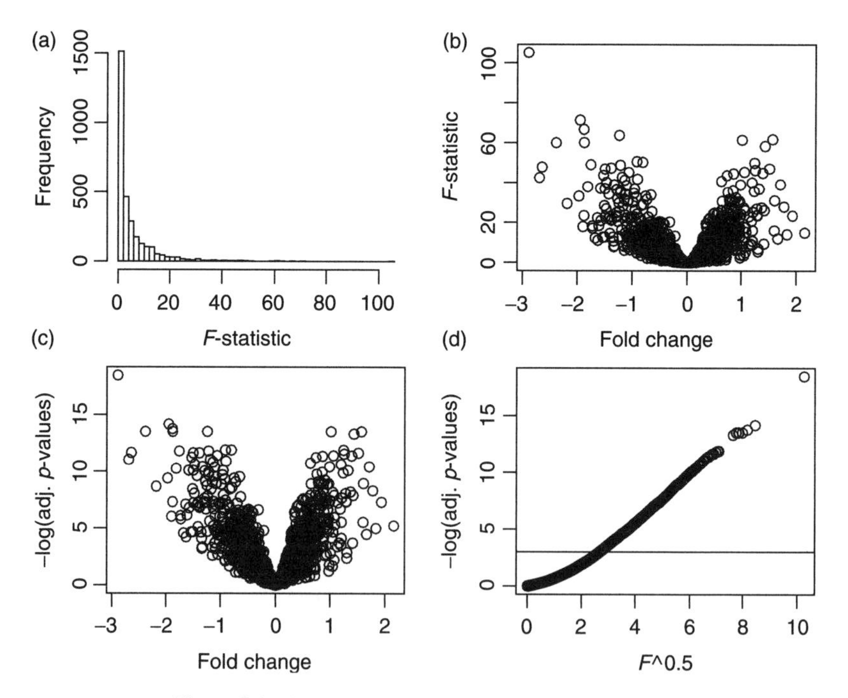

Figure 8.1 One-way ANOVA model for the Golub data.

changes. Figure 8.1d shows the F-statistic versus $-\log$ (adjusted p-values). Note that all genes with test statistics below the vertical line of $-\log(0.05)$ are significant.

Significance Analysis of Microarrays (SAM)

As we mentioned in Section 8.1, the SAM approach can be implemented for the above linear model by using the modified F-test statistic,

$$F = \frac{\mathrm{MS(V)}}{\mathrm{MS(E)} + c}.$$

For the Golub data, $c = 0.6064$. The impact of the fudge factor on the test statistics can be clearly seen in Figure 8.2A, which shows the observed test statistics with and without fudge factor. Note that the observed test statistics without the modification of the fudge factor is identical to the F-test statistic in the previous section and it is higher than the observed test statistic with fudge factor. Figure 8.2B (panel a) shows that a choice of $\Delta = 1.0139$ results in 90% FDR of approximately 5% and to 710 rejected null hypotheses. Panel c shows the observed versus the expected test statistics. All genes for which the observed test statistic is above the upper dashed line are declared differentially expressed.

Conditional F

The conditional t method that was discussed in Section 7.11 can be directly generalized from the case of two groups to the case of multiple groups, resulting in *conditional* F (Cabrera, 2010). The approach is essentially identical, with the critical values for the F-statistics being determined by generating a null distribution for F by resampling and then studying this null distribution as a function of the cubic root of the MS(E). Conditioanl F is implemented in the R package DNAMR.

8.7.2 Linear Models for Microarray Data (Limma)

In Section 7.12.2, we discussed a Bayesian approach for the analysis of gene expression data. Limma, linear models for microarray data (Smyth, 2004) uses a similar approach to fit a hybrid frequentist empirical Bayes (eBayes) linear model (Smyth, 2004; Efron et al., 2001) for the expression levels of the genes in the array. We illustrate the main concepts of Limma using the Golub data. For an experiment with two conditions, the linear model presented in Section 8.7.1 can be reparameterized as

$$Y_{gij} = \alpha_{gi} + \varepsilon_{gij},\ g = 1, \ldots, 3051,\ j = 1, \ldots, 38, i = 1, 2.$$

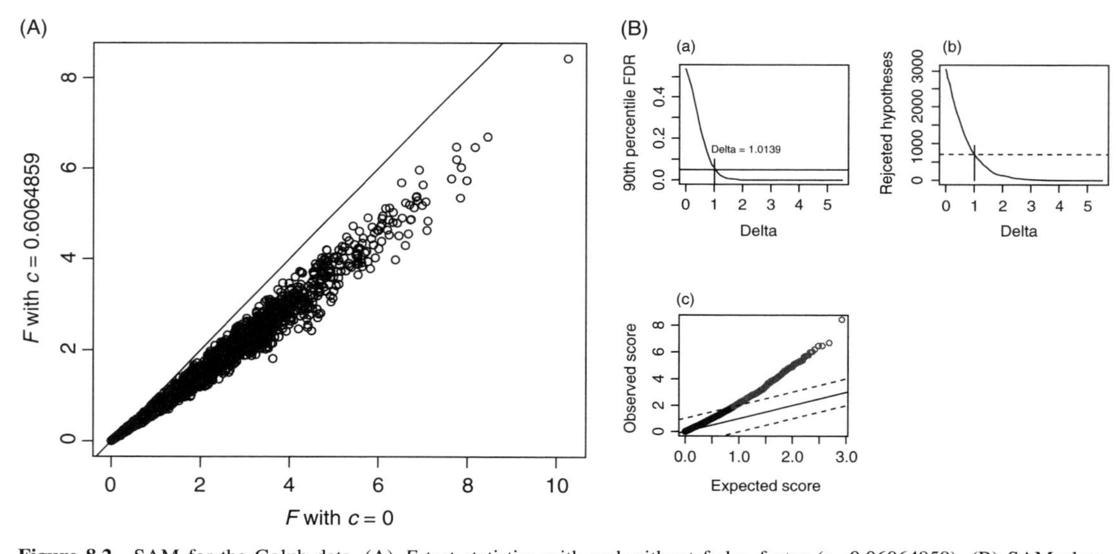

Figure 8.2 SAM for the Golub data. (A) F-test statistics with and without fudge factor (c=0.06064859). (B) SAM plots. (a) Δ versus 90% FDR. (b) Δ versus the number of rejected null hypotheses. (c) observed versus the expected test statistics. Note that for this example $\Delta = 1.0139$.

Here, α_{gi} is the mean gene expression under the ith condition and therefore the primary interest is to estimate the log(fold change), $\alpha_{g1} - \alpha_{g2}$ and to test the null hypothesis $H_0 : \alpha_{g1} = \alpha_{g2}$. In matrix notation, the above model can be written as

$$\mathbf{Y} = X\alpha + \varepsilon.$$

Here, X is a known design matrix and $\alpha = (\alpha_1, \alpha_2)$ is the parameter vector to be estimated. For the Golub data, the design matrix X is a 37×2 matrix in which the ijth entry is given by

$$X_{ij} = \begin{cases} 1 & \text{sample } j \text{ belong to tumor class } i, \quad i = \text{ALL,AML}, \\ 0 & \text{otherwise} \end{cases}$$

and α_1 and α_2 is the mean gene expression in the ALL and AML groups, respectively. It follows that $E(Y_g) = X\alpha$ and $\text{var}(Y_g) = W_g\sigma^2$. As mentioned above, the primary interest is to estimate and test the log(fold change), which can be defined as a contrast of the parameter vector, $\beta_g = C^T\alpha$. For the Golub data, $C^T = (-1, 1)$ and it follows that

$$\beta_g = (-1, 1)(\alpha_1, \alpha_2)^T = \alpha_2 - \alpha_1.$$

Let $\text{var}(\hat{\alpha}) = V_g\sigma_g^2$ be the covariance matrix for $\hat{\alpha}$ then, the covariance matrix for the contrast $\text{var}(\hat{\beta}) = C^T V_g C\sigma_g^2$ with $v_{ij}\sigma_g^2$ the diagonal element of $C^T V_g C\sigma_g^2$. For the classical frequentist approach, the distribution of the maximum likelihood estimates for β_g and σ_g^2 are given, respectively, by

$$\hat{\beta}_g \sim N(\beta_g, v_{ij}\sigma_g^2) \quad \text{and} \quad s_g^2 \sim \frac{\sigma_g^2}{d_g}\chi^2_{dg}.$$

The t-test statistic in this case is

$$t_g = \frac{\hat{\beta}_g}{s_g\sqrt{v_g}}.$$

The Limma method defines a prior distribution for the gene-specific variance $\sigma_1^2, \ldots, \sigma_G^2$ and assumes a scaled inverse χ^2 as marginal prior density,

$$\sigma_g^{-2} \sim \frac{1}{d_0 s_0^2}\chi^2_{d_0}.$$

The hyperparameters of this prior distribution, s_0^2 is the prior variance and d_0 is the prior degrees of freedom, are estimating using empirical Bayes methods to the sample variances $s_1^2 \cdots s_G^2$. The Limma method produces *moderated* test statistics, $\tilde{t}_g$, computed by dividing the standard frequentist numerator with a denominator in which the sample variance s_g^2 is replaced, similar to the concept we discussed in Section 7.12.2, with the posterior mean of $\sigma_g^2|s_g^2$ given by

$$\tilde{s}_g^2 = \frac{d_0 s_0^2 + d_g s_g^2}{d_0 + d_g}.$$

The moderated test statistic (Smyth, 2003) is given by

$$\tilde{t} = \frac{\hat{\beta}_g}{\tilde{s}_g^2 \sqrt{v_g}}.$$

Note that under the null hypothesis, $\tilde{s}_g^2 \sim t_{(d_0+d)}$.

Example. We reanalyzed the Golub data using the limma approach. Figure 8.3A shows the effect of the adjustment of the standard error on the moderated test statistic. Note how the moderated test statistics create a critical envelope compared to the two-sample t-test statistics. This is similar to the critical envelope generated by the conditional t approach of Section 7.11 and, in cases where the limma distributional assumptions hold, the two methods appear to produce very similar critical envelopes (Wijesinha and Amaratunga, 2011). The raw and adjusted p-values are shown in Figure 8.3B. After multiplicity adjustment using the BH-FDR method, 691 genes are found to be significant, similar to 710 genes for the two-sample t-test (see also panel c in Fig. 8.3b).

Smyth (2003) shows that

$$\tilde{t}_g = \left(\frac{d_0 + d_g}{d_g}\right)^{\frac{1}{2}} \frac{\hat{\beta}_g}{\sqrt{s_{*,g}^2 v_g}},$$

with $s_{*,g}^2 = s_g^2 + (d_0/d_g)s_0^2$. This implies that if all d_g are equal, the moderate statistics is proportional to a t-statistic in which the sample variance s_g^2 is adjusted by s_0^2. Recall that the SAM t-test statistic is given by

$$t_g^{\mathrm{SAM}} = \frac{\hat{\beta}_g}{(s_g + c)\sqrt{v_g}}.$$

As pointed out by Symth (2003), the adjustment in t_g^{SAM} is done on the level of the standard deviation, while in $\tilde{t}_g$ on the level of the sample variance. Figure 8.4 shows the test statistics obtained from a two-sample t-test, SAM and limma for the Golub data and shows that, in this case study, the two moderated test statistics are highly correlated.

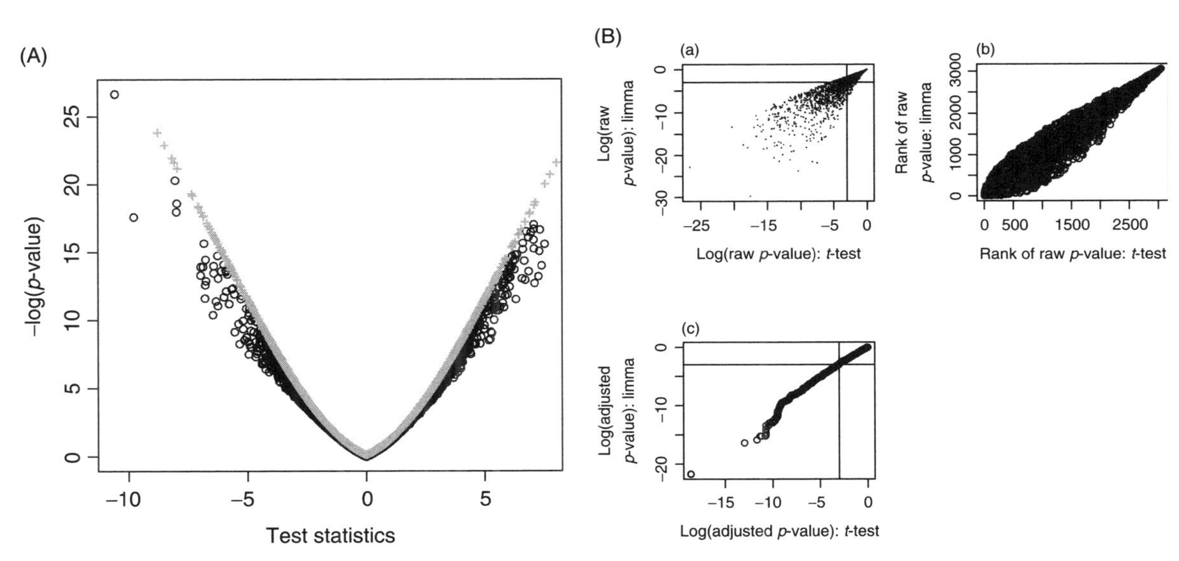

Figure 8.3 Golub data. Comparison between limma and t-test. (A) t-test statistics (circles) and moderate test statistics (pluses in gray) versus $-\log(p\text{-value})$. (B) (a) raw p-values comparison in log scale , (b) raw p-values in comparison in the regular scale (c) adjusted p-values comparison in the log scale.

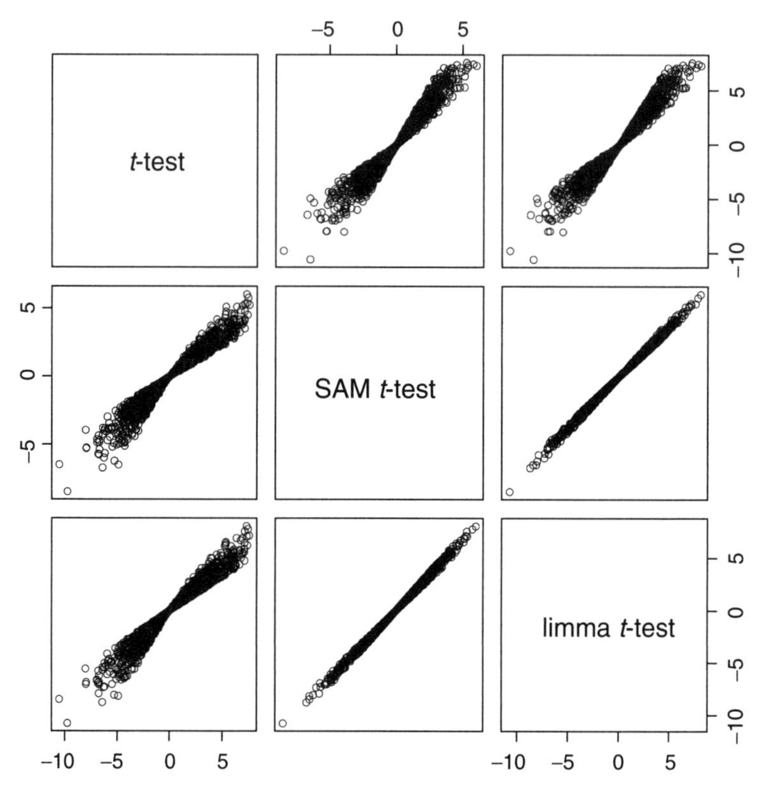

Figure 8.4 Golub data. Scatterplot matrix for the test statistics obtained by the two-sample t-test, SAM, and limma.

8.7.3 A Joint Model for Gene Expression and Response

So far in this book, we have discussed the gene-specific models for gene expression data. In this section, we focus on a microarray setting in which data are available from a single experiment. For each subject (sample), gene expression data (X) is available and, in addition, a response variable (Y) is available as well. In what follows, we focus on continuous responses.

Example. The data we analyzed were obtained from the behavioral experiment in which 24 rats were randomized to one of two treatment groups: placebo and new active compound (12 rats in each group). After the administration of the drug, the rats had to complete a behavioral test, the response of primary interest being the distance traveled by the rat during the experiment. The active drug is expected to increase this distance. After completing the test, a sample was taken from each rat and a microarray with 5644 genes was obtained. Figure 8.5a shows the boxplot for the total distance by treatment group and reveals the difference between the response level in the two treatment groups. Figure 8.5b and c shows scatterplots of the distance traveled versus expression levels of gene 2841 and 3451, respectively.

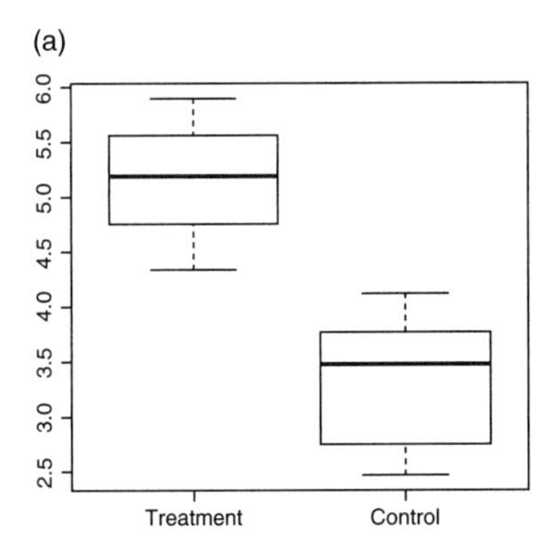

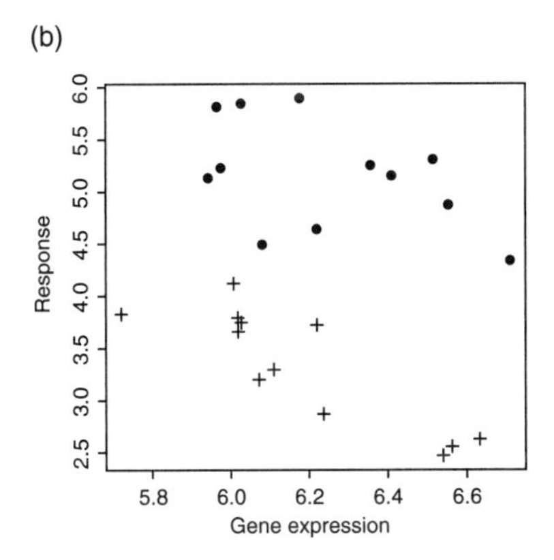

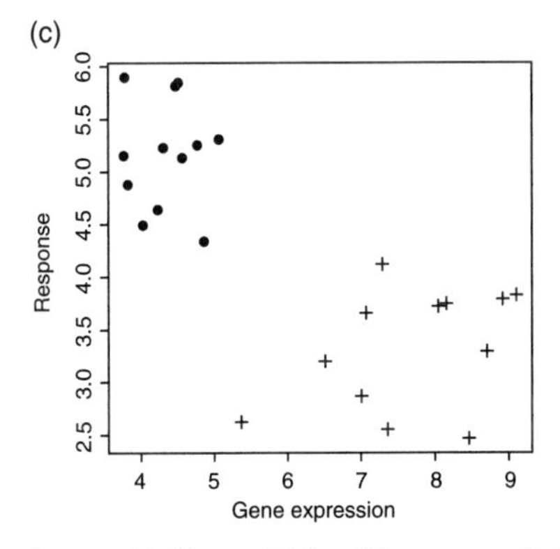

Figure 8.5 Behavioral experiment with 24 rats. (a) Log(distance traveled by the rat). (b) Gene 2841. (c) Gene 345.

Note that panel b reveals a pattern in which the gene is not differentially expressed, while the association between the gene expression and the response seems to be a linear relationship while panel c reveals a pattern in which the gene is differentially expressed but, conditional on the treatment group, the association between the gene expression and the response does not have a linear form. There are two questions of primary interest: (i) which genes are differentially expressed, that is, the treatment has a significant impact on the gene expression and (ii) which genes are correlated with the response. Both these questions addressed in the following section.

Model Formulation

Let X_{ig} be the gth gene expression $g = 1, \ldots, G$, of the ith subject, $i = 1, \ldots, n$, and denote the measurement for the response of primary interest by Y_i. Let Z_i be an indicator variable that takes value 1 if the ith subject was randomized into the active drug group and 0 otherwise. Finally, we denote by $\hat{\alpha}_g$ and $\hat{\beta}$ the ML estimates of the treatment effects for the gth gene expression and the response, respectively. We define a gene-specific joint model in which the linear predictors of the response and the gene expression are given by

$$\begin{aligned} E(X_{ig}|Z_i) &= \mu_g + \alpha_g Z_i, \quad j = 1, \ldots, G\,; \; i = 1, \ldots, n, \\ E(Y_i|Z_i) &= \mu_Y + \beta Z_i. \end{aligned}$$

Note that the above model is a gene-specific model and in practice is fitted for each gene separately. The parameters α_g are gene-specific treatment effects and μ_{X_g} are gene-specific fixed intercepts. It is further assumed that the two variables are normally distributed:

$$\begin{pmatrix} X_{ig} \\ Y_i \end{pmatrix} \sim \mathrm{N}\left(\begin{pmatrix} \mu_{X_g} + \alpha_g Z_i \\ \mu_Y + \beta Z_i \end{pmatrix}, \Sigma_g \right),$$

where Σ_g is given by

$$\Sigma_g = \begin{pmatrix} \sigma_{gg} & \sigma_{gY} \\ \sigma_{gY} & \sigma_{YY} \end{pmatrix}.$$

The adjusted association is a coefficient derived from the covariance matrix of the gene-specific joint model

$$\rho_g = \frac{\sigma_{gY}}{\sqrt{\sigma_{gg}\sigma_{YY}}}.$$

Indeed, $\rho_g = 1$ indicates perfect correlation in the sense that, given the gene expression level, a perfect prediction of the response is possible. Note that ρ_g can be equal to 1 even if the gene is not differently expressed.

Inference

In the first step, we test which genes are differentially expressed. Hence, for each gene, we wish to test the hypotheses

$$H_{0_g} : \alpha_g = 0,$$
$$H_{1_g} : \alpha_g \neq 0.$$

For a microarray with G genes, there are G null hypotheses to be tested, which implies that an adjustment for multiple testing should be applied. Throughout this section, we applied the FDR approach proposed by Hochberg and Benjamini (1995). Testing whether the treatment has a significant effect on the response consists of testing $H_0 : \beta = 0$, versus $H_1 : \beta \neq 0$. A second hypothesis of interest is related to the correlation between the gene expression and the response. Thus, in addition to the hypotheses mentioned above, one needs to test the hypotheses

$$H_{0_g} : \rho_g = 0,$$
$$H_{1_g} : \rho_g \neq 0.$$

Example. For the analysis of the behavioral study, using the BH-FDR method for multiplicity adjustment (with error rate of 5%), none of the null hypotheses for the correlation was rejected and 20 genes were declared differentially expressed for treatment effect. Figure 8.6 shows examples of two genes for which the treatment effect is found to be statistically significant. We notice that, for these genes the association between gene expression and the distance traveled by the rat is derived by the treatment and after adjusting for treatment effects (right panels) the residuals are not correlated. Figure 8.7 shows examples of two genes that are not differentially expressed. These genes reveal a pattern in which the association between the gene expression and the response seems to be linear (although, as we mentioned before, not significant) while the treatment does not have a significant effect on the gene expression.

8.7.4 Analysis of Dose–Response Microarray Experiments

The experimental design we consider in this section is a dose–response experiment in which gene expression data are available at a $K + 1$ increasing dose levels $d_0, \ldots, d_K$. The first dose level d_0 is a control group. The aim of the analysis is to detect genes with monotone (increasing or decreasing) relationship with dose.

Testing for Homogeneity of the Means Under Order-Restricted Alternatives

Let us consider the following one-way ANOVA model,

$$Y_{ij} = \mu(d_i) + \varepsilon_{ij}, \; i = 0, 1, \ldots, K, \; j = 1, 2, \ldots, n_i,$$

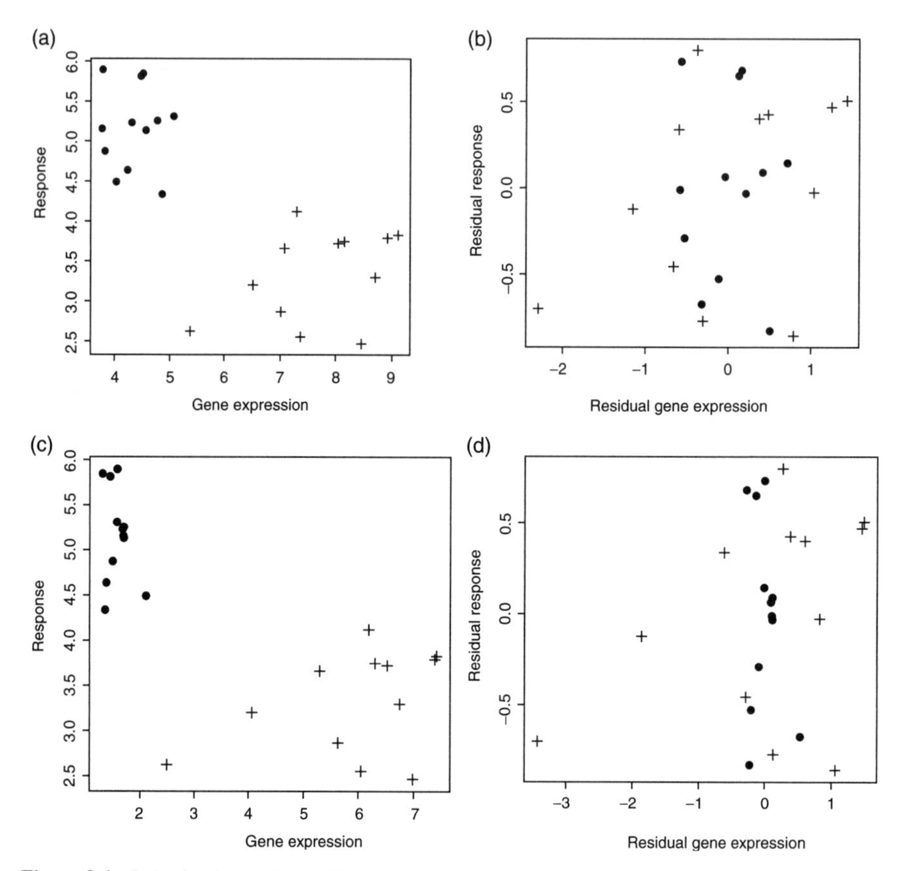

Figure 8.6 Behavioral experiment. Example of two genes: (a, b) gene 345 and (c, d) gene 1962. Left panels: gene expression versus the distance travel by the rat. Right Panels: residuals after adjustment for treatment effects.

where Y_{ij} is the jth response at the ith dose level, d_i are the $K+1$ dose levels, d_0 is the zero dose level (i.e., the control group), $\mu(d_i)$ is the mean gene expression at ith dose level, and $\varepsilon_{ij} \sim N(0, \sigma^2)$ independent of one another. The null hypothesis of no dose effect is given by

$$H_0 : \mu(d_0) = \mu(d_1) = \cdots = \mu(d_K).$$

A one-sided alternative hypothesis of a positive dose effect for at least one dose level (i.e., an increasing trend) is specified by

$$H_1^{Up} : \mu(d_0) \leq \mu(d_1) \leq \cdots \leq \mu(d_K),$$

with at least one strict inequality. When testing the effect of a drug for a positive outcome, the researcher may be able to specify a positive effect as the desirable

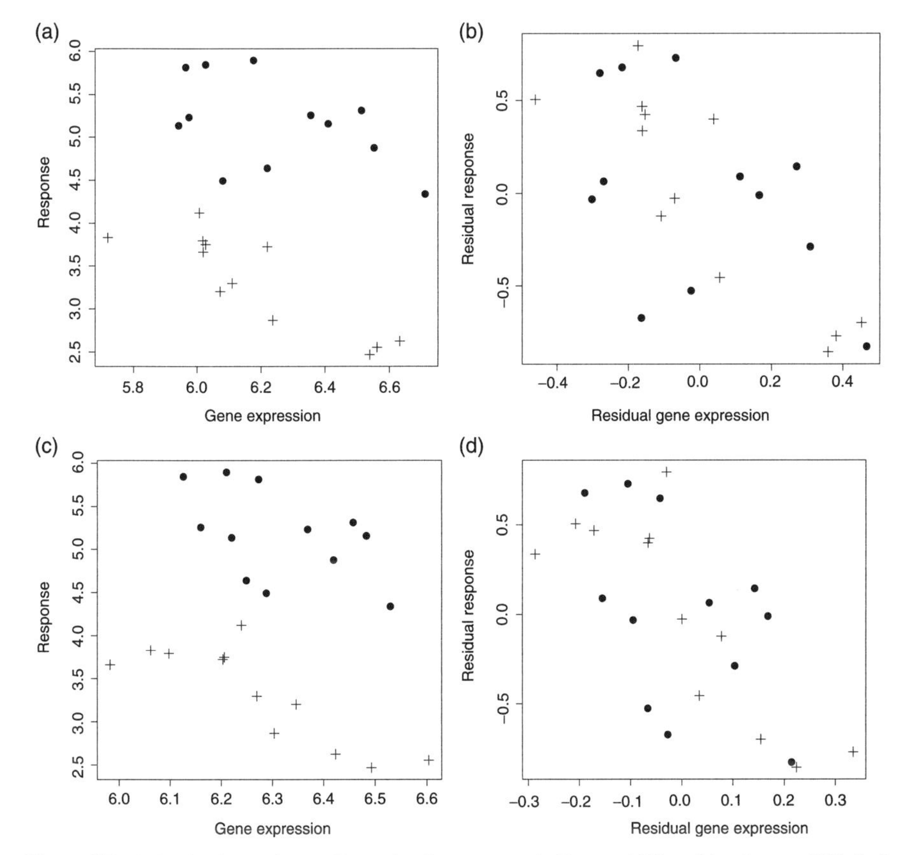

Figure 8.7 Behavioral experiment. Example of two genes: (a, b) gene 2841 and (c, d) gene 4955. Left panels: gene expression versus the distance travel by the rat. Right Panels: residuals after adjustment for treatment effects.

alternative. However, without prior knowledge, it seems reasonable to assume that the expression levels may increase or decrease in response to increasing dose, but with the direction of the trend not known in advance. Thus, we must also consider an additional alternative:

$$H_1^{\text{Down}} : \mu(d_0) \geq \mu(d_1) \geq \cdots \geq \mu(d_K),$$

with at least one strict inequality.

Testing H_0 against H_1^{Down} or H_1^{Up} requires estimation of the means under both the null and the alternative hypotheses. Under the null hypothesis, the estimator for the mean response $\hat{\mu}$ is the sample mean across all the data in all the dose groups. Under the alternative, the maximum likelihood estimate for the means (at each dose level) is the isotonic (antitonic) regression $\hat{\mu}_0^*, \hat{\mu}_1^*, \ldots, \hat{\mu}_K^*$ (Robertson et al., 1988; Lin et al., 2012).

***t*-Type Test Statistics: Williams' (1971, 1972)**

Williams' procedure defines H_0 as the null hypothesis and either H_1^{Up} or H_1^{Down} as the one-sided alternative. Williams' (1971, 1972) test statistic was suggested for a setting in which n observations are available at each dose level. Each dose level is compared with the control level using the test statistic:

$$t_i = \frac{\hat{\mu}_i^* - \overline{y}_0}{\sqrt{2s^2/n}}.$$

Here, $\overline{y}_0$ is the observed mean gene expression at the zero dose level (control), $\hat{\mu}_i^*$ is the estimate of the mean gene expression at the ith dose level under the ordered alternative, and s^2 is an estimate of the variance. For the $\hat{\mu}_i^*$, Williams (1971, 1972) used the isotonic regression estimates of the observed means with respect to dose. In case the number of observations at dose i $n_i \neq n$, the denominator of Williams' test statistic can be adjusted as a two-sample t-test. Marcus (1976) proposed a modification for the test statistics in which $\overline{y}_0$ is replaced with the isotonic mean of the first dose level $\hat{\mu}_0^*$.

Likelihood Ratio Test Statistic for Monotonicity

Testing the equality of ordered means using a likelihood ratio test, for the case that the response is assumed to be normally distributed, was discussed by Barlow et al. (1972) and Robertson et al. (1988) in a general setting and by Lin et al. (2012) for the setting of dose–response microarray experiments. The likelihood ratio test works out to be the ratio of the error variances under the null and the alternative hypotheses:

$$\Lambda_{01}^{\frac{2}{N}} = \frac{\hat{\sigma}_{H_1}^2}{\hat{\sigma}_{H_0}^2} = \frac{\sum_{ij}(y_{ij} - \hat{\mu}_i^*)^2}{\sum_{ij}(y_{ij} - \hat{\mu})^2},$$

where $\hat{\sigma}_{H_0}^2$ and $\hat{\sigma}_{H_1}^2$ are the ML estimates for the error variance under the null and the alternative hypothesis, respectively. The null hypothesis is rejected for a small value of $\Lambda_{01}^{\frac{2}{N}}$. Equivalently, H_0 is rejected for large value of $\overline{E}_{01}^2$, where

$$\overline{E}_{01}^2 = 1 - \Lambda_{01}^{\frac{2}{N}} = \frac{\sum_{ij}(y_{ij} - \hat{\mu})^2 - \sum_{ij}(y_{ij} - \hat{\mu}_i^*)^2}{\sum_{ij}(y_{ij} - \hat{\mu})^2}.$$

Estimating the parameters $\mu(d_i)$ using isotonic regression requires knowledge of the direction of the trend. In practice, the direction of the trend may not be known in advance. In such a case, one can maximize the likelihood twice, for a monotone decreasing trend and for a monotone increasing trend, and choose the trend with the higher likelihood. In practice, we can calculate $\overline{E}_{01}^2$ for each direction and choose the higher value of $\overline{E}_{01}^2$ (Barlow et al., 1972).

Example. We use the human epidermal squamous carcinoma cell line A431 experiment, discussed in Chapter 1, for illustration. The experiment consists of four

Table 8.13 Number of Rejected Null Hypotheses for Various Testing Procedures at the Significance Level of 0.05

Method	$\overline{E}^2_{01}$	Willams	Marcus
Unadjusted	5457	5238	5465
Bonferroni	1814	1592	1669
Holm	1814	1592	1669
FDR-BH	3613	3209	3533
FDR-BY	1814	1592	1669

dose levels with three arrays per dose. Table 8.13 shows the number of rejected null hypotheses for the three test statistics mentioned above using different adjustment methods. As expected the combination of the LRT and BH-FDR methods leads to the highest number of rejected null hypotheses (3613), while the results obtained from the other adjustment methods seems to be more conservative and lead to a lower number of rejections. Figure 8.9 shows (solid line) three examples of genes for which a monotone trend was detected. For an elaborate discussion about dose–response microarray analysis and the application of the SAM method within this setting, we refer to Lin et al. (2012).

8.7.5 Analysis of Time Course Data

Dose–response modeling of microarray experiments is a special case of the analysis of gene expression studies for with the experimental designs are ordered (such as dose, time, age, and temperature). In this section we discuss the setting of time course microarray experiment. An elaborate overview for this setting can be found in Peddada, Umbach, and Harris (2012).

Testing H_0 Versus a Simple Order Alternative

Similar to the previous section, we consider a gene-specific one-way ANOVA model and assume heteroscedastic variances,

$$Y_{ij} \sim \mathrm{N}(\mu(t_i), \sigma_i^2),\ i = 0, 1, \ldots, T,\ j = 1, 2, \ldots, n_i.$$

Our primary interest is to test the null hypothesis of no time effect

$$H_0 : \mu(t_0) = \mu(t_2) = \cdots = \mu(t_T)$$

against the simple order alternatives

$$H_1^{Up} : \mu(t_0) \leq \mu(t_t) \leq \cdots \leq \mu(t_T)$$

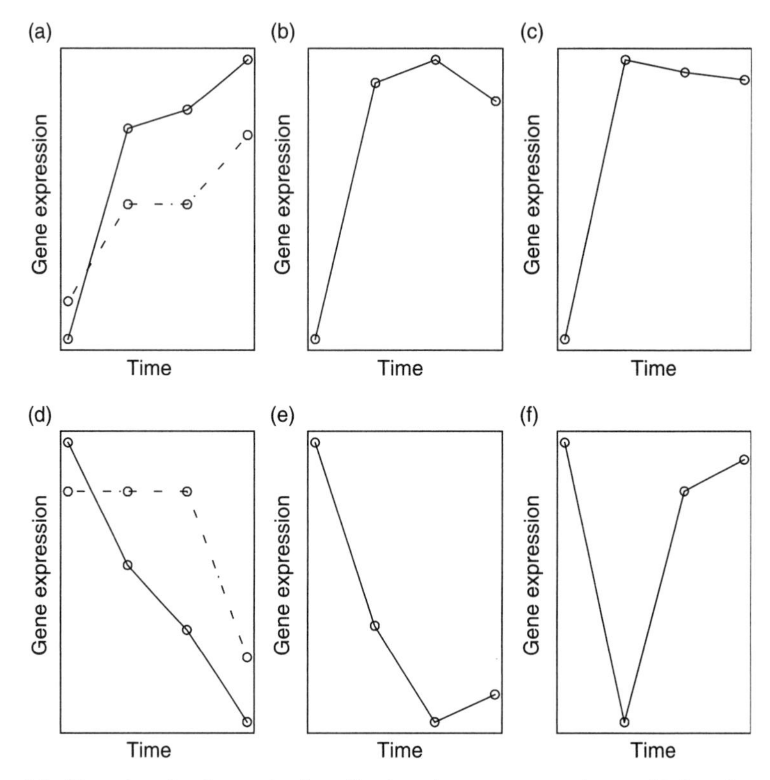

Figure 8.8 Examples of order-restricted profiles in a time course experiment with four time points. (a) Increasing profiles. (b) An umbrella profile with downturn at the third time point. (c) An umbrella profile with downturn at the second time point. (d) Decreasing profiles. (e) An inverted umbrella profile with upturn at the third time point. (f) An inverted umbrella profile with upturn at the second time point.

or

$$H_1^{\text{Down}} : \mu(t_0) \geq \mu(t_1) \geq \cdots \geq \mu(t_T)$$

with at least one strict inequality. To test the null hypothesis against simple order alternatives the ORIOGEN 3.0 package performs a resampling-based SAM analysis using a SAM t-type test statistics given, respectively, for increasing and decreasing profiles by

$$l_{\text{Up}}^{\infty} = \frac{\hat{\mu}_T^* - \hat{\mu}_0^*}{(s_0 + s)\sqrt{\dfrac{1}{n_T} + \dfrac{1}{n_0}}} \quad \text{and} \quad l_{\text{Down}}^{\infty} = \frac{\hat{\mu}_0^* - \hat{\mu}_T^*}{(s_0 + s)\sqrt{\dfrac{1}{n_0} + \dfrac{1}{n_T}}}.$$

Note that for a given value of the fudge factor s_0 this specific analysis is similar to the SAM analysis discussed in the previous section. The main difference is that

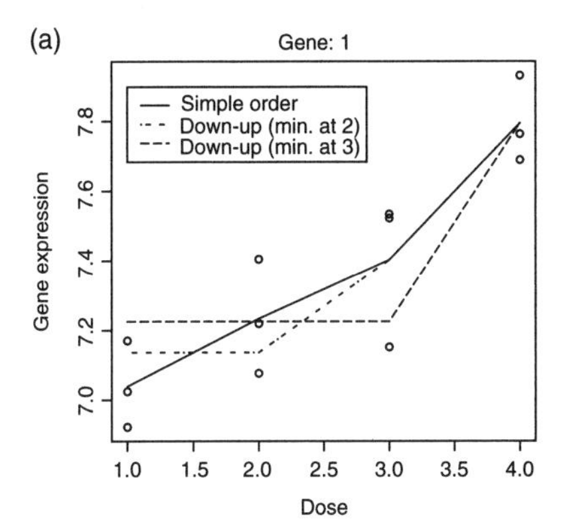

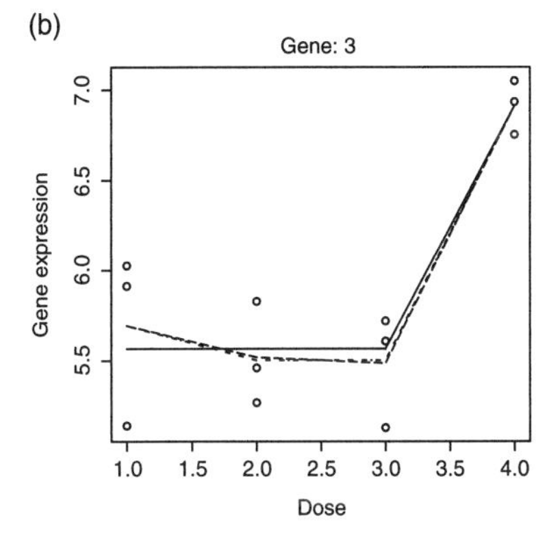

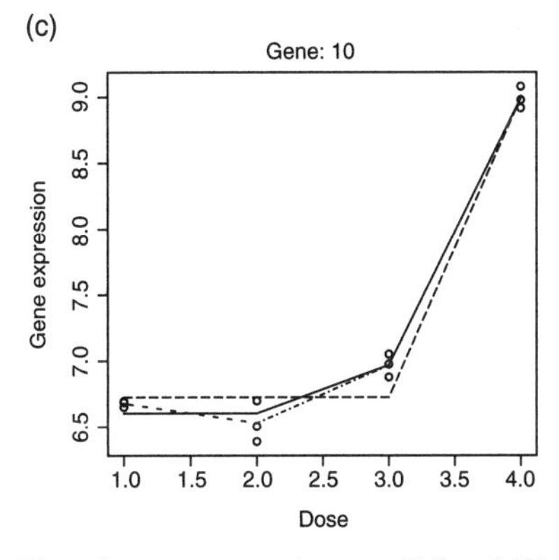

Figure 8.9 The human epidermal squamous carcinoma cell line A431 experiment. Testing the null hypothesis against simple order alternative Example of three genes with significant dose–response relationship. (a) Gene 1. (b) Gene 3. (c) Gene 10. Solid line: the estimated mean expression under simple order restriction. Dashed line: inverted umbrella with turn point at the third dose level. Dotted-dashed line: inverted umbrella with turn point at the second dose level.

the analysis in the previous section uses permutation-based inference of the actual expression data in which the columns of the expression matrix are permuted (and therefore assumes variance homogeneity across the dose levels), while the analysis presented here approximates the distribution of the test statistic by bootstraping residuals. The bootstrap algorithm is discussed in Simmons and Peddada (2007) and Peddada, Harris, and Davidov (2010).

Example. For the human epidermal squamous carcinoma cell line A431 experiment using FDR level equal to 5% and $s_0 = s_{10\%}$ (i.e., s_0 equals to 10th percentile of the standard errors of the test statistics), we obtained 3459 significant genes from which 1187 and 2272 are clustered as increasing and decreasing profiles, respectively. We consider a second analysis (with 1000 bootstraps) without the fudge factor, that is, s_0 =0. The numbers of significant genes is equal to 3151 from which 1716 and 1435 are clustered as increasing and decreasing profiles, respectively. In the previous section, for Marcus' test statistic, 3533 genes were found to be significant (using permutation-based inference with BH-FDR = 5%). In total, 2957 significant genes are found to be common for the two approaches. An example of three genes found to be significant is shown in Figure 8.9.

Testing H_0 Against Partial Order (Umbrella) Alternatives

The main advantage of the ORIOGEN algorithm is that it allows one to test the null hypothesis against any ordered alternative of interest (Peddada, Umbach, and Harris, 2012). To keep notation in line with Peddada et al. (2003), we denote C_r as a possible order-restricted profile. For a study with four time points (or four ordered experimental conditions) $(T + 1 = 4)$, there are six noncyclical order-restricted profiles given by

$$\begin{array}{lll}
C_1 = \{\mu \in R^{T+1} & : \mu_0 \le \mu_1 \le \mu_2 \le \mu_3\}, & \text{Increasing profile,} \\
C_2 = \{\mu \in R^{T+1} & : \mu_0 \le \mu_1 \ge \mu_2 \ge \mu_3\}, & \text{Umbrella profile, downturn at 2,} \\
C_3 = \{\mu \in R^{T+1} & : \mu_0 \le \mu_1 \le \mu_2 \ge \mu_3\}, & \text{Umbrella profile, downturn at 3,} \\
C_4 = \{\mu \in R^{T+1} & : \mu_0 \ge \mu_1 \ge \mu_2 \ge \mu_3\}, & \text{Decreasing profile,} \\
C_5 = \{\mu \in R^{T+1} & : \mu_0 \ge \mu_1 \le \mu_2 \le \mu_3\}, & \text{Inverted umbrella profile, upturn at 2,} \\
C_6 = \{\mu \in R^{T+1} & : \mu_0 \ge \mu_1 \ge \mu_2 \le \mu_3\}, & \text{Inverted umbrella profile, upturn at 3.}
\end{array}$$

The profiles C_1 and C_4 are the simple order profiles that were tested in the previous section. The algorithm implemented in the ORIOGEN package consists of the following steps:

- Specify the set of candidate profiles of primary interest $C_1, C_2, \ldots, C_R$.
- For each gene, estimate the mean under each candidate profile.
- Calculate the goodness of fit statistic, $l_\infty^1, \ldots, l_\infty^R$ for each candidate model.
- Use a bootstrap algorithm to approximate the distribution of the test statistic (the goodness of fit statistic) $l_\infty^r = \max(l_\infty^1, \ldots, l_\infty^R)$ under the null hypothesis.

- Once a gene is declared significant, assign a gene to the profile that has the largest goodness of fit statistic.

The methodology used in each step was discussed in details by Peddada et al. (2003), Simmons and Peddada (2007), and Peddada, Harris, and Davidov (2010).

Calculation of the Test Statistic

Let us consider a time course experiment with T time points and we assume that s is the turning point for an umbrella shape profile with downturn at dose level s. Hence, we can define two subvectors

$$C_{21} = \{\mu_0 \leq \mu_1 \leq \cdots \leq \mu_s\},$$
$$C_{22} = \{\mu_T \leq \mu_{T-1} \leq \cdots \leq \mu_s\},$$

for which all the parameters in C_{21} are linked and all the parameters in C_{22} are linked but the parameters in C_{21}, except μ_s, are not linked with the parameters in C_{22}. The parameter μ_s is linked with all the parameters in the profile and it is called a *nodal* parameter (Peddada et al., 2003).

For the umbrella shape profile, the goodness of fit statistic is the maximum between the standardized difference of the farthest parameter estimates of C_{21} and C_{22}, that is,

$$l_2^{\infty} = \max\left(\frac{\hat{\mu}_s^* - \hat{\mu}_0^*}{\sqrt{\frac{\hat{\sigma}_s^2}{n_s} + \frac{\hat{\sigma}_0^2}{n_0}}}, \frac{\hat{\mu}_s^* - \hat{\mu}_T^*}{\sqrt{\frac{\hat{\sigma}_s^2}{n_s} + \frac{\hat{\sigma}_T^2}{n_T}}}\right).$$

Hence, for an umbrella with a downturn point at dose level s the goodness of fit statistic is the maximum of Marcus' statistics calculated for each subgraph. Under the assumption of homoscedastic variance, the parameter estimates for dose-specific variance can be replaced by the pooled sample variance in both l_1^{∞} and l_2^{∞}. Both test statistics can be modified as SAM test statistics as discussed in the previous section.

Example. We use the breast cancer data, discussed in Chapter 1 for illustration. The data consists of six time points with eight replicates at each time point. For an analysis with FDR= 5%, s_{25} as the fudge factor and using 5000 permutations, we obtained 292 significant genes. Figure 8.10 shows an example of four genes found to be significant.

SUPPLEMENTARY READING

There is extensive literature on statistical linear models and statistical experimental designs, dating back to Sir R. A. Fisher, a renowned geneticist and statistician, who,

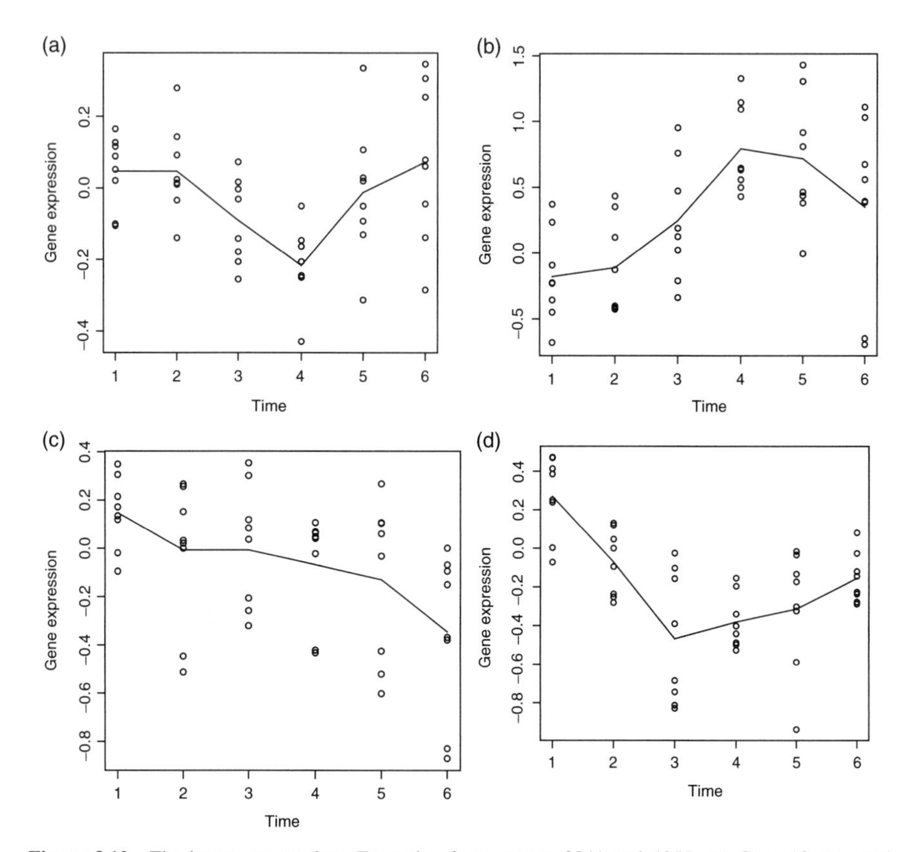

Figure 8.10 The breast cancer data. Example of two genes: 2841 and 4955. (a) Gene 12. Inverted umbrella profile, upturn at 4. (b) Gene 55. Umbrella profile, downturn at 4. (c) Gene 307. Decreasing profile. (d) Gene 1283. Inverted umbrella profile, upturn at 3.

motivated largely by problems that arose from agricultural experiments, pioneered work in these areas. Fisher (1951) remains, to this day, the best exposition of the philosophy behind practical experimental design. Cochran and Cox (1992) is another classical textbook on this topic. McCulloch and Searle (2001) is an up-to-date treatment of the theory of linear models.

SOFTWARE NOTES

`Conditional` *F*

`R` function implementing for Conditional *F* is available in DNAMR.

`ORIOGEN` 3.0

`ORIOGEN` 3.0 (Peddada, Harris, and Harvey, 2005) is a java-based interface which can be used to test the null hypothesis of no time/dose effect against order-restricted alternatives. The methodology implemented in `ORIOGEN` is discussed in Peddada et al. (2003, 2005). The package can be downloaded freely from `http://dir.niehs.gov/dirbb/oriogen/index.cfm`.

`limma`

The Bioconductor `Limma` package fits a hybrid frequentist/eBayes linear model for the expression levels of the genes in the array. The package can be used to analyze gene expression data obtained from several microarray platforms such as two-color cDNA (including normalization function for data preprocessing) and Affymetrix.

`IsoGene`

A CRAN R package for testing monotone trends in dose–response microarray experiments. The package provides several testing procedures discussed in Lin et al. (2007). Inference is based on either the asymptotic distribution of the likelihood ratio test statistic or resampling-based inference for the t-type test statistics. Adjustment for multiplicity is based on either the BH-FDR procedure or SAM.

`IsoGeneGUI`

A graphical user interface for the `IsoGene` package that does not require an extensive knowledge of R. The package performs all the statistical tests implemented in the `IsoGene` and provides several default and user-defined graphical and numerical output. The capacity of the package is discussed Pramana et al. (2010).

EXERCISES

8.1. Consider only the 0-, 1-, and 2-h data Experiment E8.

- **(a)** Carry out gene-specific F-tests to determine which genes are significantly differentially expressed across the three groups at the 5% level (i) without any adjustment for multiplicity and (ii) with Holm's adjustment for multiplicity.
- **(b)** Calculate the FDR for the results in (a).
- **(c)** For the analysis in (a), draw a scatterplot of log (MS(V)) versus log (MS(E)). Comment.
- **(d)** Fit the linear models suggested in Section 8.2 to the data. Compare the results here with those in (a).
- **(e)** Use the limma approach described in Section 8.7.2 to analyze the data. Compare the results here with those in (a).
- **(f)** Carry out gene-specific t-tests to determine which genes are not significantly differentially expressed at 1 h compared to the control but are significantly differentially expressed at 2 h compared to the control. Compare these genes with those picked out in (a).

8.2. Lee et al. (2002) mention a two-channel microarray experiment that was run to compare two types of kidney tissue, wild type (W) and mutant (M). The experiment had the following design.

	Array A_1	Array A_2	Array A_3	Array A_4
Channel R	W	W	M	M
Channel G	W	M	W	M

Compare this design with the following alternative design:

	Array A_1	Array A_2	Array A_3	Array A_4
Channel R	W	W	M	M
Channel G	M	M	W	W

8.3. Compare the loop design:

	Array A_1	Array A_2	Array A_3	Array A_4
Channel R	A	B	C	D
Channel G	B	C	D	A

to the *modified loop design* also suggested by Kerr and Churchill (2001b).

	Array A_1	Array A_2	Array A_3	Array A_4
Channel R	A	A	B	B
Channel G	C	D	C	D

8.4. Use the Golub Data to investigate the different between SAM, One-way ANOVA and limma.

(a) For each gene, calculate the mean difference (the fold change) and plot it versus the F-test statistic obtained from a gene specific one-way ANOVA model.

(b) Use SAM to analyze the data and compare the F-test statistic from (a) to the modified F-test statistic obtained from SAM.

(c) Analyze the data using limma. For each analysis in (a)–(c), use FDR correction with error rate of 5% and compare the results between all methods.

8.5. In this question, use the behavioral study in order to select genes correlated with the response variable log(distance travel by the rat).

1. Fit a gene specific regression model of the form

$$Y_i = \beta_0 + \beta_1 X_{ij} + \varepsilon_{ij}.$$

Here Y_i is the log(distance) traveled by the ith rat and X_{ij} is the corresponding gene expression. Plot the top 10 genes versus the response variable.

2. Use SAM to obtained the moderate test statistics for β_{1j} and plot it versus the test statistics in (a). What is the influence of SAM on the test statistics?

8.6. In this question we use the XXXX dataset for dose-response modeling. The XXXX data is publicly available data set and it is a part of the CRAN ORClust R package

1. Use the XXXX data to and test for monotone trend. Use the IsoGene package and the ORIOGEN package for inference. What is the different between the analysis implemented in the two packages?

8.7. 1. Read Chapter 9 in Lin et al. (2012) and use the XXXX dataset (see question 8.3) to cluster genes with similar dose-response curves. Note that if you use the ORICME package you first need to test for monotone trend.

2. Use the ORIClust to cluster genes with similar dose-response trends. What is the different between the clustering approach implemented in ORCME and ORIClust?

CHAPTER 9

Analysis of Gene Sets

In Chapters 7 and 8, we discussed methods for identifying genes that were statistically significantly differentially expressed across two or more groups. In this approach, data analysis proceeds in a gene-specific manner with a t-type test or an F-type test applied to each gene. The upshot of this testing procedure is that each gene is assigned a p-value, resulting in a long list of p-values. Of interest are the genes with small p-values.

While it is indeed important to identify individual differentially expressing genes, interpretation of the findings of this analysis is often facilitated by taking into account the fact that biological phenomena occur through the actions and interactions of multiple genes, via signaling pathways or other functional relationships. Thus, what typically happens is that once the data analyst generates a ranked list of genes with small p-values and presents it to the biologists, they will study preexisting information about the genes, which is now available for many genes, to seek patterns of differential gene expression, such as a series of functionally related genes exhibiting differential gene expression. If a set of such functionally interrelated genes contains a large proportion of small p-values, it is reasonable to infer that the function associated with those genes is potentially involved with the phenomenon being studied. Such gene sets are said to be "enriched."

It is helpful for the interpretation of the findings to formalize this step of determining whether any predefined gene sets are enriched, where a predefined gene set is a compilation of genes that are putatively related to one another, such as a set of genes involved in a particular biological process or pathway or a set of genes that belong to the same complex. Analysis of gene sets is often able to elicit a more understandable view of the biology than is immediately possible with the gene-specific analysis that we have been discussing so far.

Another consideration is that the individual genes in a significantly enriched gene set may not even have particularly significant individual p-values; the genes that comprise that gene set may be acting in concert with each other to regulate certain

Exploration and Analysis of DNA Microarray and Other High-Dimensional Data, Second Edition.
Dhammika Amaratunga, Javier Cabrera, Ziv Shkedy.

molecular mechanisms and biological pathways and thus playing an important role in the phenomenon of interest but each with having relatively small changes in expression. This consideration is important given that microarray experiments often have small sample sizes and therefore the power of the gene-specific tests tends to be quite low.

Gene sets can be compiled by using one of a number of repositories that store a wide range of current knowledge regarding the network of complex molecular interactions and regulations that constitute living organisms. Because the volume of such data is enormous, the construction of the ontologies that make up these repositories enables biological information to be organized and stored in such a way that they constitute a structured and accessible representation of the current knowledge base. In these repositories, an ontology of a domain may represent the genes that belong to that domain, the functions of these genes, the relationships between these genes, and the relationships between the domains, provided that the knowledge is available. These ontologies are regularly curated and updated as new knowledge becomes available. Some repositories of this kind that can be used for compilation of gene sets are

- *Gene Ontology* (*GO*). The Gene Ontology Consortium (2000) has developed an extensive taxonomy of gene annotations for three separate ontologies: biological process, cellular component, and molecular function. Each ontology is structured as a directed acyclic graph, with a hierarchy of terms that vary from broad levels of classification down to more narrowly defined levels.
- *The Kyoto Encyclopedia of Genes and Genomes* (*KEGG*). KEGG (Kanehisa and Goto, 2000) is a collection of online databases dealing with genomes, enzymatic pathways, and biological chemical pathways generated from publicly available resources.
- *Reactome*. It is an open access manually curated database of biological pathways.
- *Biocarta*. It is a database of mappings of genomic and proteomic relationships.
- *WikiPathways*. It is an open collaborative platform for the curation of biological pathways.

Note that when gene sets are compiled, it is possible that some genes will be categorized into multiple gene sets, so that gene sets will have non-null intersection. In fact, in hierarchies, a gene set at a lower level of the hierarchy will be a subset of a gene set at the next higher level. It is helpful to take these structures into account when interpreting gene set level results.

9.1 METHODS FOR IDENTIFYING ENRICHED GENE SETS

Several methods have been proposed in the literature for identifying enriched gene sets. We now review some of the more widely used and preferred methods.

The starting point is a list of genes that are differentially expressed across the different conditions or, preferably, a list of p-values or similar statistics that quantify the degree of differential expression for all the genes probed by the experiment. We will assume the latter; that is, we will assume that an adequate gene-level analysis has been performed (as in Chapter 7 or 8) and begin with gene-level p-values $\{p_i : i \in G\}$ where p_i is the p-value of the ith gene and G is the set of all genes.

Now the idea is to examine the set of p-values $\{p_i : i \in G\}$ associated with a particular gene set GS to see whether they are, in general, smaller in magnitude than the overall set of p-values (i.e., the set of p-values for all the genes in G). This involves use of (i) a test statistic to quantify the extent of the difference between the p-values in GS and the p-values in G and (ii) a significance test to judge whether the difference is possibly real or attributable to chance. This process can be repeated for all gene sets of interest.

Many different methods for doing this have been proposed in the literature. They can, however, be roughly pigeonholed as follows:

- *Functional Scoring (FS) Methods*. These methods use test statistics that summarize the p-values in the gene set.
- *Overrepresentation Analysis (ORA)*. These methods use test statistics based on the proportion of genes in the gene set that are declared significant.

Now, we will review three methods in detail. We will use n to denote the number of genes in GS and N to denote the number of genes in G.

9.1.1 MLP and Fisher's Test

This is a FS method. One way to summarize the p-values in a gene set in such a way that small p-values are highlighted is to take the mean of the log-transformed p-values. This is the mean log P (MLP) statistic (Pavlidis et al., 2004; further extensively studied by Raghavan et al. (2006) and Raghavan et al., 2007):

$$\text{MLP} = Mean(-\log(p_i)) = \frac{\sum_{i \in \text{GS}} (-\log(p_i))}{n}.$$

Note that this is entirely equivalent to Fisher's statistic for combining p-values (Fisher, 1925):

$$F = \sum_{i \in \text{GS}} (-2\log(p_i)).$$

Generally, the p-values of the nondifferentially expressed genes would be expected to follow a uniform distribution (i.e., $p_i \sim Unif(0, 1)$). If this was the case, MLP $\sim$Gamma$(n, 1/n)$ and $F \sim \chi^2_{2n}$ for any null gene set and either one of these could be used as a means of identifying enriched gene sets. However, it has been observed that, in most microarray experiments, the null p-values do not appear to be uniformly distributed, perhaps due to correlation among genes and/or among samples (Efron, 2009). As a consequence, this approach cannot be used to identify enriched gene sets.

The alternative that is generally used is to apply a gene permutation procedure. This is carried out as follows:

1. Evaluate the MLP statistic for each gene set GS.
2. Randomly permute the N p-values among the list of genes and map them back to the respective gene sets. Again evaluate the MLP statistic for each gene set GS with these random p-values; call these MLP*.
3. Repeat step 2 for a large number of times.
4. The proportion of times that MLP* is larger than the observed value MLP is the p-value for the significance of that gene set.

Note that the way the gene permutation is carried out in step 2 ensures that the correlational structure among the gene sets is preserved. For instance, consider two gene sets that have four genes in common; every permutation will preserve these four shared genes, and the p-values will be identically permuted. Thus, their permutation distributions will retain the correlation. Preserving this correlation is important so that correlated significant gene sets are identified in a manner that is consistent.

A drawback to this permutation approach is that it is highly computationally intensive. In order to obtain reasonable accuracy for the gene set p-values that are calculated in step 4, a very large number of permutations (several thousand) would have to be performed. This can make the procedure very time consuming. The computational complexity that is involved can be reduced in one of two ways.

Before describing these approaches, it is useful to recognize that when we draw random samples of gene p-values from G, we are actually performing finite population sampling (Newton et al., 2007; Amaratunga et al., 2012). If we let X_i= -log(p_i), we can, from finite population sampling theory, determine the mean and variance of the null distribution of MLP:

$$E(\text{MLP}) = \mu \text{ and } \text{var}(MLP) = \frac{((1-f)\sigma^2)}{((N-1)f)},$$

where $\mu = \sum_{i \in G} X_i/N$, and $\sigma^2 = \sum_{i \in G}(X_i - \overline{X})^2/N$ are the mean and variance of X_i in G and $f = n/N$ is the sampling fraction (Cochran, 1977).

The first approach to reduce the computational complexity of the permutation approach is to observe that the null distribution of the test statistics all have the same mean μ but have variances that are dependent on the size of the gene set in an $O(1/n)$ manner. Thus, in order to determine the p-values, step 4 of the procedure could be modified as follows:

Step 4′: Plot MLP* versus n. For several values of α, run quantile smoothers, $q(\alpha, n)$, through the MLP* versus n relationship so that a proportion α of the observations lie above the smoother. This produces a 100(1−α)% critical region for the set of all MLP values α_0. If MLP_0, the value of MLP for a particular gene set GS_0 lies on a quantile smoother corresponding to α_0, then the p-value for GS_0 is α_0. If MLP_0 lies in between the quantile smoothers corresponding to α_1 and α_2, then its p-value can be found by interpolating between α_1 and α_2.

An added bonus of this procedure is that we are borrowing strength across all gene sets of the same size, as well as across gene sets of different sizes. As a result, this procedure will yield a uniform critical value for all gene sets of a given size and gene sets of similar sizes will have critical values close to each other and will require fewer permutations.

The second approach to reduce the computational complexity of the permutation approach is to approximate the null distribution of MLP. For large gene set sizes, the central limit theorem implies that MLP is normally distributed with mean μ and variance σ^2. The p-value for the significance of a gene set can then be determined as

$$p_{\text{MLP}} = 1 - \Pr[Z_f \leq z_f] = 1 - \Phi(z_f),$$

where

$$Z_f = \sqrt{(N-1)f}(\text{MLP} - \mu)/(\sigma\sqrt{1-f})$$

is a standardized version of MLP. However, the strong skewness and kurtosis of X_i hinders the convergence of Z_i to normality, and hence, this approximation is unlikely to be adequate for small gene sets. A better approximation can be achieved by using an Edgeworth expansion (Robinson, 1978; Sugden and Smith, 1997; correction, 1998), because such expansions adjust for skewness and kurtosis:

$$p_E = 1 - \Pr[Z_f \leq z_f] = 1 - [\Phi(z_f) + \frac{p_1(z_f)\varphi(z_f)}{\sqrt{n}} + \frac{p_2(z_f)\varphi(z_f)}{n}],$$

where

$$p_1(z_f) = -\frac{\gamma_1}{6}\frac{(1-2f)}{\sqrt{(1-f)}}(z_f^2 - 1),$$

$$p_2(z_f) = (-\gamma_2\frac{1-6f(1-f)}{24(1-f)} + \frac{f}{4}(z_f^3 - 3z_f) - \frac{\gamma_1^2}{72}\frac{(1-2f)^2}{1-f}(z_f^5 - 10z_f^3 + 15z_f),$$

$$\gamma_1 = \frac{\sum_{i=1}^N (X_i - \overline{X})^3}{N\sigma^3},$$

$$\gamma_2 = \frac{\sum_{i=1}^N (X_i - \overline{X})^4}{N\sigma^4} - 3.$$

Amaratunga et al. (2013) show that this approximation works well.

The above gene-based permutation scheme assesses whether or not a gene set is enriched conditional on the observed p-values. If necessary, it is possible to also include a sample-based permutation to assess the unconditional significance of the enrichment. This, however, exacerbates the computational complexity of the procedure and it remains unclear as to whether it adds substantive information.

9.1.2 GSEA and the Kolmogorov–Smirnov Test

This is another FS method. In this approach, a form of the Kolmogorov–Smirnov test is used to compare the p-values in GS with the p-values in G. This is implemented in the software GSEA (gene set enrichment analysis).

The original version of GSEA (Mootha et al., 2003) used the Kolmogorov–Smirnov (KS) test statistic itself:

$$\text{KS} = \max\left\{\left|\hat{F}_{\text{GS}} - \hat{F}_{G-\text{GS}}\right|\right\},$$

where $\hat{F}_{\text{GS}}$ and $\hat{F}_{G-\text{GS}}$ are the empirical distribution functions of G and $G-$ GS respectively.

Later versions of GSEA modified the KS test statistic (Subramanian et al., 2005) because of its propensity to pick up gene sets that have modest p-value differences in the center of the distribution rather than in the tails (i.e., small p-values), a well-known characteristic of the KS test, but one that is undesirable for this application. The modified KS test statistic, KSW, is similar to the KS test statistic but assigns greater weight to small p-values

$$\text{KSW} = \max_i(P_{\text{hit}}(i) - P_{\text{miss}}(i)),$$

where $P_{\text{hit}}(i) = \sum \frac{|r_j|^p}{N_R}$, $P_{\text{miss}}(i) = \sum \frac{1}{N-N_R}n$, r_j is a measure of the signal in gene g_j (e.g., $r_j = -\log(pj)$), and all summations are over the set g_j, where $j \leq i$. Note that the KSW statistic is the same as the KS statistic when $p = 0$. GSEA uses KSW with $p = 1$.

The significance of KS and KSW can be assessed using the permutation procedure outlined in Section 9.2.1. Amaratunga et al. (2012) show that, while KSW is indeed far superior to KS for analyzing gene sets, it is weaker than MLP.

However, while GSEA also uses a permutation procedure to assess the significance of gene sets, it uses permutations of samples (as outlined in Section 9.1.1) instead of permutations of genes.

9.2 ORA AND FISHER'S EXACT TEST

This is the most commonly used ORA method. It involves testing whether small p-values are overrepresented in GS. This approach applies a p-value threshold (such as 5%) and labels each gene as "significant" or "not significant" based on whether its p-value is below or above the threshold. The proportion of significant genes in GS is then compared to the proportion of significant genes in G using Fisher's exact test (Fisher, 1922), which uses a hypergeometric distribution to test whether or not the gene set GS is enriched with significant genes.

Raghavan et al. (1996) show that the performance of this method depends on the choice of p-value threshold. As it is generally impossible to know what value would give the best overall performance, this method usually tends to be weaker than MLP.

9.3 INTERPRETATION OF RESULTS

The result of a gene set analysis through any of the methods described above would be a list of gene set p-values. The gene sets with low p-values would correspond to the biological functions most likely to be affected and therefore of most interest.

However, even here there could still be a long list of results (now it would be the list of gene set p-values). The fact that there is substantial redundancy between gene sets should also be kept in mind. It is therefore often useful to organize the results and represent them as a network or hierarchy to facilitate the exploration of these findings to discover general functional themes that may be of interest. The example below shows one way to do this.

9.4 EXAMPLE

The Sialin experiment was described in Moechars et al. (2005) and Raghavan et al. (2007). This experiment used Affymetrix Mouse430_2 GeneChips to profile the gene expressions of 12 RNA samples drawn from 18-day-old mice; 6 were from wild-type mice and 6 were from mice whose SLC17A5 gene had been knocked out. Genes were tested for differential expression using `limma`; the resulting p-values were analyzed using the MLP method.

The MLP method identified five top gene sets, all of which lie along one GO hierarchy (Figure 9.1a) and are known to be contextually relevant (Raghavan et al., 2007). The smallest of the five is gene set GO:0042552 (myelination), which has 35 genes and is a biological process known to be affected by absence of sialin. A heat map of the 35 genes (Figure 9.1b) shows patterns indicating some differential expression and co-expression. Exploring this further, a hierarchical cluster analysis of these 35 genes using Ward's method revealed a cluster of 12 genes that are quite highly significant and correlated to one another (Figure 9.1c shows a dendrogram of the clustering and Figure 9.1d shows a line plot of these 12 genes). If GS* denotes this cluster of 12 genes, MLP run on GS* shows it to highly significant with a p-value that is almost zero while *MLP* run on GO:0042552 without the GS* genes shows it to be nonsignificant with a p-value of 0.12. This implies that the genes in GS* are the main genes responsible for the significance of GO:0042552. Even though these 12 genes appear to be individually quite significant ($p < 0.00001$ for all of them), none are among the top 10 genes when all the genes in the data set are sorted according to p-value and only 2 are among the top 50 genes; thus they could be easily overlooked in an analysis that did not take gene sets into account; it is only when considered together that their possible importance emerges.

SOFTWARE NOTES

`mlp`

The `R` package `mlp` available from the authors implements the MLP method described in Section 9.1.

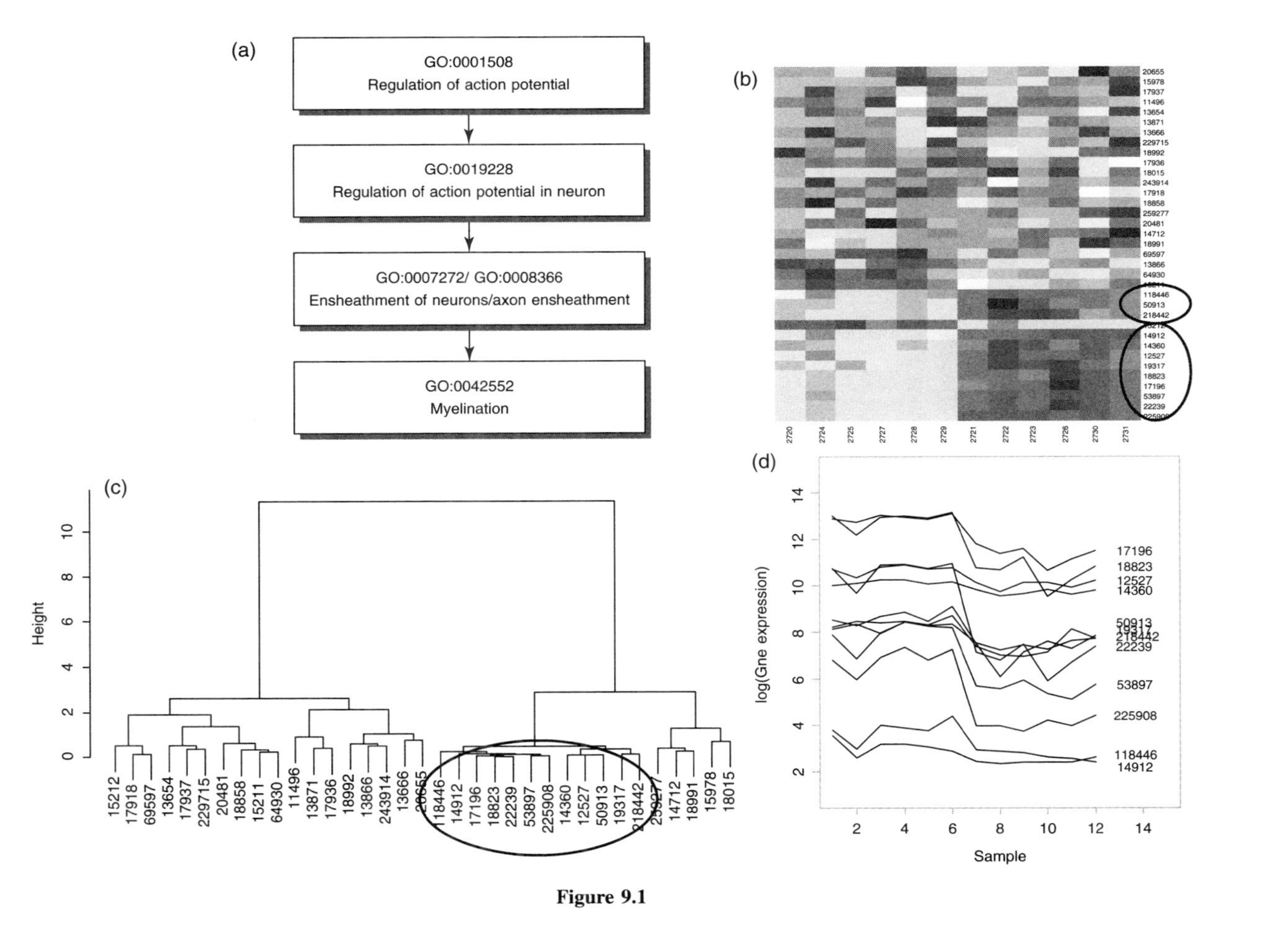
(a)
GO:0001508
Regulation of action potential
GO:0019228
Regulation of action potential in neuron
GO:0007272/ GO:0008366
Ensheathment of neurons/axon ensheathment
GO:0042552
Myelination
(b)
(c)
Height
(d)
log(Gne expression)
Sample
17196
18823
12527
14360
50913
19317
218442
22239
53897
225908
118446
14912

Figure 9.1

`GSEA`
The `GSEA` software that implements the modified Kolmogorov–Smirnov (KS) test is available from the Broad Institute.

`GOstats`
The GOstats packagefrom Bioconductor implements tools for obtaining GO information form microarrays and for manipulating and visualizing GO information and microarrays.

`GO.db`
This package contains the annotation information for the entire Gene Ontology.

The Fishers exact test is available in most standard statistical packages including `R`, `GoMiner`, `MAPPFinder`, OntologyTraverser, EASE [DAVID], FatiGO, FunSpec, GFINDer, GOTM, and IPA (Ingenuity Pathway Analysis).

EXERCISES

9.1. Suppose that a data set comprising 25 genes was analyzed and that the p-values for a test of differential expression for these 25 genes are

```
0.0012 0.6103 0.4441 0.0442 0.0724
0.1230 0.6044 0.8094 0.2045 0.0466
0.0768 0.4026 0.1330 0.3664 0.7003
0.9743 0.7919 0.8487 0.5468 0.9753
0.9877 0.2019 0.6398 0.6570 0.4599
```

(a) Suppose that the genes in the first row comprise a gene set according to GO. How many genes in this gene set are significant at the 5% level? Apply the MLP method to determine whether the gene set is significantly enriched.

(b) Suppose that the genes in the first two row comprise a gene set according to GO; that is, it is a GO term that is a parent of the GO term in (a). How many genes in this gene set are significant at the 5% level? Apply the MLP method to determine whether the gene set is significantly enriched.

(c) What additional factors should a biologist consider when assessing these findings?

9.2. Give examples as follows:

(a) Give an example of a data set G and a gene set GS, which are such that GS that consists of genes that are all significantly differentially expressed with p-values less than 0.05 for MLP, yet GS itself is not significantly enriched.

(b) Give an example of a data set G and a gene set GS, which are such that none of the genes in GS is significantly differentially expressed with p-values greater than 0.05 for MLP, yet GS itself is significantly enriched.

(c) Give an example of a data set G and a gene set GS, which are such GS is significantly enriched according to Fisher's exact test but not significantly enriched according to MLP.

(d) Give an example of a data set G and a gene set GS in which GS is not significantly enriched according to Fisher's exact test but significantly enriched according to MLP.

9.3. This excersise is about comparing MLP with Fisher's exact test in the GOLUB dataset.

(a) Obtain the GOLUB data from Bioconductor package golubEsets and the corresponding chip package hu6800.

(b) Extract the list of all gene sets for this data and calculate the MLP statistic and the corresponding p-values.

(c) Calculate the p-values for all gene sets just like in (b) but using Fisher exact test and compare them to the p-values from MLP in part (b).

9.4. In this question we use the the Breast Cancer Data discussed in Chapter 1. The aim of the analysis is to identify genes with monotone trend with respect to time as discussed in Section 8.7.4 (note that the predictor in this data is time and not dose).

(a) How many genes are declared differently expressed in this analysis (use BH-FDR with error rate of 5%).

(b) Read Chapter 12 in the book "Modeling Dose-Response Microarray Data in Early Drug Development Experiments Using R" by Lin et al. (2012) and use the R package `MLP` to preform gene set analysis.

9.5. Use the SAM method, discussed in Chapter 7, in order to identify differentially expressed genes in the Golub data.

(a) How many genes are declared differentially expressed for FDR = 1%?

(b) Use the R package `MLP` to preform gene set analysis. Give an example of a gene which was not found to be differentially expressed by belong to significant pathway.

CHAPTER 10

Pattern Discovery

Thus far, we have been discussing statistical techniques for identifying those genes that are differentially expressed across a series of conditions. Essentially, all these analyses were conducted on a gene-by-gene basis. While there is little doubt that these analyses yield useful results, they do suffer from one basic shortcoming: they neither expose nor exploit the correlated patterns of gene expression displayed by genes behaving jointly, such as genes performing similar functions or genes operating along a genetic pathway. As a result, they fail to make use of what should ideally be the full potential of multigene experiments. This can be resolved by applying multivariate analysis techniques to elicit more complex structures from microarray data.

Multivariate methods can be used for both finding multivariate patterns in data (called *pattern discovery* or *unsupervised classification* or *cluster analysis*) and for predicting classes (called *class prediction* or *supervised classification* or *discriminant analysis*). We discuss pattern discovery in this chapter and class prediction in Chapter 11.

10.1 INITIAL CONSIDERATIONS

When taking a multivariate approach, it is customary in the microarray literature to organize the data as a *gene expression matrix*, a $G \times p$ matrix, $<X = x_{gi}>$, whose G rows and p columns represent the G genes and p samples, respectively. Depending on the experiment, the p samples may correspond to p tissue types, cell lines, times, patients, treatments, experimental conditions or something else. The values x_{gi} that make up the gene expression matrix could be either the measured gene expression level for the gth gene in the ith sample, suitably transformed and normalized, or, particularly in two-channel experiments, the log of the ratio of the

Exploration and Analysis of DNA Microarray and Other High-Dimensional Data, Second Edition.
Dhammika Amaratunga, Javier Cabrera, Ziv Shkedy.

normalized gene expression level for the gth gene in the ith sample relative to its corresponding value in a reference sample.

When it comes to analysis, there is a dichotomy of approaches. Depending on the goal of the analysis, the columns may be regarded as the variables and the rows as the observations as in traditional multivariate statistical analysis, or the roles of the rows and the columns could be reversed. If the objective of the analysis is to identify groups of genes that have similar regulatory mechanisms, the columns (i.e., the samples) are regarded as the variables and the rows (i.e., the genes) are regarded as the observations. However, if the objective of the analysis is to classify the samples on the basis of their gene expression profiles, the rows (i.e., the genes) are regarded as the variables and the columns (i.e., the samples) are regarded as the observations. In this latter case, not only is the notation diametrically opposite to traditional multivariate statistical analysis notation, but also unlike traditional multivariate statistical analysis, the number of variables, G, greatly exceeds the number of observations, p, whereas almost all traditional multivariate data analysis methods were developed with the expectation that the number of cases would exceed the number of variables.

We discuss both the multivariate approaches in this chapter. However, to discuss methods of clustering genes in Section 10.2, we will use traditional multivariate statistical analysis notation, that is, the columns are the variables and the rows are the observations. In Section 10.3, where the goal is to summarize the information provided by a large pool of genes into a few variables that are more manageable, the genes are treated as variables and the samples as cases, contrary to classical statistical notation.

In many applications, besides the gene expression data, there is also auxiliary information available about the individual rows and/or columns. This information can be stored as *covariates* for the rows and/or columns. For example, we may know that the samples can be categorized as treatment or control, or that they come from different patients (perhaps demographic information, such as age and gender, is also available), or that they are from different tissue types. On the other hand, for some, if not all genes, we may have some information regarding their functionality; certainly their sequences will be available. In this chapter, we discuss *unsupervised* methods that do not consider the covariate information directly in the analysis, although it may be used for interpreting the findings of the analysis. In Chapter 11, we will discuss *supervised* methods that do take covariate information into account.

The definitions of sample variance covariance and sample correlation between two genes were given in Section 5.5. These two definitions are applied for the definitions of the sample variance-covariance and correlation matrices:

$$S = \begin{pmatrix} s_1^2, s_{12}, \ldots, s_{1G} \\ s_{21}, s_2^2, \ldots, s_{2G} \\ \ldots\ldots\ldots\ldots\ldots \\ s_{G1}, s_{G2}, \ldots, s_G^2 \end{pmatrix} = (X^tX - G^{-1}X^t11^tX)/(G-1)$$

and

$$R = \begin{pmatrix} 1, r_{12}, \ldots, r_{1G} \\ r_{21}, 1, \ldots, r_{2G} \\ \ldots\ldots\ldots\ldots\ldots \\ r_{G1}, r_{G2}, \ldots, 1 \end{pmatrix},$$

where s_{ij} and r_{ij} are the sample covariance and correlation coefficients between the ith and jth genes, respectively. These two $G \times G$ matrices are of rank $p - 1$ and, given the fact that in most experiments, G is normally in thousands, justifies the need for the dimension reduction methods described in Section 10.3. If we consider the microarray as a data set where the genes are the observations and the samples are the variables then the dimension of the correlation and covariance matrices is $p \times p$ and, because p is typically much smaller than G, there is less of a problem with the dimensions (unless, of course, when p is very large).

Example. We will use a subset of the data of Khan et al. (2001) to illustrate the methods of this chapter. The data set contains gene expression measurements, obtained using cDNA microarrays, from four types of pediatric small round blue cell tumors SRBCT. Here, we concentrate on the subset with types: rhabdomyosarcoma (RMS) and the Ewing family of tumors (EWS). This data was filtered to remove any gene that consistently expressed below a certain minimum level of expression, leaving expression data for 2308 genes ($G = 2308$). A subset of 43 cells is considered here (23 EWS, 20 RMS so $p = 43$).

Working with 2308 genes is too many for the purpose of the illustrations that will be presented throughout this chapter. For this reason, we will concentrate only on 100 genes that were selected because they produced the highest t-values for comparing the means of the two groups of samples for each individual gene. The complete set will be described more thoroughly in Chapter 11.

10.2 CLUSTER ANALYSIS

Broadly speaking, *cluster analysis*, a significant branch of *unsupervised learning*, refers to a hodgepodge collection of algorithms and procedures that have been developed over the years and across a variety of disciplines for organizing a given multivariate data set into an assortment of *clusters* in such a way that the observations within each cluster are more or less similar to each other.

As might be expected, cluster analysis was one of the first multivariate data analysis techniques employed for an analysis of microarray data (the seminal paper in this regard is Eisen et al. (1998)). There is a compelling argument for using cluster analysis for analyzing gene expression data. It is reasonable, after all, to expect that a set of genes operating in a particular genetic pathway would behave fairly similarly across a series of conditions. For this reason, their expression levels are likely to be relatively highly correlated and, in a cluster analysis, should all fall into a single cluster. A cluster analysis will sort the entirety of genes (or a suitably selected subset of them) into a series of clusters in such a way that those genes that behaved the most similarly in the experiment will be members of the same cluster, while genes that behaved differently will be members of separate clusters. The hope, of course, is that genes performing similar functions or participating in the same genetic pathway would all congregate in the same cluster.

The gene clusters generated by the cluster analysis can then be assessed in the context of known or putative genetic pathways, such as metabolic pathways, gene families, and subcellular components, in order to deduce functional relationships. For example, if a gene is known to code for a particular enzyme, it can be mapped onto the reaction that is catalyzed by that enzyme. By exploring constructs of all qualitatively feasible metabolic pathways from a set of biochemical reactions, inferences can be made regarding the pathway. As another example, in experiments involving normal and diseased subjects, the findings from a cluster analysis could lead to the discovery of a genetic pathway (or the disruption of one) that causes a disease. Of course, cluster analysis cannot reveal functionally related genes if they do not display similar expression patterns or if they express with a time delay. Still, with technology having evolved to such a state that it is possible to array almost an entire genome onto a microarray, cluster analysis has emerged as one of the most valuable tools for gathering information about how genes work in combination.

Both the statistics and data mining literature are replete with clustering methods that are mostly algorithmic in nature. Most clustering algorithms can be classified as being either hierarchical or partitioning. We discuss these in the following sections. However, all clustering methods depend on either a dissimilarity or a similarity measure, which quantifies how far, or how close, two observations (in this case, genes) are from each other. We discuss such measures first.

For the clustering approach, we treat the gene expression levels from a gene (i.e., the *expression profile* of gene over the samples) as multivariate observations. This does not mean that we cannot use clustering methodology when we believe that genes are treated as variables, but conceptually, it is more rigorous to think of genes as multivariate observations in the remainder of this section.

10.2.1 Dissimilarity Measures and Similarity Measures

Given data for two genes, g and h, with corresponding data $x_g = (x_{gj})$ and $x_h = (x_{hj})$ (i.e., the gth and hth rows of X), a *dissimilarity measure* (sometimes referred to as a *distance*), $D(x_g, x_h)$, is a statistic that states quantitatively how dissimilar x_g and x_h are to each other. There are many choices for D and many of the better choices satisfy the following *dissimilarity axioms*: (i) $D \geq 0$, (ii) $D = 0$ if and only if $x_g = x_h$, (iii) D gets larger the further x_g and x_h are apart, and (iv) $D(x_g, x_h) = D(x_h, x_g)$. Some choices for D also satisfy either (v) the *triangle inequality*, $D(x_g, x_h) \leq D(x_g, x_i) + D(x_i, x_h)$ or (vi) the *ultrametric inequality*, $D(x_g, x_h) \leq \max\,(D(x_g, x_i), D(x_h, x_i))$.

The most widely used dissimilarity measure is the *Euclidean distance*, D_{E}. $D_{\mathrm{E}}(x_g, x_h)$ is the geometrical distance between x_g and x_h in the p-dimensional space in which they lie:

$$D_{\mathrm{E}}(x_g, x_h) = \sqrt{\sum_{j=1}^{p} (x_{gj} - x_{hj})^2}.$$

D_{E} satisfies all the dissimilarity axioms above but has the drawback wherein changing the column variances could substantially change the ordering of the distances between the genes and, as a result, change the clustering. Of course, one may hope that the normalization step would have relegated this to a nonissue by bringing the column variances into close alignment with one another. Otherwise, one way to reduce this effect is to divide each column by its standard deviation or median absolute deviation. This gives the *standardized Euclidean distance*:

$$D_{\mathrm{SE}}(x_g, x_h) = \sqrt{\sum_{j=1}^{p} \left(\frac{x_{gj} - x_{hj}}{s_j} \right)^2}.$$

However, some care is necessary when rescaling the data this way as it could also dilute the differences between the clusters with respect to the columns that are intrinsically the best discriminators. Skewness could also exacerbate the effect of scaling on the data.

Two other dissimilarity measures that have been used for clustering are the *Manhattan* or *city block distance*

$$D_M = \sum_{j=1}^{p} |x_{gj} - x_{hj}|$$

and the *Canberra distance*

$$D_{CAN} = \sum_{j=1}^{p} \frac{|x_{gj} - x_{hj}|}{x_{gj} + x_{hj}}.$$

Clustering can also be based on similarities between pairs of observations rather than dissimilarities between pairs of observations. A measure of similarity, $C(x_g, x_h)$, between two objects, x_g, x_h, must comply with the conditions: (i) $C(x_g, x_h) = C(x_h, x_g)$; (ii) $C(x_g, x_h) \leq C(x_g, x_g)$ for all g, h; and (iii) C gets smaller the further apart x_g and x_h are. A similarity measure can be converted to a dissimilarity measure by the standard transformation (Mardia, Kent, and Bibby, 1979):

$$D_C(x_g, x_h) = \sqrt{C(x_g, x_g) + C(x_h, x_h) - 2C(x_h, x_g)}.$$

One popular example of a similarity measure is Pearson correlation coefficient, R:

$$R\left(x_g, x_h\right) = \frac{\sum_{j=1}^{p}(x_{gj} - \overline{x}_{g.})(x_{hj} - \overline{x}_{h.})}{\sqrt{\sum_{j=1}^{p}(x_{gj} - \overline{x}_{g.})^2 \sum_{j=1}^{p}(x_{hj} - \overline{x}_{h.})^2}}.$$

R measures how linearly correlated x_g and x_h are to each other. It lies between -1 and $+1$, and the closer it is to these values, the more linearly correlated x_g and x_h are to each other, with negative values indicating negative association. Values near zero connote the absence of a linear correlation between x_g and x_h.

R can be converted to a dissimilarity measure using either the standard transformation

$$D_{C2}(x_g, x_h) = \sqrt{1 - R(x_g, x_h)^2}$$

or the transformation

$$D_{C1}(x_g, x_h) = 1 - |R(x_g, x_h)|.$$

Note that neither D_{C1} nor D_{C2} quite satisfies the dissimilarity axioms. For instance, instead of axioms (ii) and (iii), $D_{C1} = 0$ if and only if x_g and x_h are linearly correlated (rather than if and only if $x_g = x_h$) and D_{C1} increases toward its maximum value of 1, the less linearly correlated x_g and x_h are. Nevertheless, it is a useful measure to use with microarray data as coexpressing genes may have expression values that are highly correlated to each other, even though their raw values may be far apart as they express at quite different levels.

When the observations have a natural reference value, c, the observations may be centered at c rather than at the mean:

$$R_c(x_g, x_h) = \frac{\sum_{j=1}^{p}(x_{gj} - c)(x_{hj} - c)}{\sqrt{\sum_{j=1}^{p}(x_{gj} - c)^2 \sum_{j=1}^{p}(x_{hj} - c)^2}}.$$

For example, when clustering gene expression ratios, and the observations are log expression ratios, $c = \log_2(1) = 0$ is a natural reference value.

The *Spearman correlation coefficient*, which is the Pearson correlation coefficient calculated on the ranks of the data, measures closeness in terms of whether two observations are monotonically related to each other.

10.2.2 Guilt by Association

When a set of genes is known to be associated with a disease (or other factor), discovering that there is a novel gene whose expression profile closely matches that of one of the known genes could prove to be a very valuable piece of information about the genetic pathway involved in the disease process. Besides assisting in better understanding of pathways, medical applications are also possible; for example, if the novel gene is one that is expressed earlier in the progression of the disease than any of the known genes, it could perhaps be used as a disease marker allowing for earlier diagnosis and treatment of the disease. Walker et al. (1999) call this concept *guilt by association* (see also Oliver, 2000).

Any of the dissimilarity or similarity measures mentioned in Section 9.2.1 could be used for searching through a database of gene expression profiles that includes data for both known genes and novel genes. Thus, for example, if gene d is a known gene, any novel gene g that is such that $R(x_d, x_g)$ is relatively very high would be considered "guilty by association" and subjected to closer scrutiny to assess its involvement in the disease process.

On the other hand, because many genes tend to express only under specific circumstances, it is possible that these measures would be dampened by the many genes that are not expressed. Also, when the database has been derived from diverse sources, there may be some doubt as to whether the data are directly comparable. For these reasons, it may be preferable to dichotomize the data (i.e., transform them to a binary variable that is set equal to 1 if the gene is expressed and 0 otherwise) and use the log odds ratio or the Fisher exact test (Agresti, 2002) as a measure or test of association.

The premise underlying guilt by association is that functionally related genes would display very similar expression patterns. This has been demonstrated to be true to some extent, as, for instance, when they are coregulated by common transcription factors. However, in other instances, they may not necessarily display similar expression patterns, and, conversely, genes having quite different functions may exhibit similar expression patterns simply due to chance. Thus, some care is necessary, particularly in view of the large number of correlations being estimated, that a novel gene with an expression profile that, just by chance, happens to look correlated to that of a known gene, is not inadvertently found "guilty" and vice versa.

10.2.3 Hierarchical Clustering

Hierarchical clustering (Sokal and Michener, 1958) is an often cited early reference, but not the earliest) is one of the most widely used clustering methods. It is not surprising that some of the key developments in this area, such as Eisen et al. (1998) and Alizadeh et al. (2000) utilized hierarchical clustering methodology. Hierarchical clustering methods can themselves be classified as being either bottom-up or top-down.

Bottom-up clustering (also known as *agglomerative hierarchical clustering*) algorithms are initiated with each gene situated in its own cluster. At the next and subsequent steps, the closest pair of clusters is agglomerated (i.e., combined). In principal, the process can be continued until all the data falls into one giant cluster.

Whenever two clusters are agglomerated, the distances between the new cluster and all the other clusters are recalculated. Different hierarchical clustering schemes calculate the distance between two clusters differently:

- In *complete linkage hierarchical clustering* (or *farthest neighbor clustering*), the distance between two clusters is taken to be the largest dissimilarity measure between any two members in different clusters.
- In *single linkage hierarchical clustering* (or *nearest neighbor clustering*), the distance between two clusters is taken to be the smallest dissimilarity measure between any two members in different clusters.
- In *average linkage hierarchical clustering*, the distance between two clusters is taken to be the arithmetic mean of the dissimilarity measures between all pairs of members in different clusters.
- In *centroid clustering*, the distance between two clusters is taken to be the dissimilarity measure between the cluster centers.
- In *Ward's clustering*, the distance between two clusters is taken to be the sum of squares between clusters divided by the total sum of squares, or, equivalently, the change in R^2 when a cluster is split into two clusters, where the *coefficient of determination*, R^2, is the percent of the variation that can be explained by the clustering.

Despite their apparent similarity, these methods have different properties and will generally cluster the data in quite different ways and may even impose a structure of their own. The complete linkage hierarchical clustering algorithm is set up to minimize the maximum within-cluster distance and hence tends to find compact clusters but may overemphasize small differences between clusters. The single linkage hierarchical clustering algorithm is set up to maximize the connectedness of a cluster and hence exhibits a highly undesirable tendency to find chain-like clusters; by creating chains, two dissimilar observations may find themselves placed in the same cluster merely because they are linked via a few intermediate observations. The average linkage hierarchical clustering algorithm and the centroid clustering algorithm are compromises between the above two; note however, that unlike the other methods, they are not invariant to monotone transformations of the distances. Nevertheless, the number of small tight clusters they usually produce can be useful for the discovery process.

Eisen et al. (1998) applied an average linkage hierarchical clustering procedure with dissimilarity measure D_c and $c = 0$ to a dataset consisting of gene expression ratios generated from an experiment in the budding yeast *Saccharomyces cerevisiae*. The data was a combination of time course data from separate experiments involving the diauxic shift (DeRisi et al., 1997), the mitotic cell division cycle (Spellman et al., 1998), sporulation (Chu et al., 1998), and temperature and reducing shocks. The goal of the exercise was to understand the genetic processes taking place during the life cycle of the yeast. The cluster analysis successfully identified patterns of genomic expression correlated with the status of cellular processes within the yeast during diauxic shift, mitosis, sporulation, and heat shock disruption. In another experiment, Alizadeh et al. (1999) applied hierarchical clustering to separate diffuse B-cell lymphomas, an often fatal type of non-Hodgkins lymphoma, into two subtypes, which corresponded to distinct stages in the differentiation of B cells and showed substantial survival differences. In yet another study, Bittner et al., (2000) applied hierarchical clustering methodology to subtype cutaneous malignant melanoma.

Top-down clustering (also known as *divisive hierarchical clustering*) algorithms are initiated with all the genes placed together in one cluster. At the next and subsequent steps, the loosest cluster is split into two. In principal, the process can be continued until each gene is alone in its own cluster. A serious computational issue that sometimes hinders the use of top-down clustering methods is that, at the early stages, there are a huge number of ways (e.g., $2^{G-1} - 1$, in the first stage) of splitting even the initial cluster. Divisive algorithms are rarely used in practice.

Typically, the hierarchical clustering process is terminated either when once a specified number of clusters has been reached or when a criterion has been optimized or has converged. Several criteria for choosing an appropriate number of clusters have been proposed, none is entirely satisfactory. Some of the criteria are

- Ward's (1963) statistic, which is R^2 of the entire configuration; an adequate clustering is gauged by graphing the change in R^2 against the number of clusters;
- the *gap statistic* (Tibshirani et al., 2000), which is the change in within-cluster dispersion compared to its expected value;
- a normalized ratio of between- and within-cluster distances (Calinski and Harabasz, 1974);
- difference of weighted within-cluster sum of squares (Krzanowski and Lai, 1985);
- a prediction-based resampling method for classifying microarray data (Dudoit and Fridlyand, 2002);
- a stability-based resampling method (Ben-Hur et al., 2002), where a stable clustering pattern is characterized as a high degree of similarity between a reference clustering and clusterings obtained from subsamples of the data.

The hierarchy of fusions in which the clusters are formed either by a bottom-up clustering algorithm or by the hierarchy of divisions in which the clusters are divided by a top-down clustering algorithm can be displayed diagrammatically as a hierarchical tree called a *dendrogram*. Each node of the dendrogram represents a cluster and its "children" are the subclusters. One reason for the popularity of hierarchical clustering is the ease with which dendrograms can be interpreted.

Example. Figure 10.1 shows dendrograms for the hierarchical decompositions obtained by applying (i) average linkage hierarchical clustering and (ii) complete linkage hierarchical clustering with dissimilarity measure D_C to the tumor example data described above. It is easy to observe that these two methods produce slightly skewed trees, whereas Ward's method, shown in Figure 10.2, produces a more balanced and clear tree.

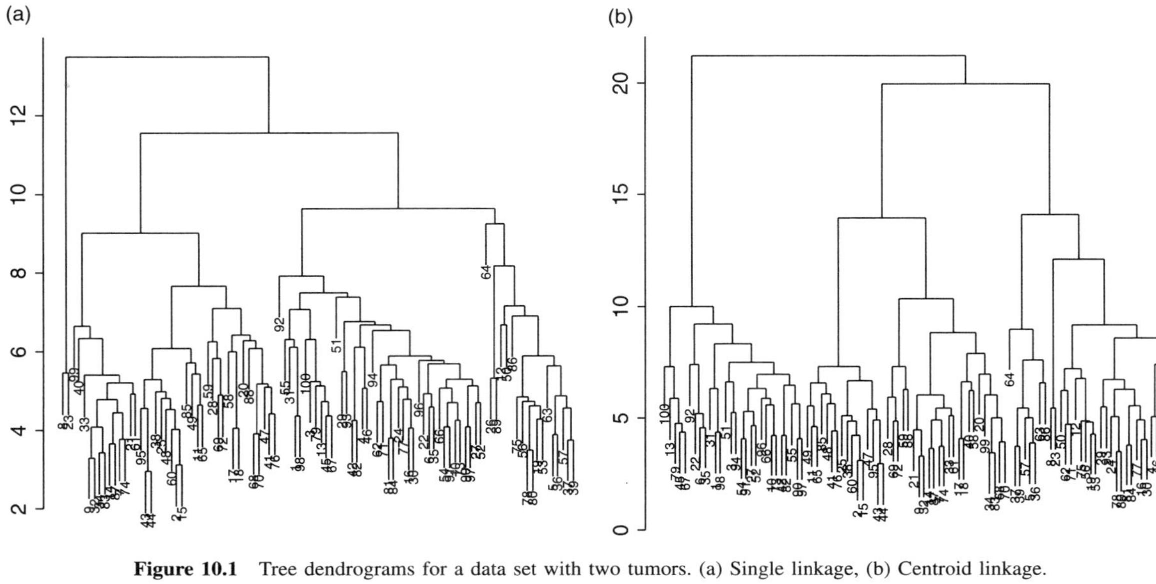

Figure 10.1 Tree dendrograms for a data set with two tumors. (a) Single linkage, (b) Centroid linkage.

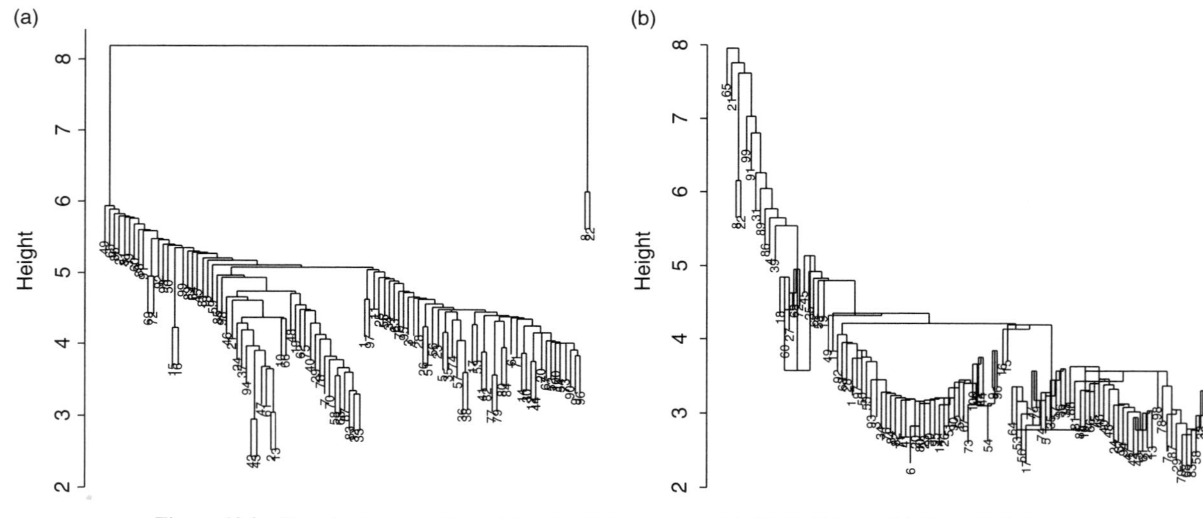

Figure 10.2 Tree dendrograms for a data set with two tumors. (a) Single linkage, (b) Centroid linkage.

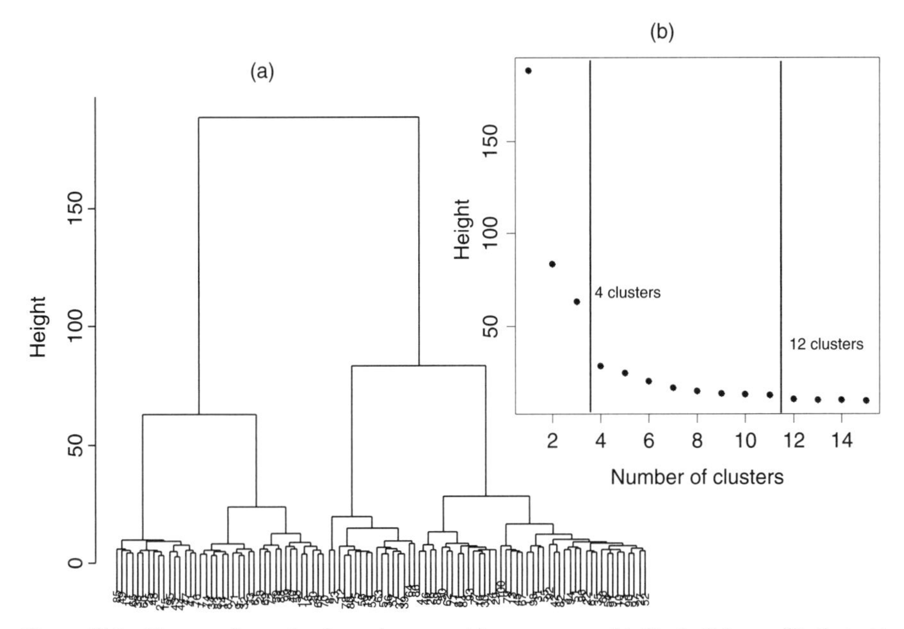

Figure 10.3 Clusters of samples for a data set with two tumors. (a) Single linkage, (b) Centroid linkage.

In general, it is known that all hierarchical clustering methods may produce unbalanced trees and, in many cases, some of the clusters could consist of single observations. Another undesirable pattern that one observes when using these methods is a big cluster with most of the data and a few small clusters around it. Nevertheless, hierarchical clustering remains a popular clustering tool.

Example. On the question of selecting the number of clusters, Figure 10.3 shows the dendrogram generated by the Ward method and next to it is a graph of Ward's statistic versus the corresponding number of clusters. From the dip in this second graph at 12, it was decided to select 12 as the number of clusters. The average profiles of these 12 clusters are displayed in Figure 10.4. The profiles clearly show that it is very easy to differentiate between the two groups of tumors (samples).

We can also apply the clustering methods to the samples (e.g., Slonim et al., 2000; Sorlie et al., 2001). In this case, the genes will act as the variables.

Example. For simplicity, we continue with the top 100 genes selected using the t-statistic. Figure 10.5 displays the dendrogram produced by Ward's hierarchical clustering procedure that clearly separates the samples into two groups. The two groups correspond to the two tumor groups. To complete the analysis, we may draw a microarray image graph combining the elements that we have seen here in Figures 10.1, 10.3, and 10.5. The graph is shown in Figure 10.6. The main panel

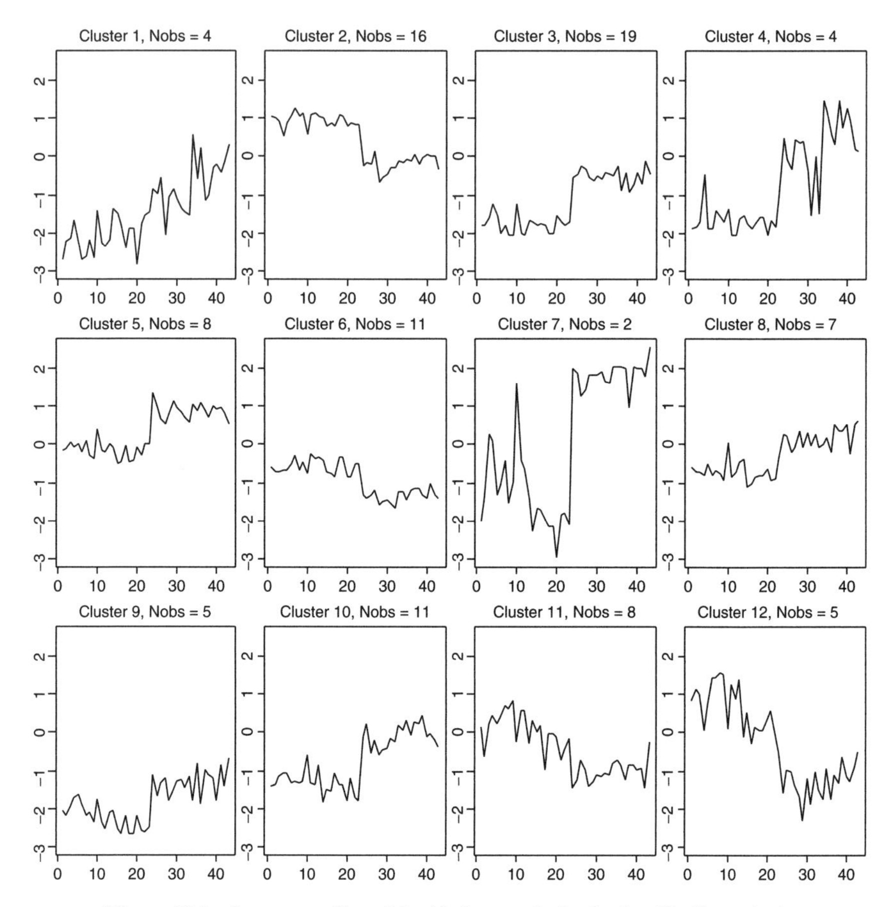

Figure 10.4 Average profiles of the 12 clusters obtained using Ward's method.

represents the image graph of the intensities for the 100 × 43 array. A horizontal and a vertical bar on the top and left side of the main image indicate the clustering of genes and samples, respectively. The right panel shows the 12 cluster profiles on a normalized scale from zero to one. Finally, the lower panel shows the color scale for the main image.

Friedman and Meulman (2004) present a distance-based clustering approach called *COSA* (which stands for "clustering objects on subsets of attributes") that attempts to identify groups of samples that exhibit preferentially close values in different, possibly overlapping subsets of genes.

10.2.4 Partitioning Methods

Partitioning methods split the data up into a specified number of nonoverlapping clusters. The general idea behind most partitioning methods is to cluster the genes

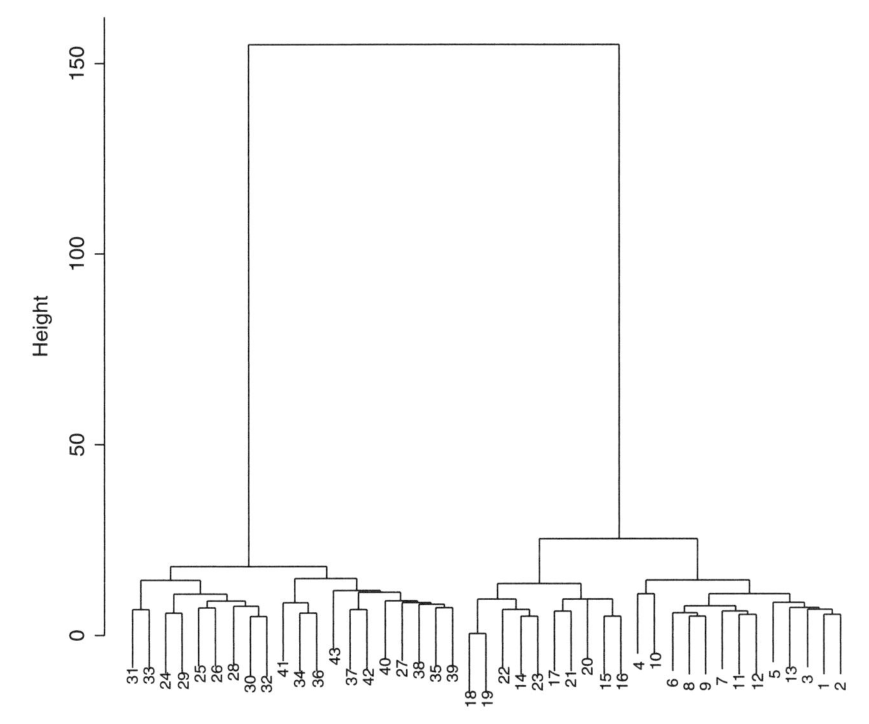

Figure 10.5 Hierarchical tree of a cluster analysis of the 43 samples using the 100 genes data set. The clustering method applied was Ward's.

so that the sum of squared dissimilarities of each gene from the closest of a set of representative central genes is minimized. Clearly, this problem cannot be solved in real time and several algorithms, three of which are k-means clustering, k-medoids clustering, and self-organizing maps (SOMs), have been developed to produce approximations.

The k-means clustering algorithm (an early version was described by MacQueen, 1967) is a procedure that clusters the G genes around k cluster centers. It is an iterative procedure that is begun with a set of k initial cluster centers. Each gene is then placed in the cluster whose center is closest in distance to the gene. The genes in each cluster are then averaged to produce a new cluster center. The procedure is repeated with the repositioned cluster centers. This process is continued until no gene is reallocated to a new cluster or a criterion function has been optimized.

At each stage, cluster statistics can be computed to assess the strength of the clusters. One such statistic is $\overline{D}$, the average intracluster distance across clusters:

$$\overline{D} = \frac{1}{G} \sum_{r=1}^{k} \sum_{s=1}^{n_r} D(x_{rs}, \overline{x}_r),$$

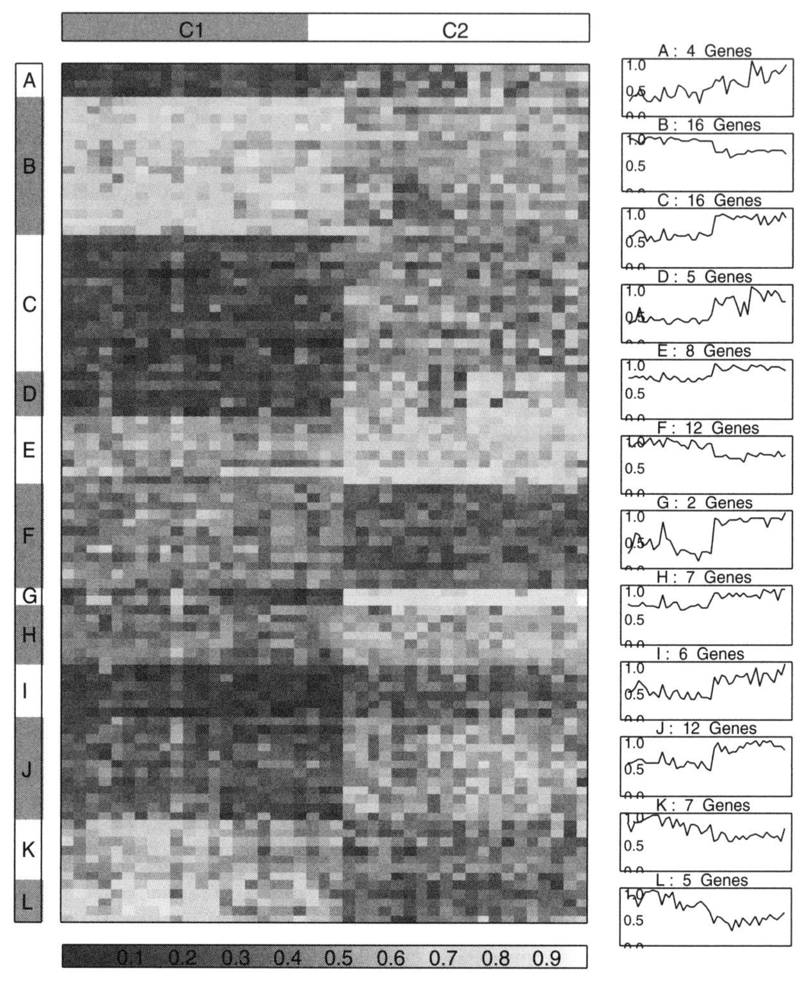

Figure 10.6 Microarray graph summarizing the gene clusters and the sample clusters. The main panel is the image plot of the intensities for the 100 × 43 array. The horizontal and vertical bars on the top and left side of the main image indicate the clustering of genes and samples, respectively. The right panel shows the 12 cluster profiles on a normalized scale from 0 to 1. Finally, the lower panel shows the color scale for the main image.

where n_r is the number of members of the rth cluster, x_{rs} is the sth member of the rth cluster, and $\overline{x}_r$ is mean of the rth cluster. $\overline{D}$ indicates the tightness of the clusters.

Another cluster statistic is S, the *total within-cluster sum of squares*

$$S = \sum_{r=1}^{k} \sum_{s=1}^{n_r} \sum_{j=1}^{p} (x_{rsj} - \overline{x}_{rj})^2,$$

where n_r is the number of members of the rth cluster, x_{rsj} is the jth coordinate of the sth member in the rth cluster, and $\overline{x}_{rj}$ is the jth coordinate of the mean of the rth cluster. A stopping rule that is sometimes used is to stop the iteration once the total within-cluster sum of squares stops reducing by appreciable amounts; in other words, until the process converges to a local minimum of the total within-cluster sum of squares.

Typically, the entire procedure is repeated with a set of different randomly generated initial cluster centers and the best solution, the one that has the smallest total within-cluster sum of squares overall, is chosen as the final partition for that value of k. As it is also impossible to know in advance how many clusters are there in the data, the procedure is generally repeated with several different values of k. For instance, Brazma and Vilo (2000) applied k-means clustering to a 6221×80 gene expression matrix, in which k was varied from 2 to 1000 and, for each k, the process was run 10 times with different random initial cluster centers. Tavazoie et al. (2000) also applied k-means clustering to gene expression data.

The k-medoids clustering algorithm (Kaufman and Rousseeuw, 1990) is identical to the k-means clustering algorithm, except that the cluster centers are taken to be the p-dimensional medians (which are sometimes called *medoids*) rather than the means. Dudoit and Fridyland (2002) use k-medoids for clustering microarray data because medoids, similar to medians, are less affected by outliers than means.

The SOM (Kohonen, 1995) is a neural network procedure that is also similar to k-means clustering. It imposes a constraint, however, that forces the cluster centers to lie in a discrete two-dimensional space. Thus, it produces a mapping of the data from a multidimensional space to a two-dimensional space, in which the clusters are sorted according to their degree of similarity. As a result, neighboring clusters are interpreted as being similar, while clusters that appear more distant in the two-dimensional space are more diverse. Tamayo et al. (1999) and Toronen et al. (1999) used SOM for clustering microarray data.

Partitioning methods are inherently nonhierarchical. In partitioning methods, unlike in hierarchical methods, the clusters obtained when the data are partitioned into k clusters cannot be constructed as a merger of the clusters obtained when the data are partitioned into $k+1$ clusters. Generally, partitioning methods will produce spherical clusters. Tibshirani et al. (2000) report finding that k-means clustering produces tighter clusters than hierarchical clustering.

Example. Consider the data set consisting of the top 100 genes, Table 10.1 shows the number of membership discrepancies between the groups produced by the various clustering methods when choosing 12 clusters. For example, there are 17 discrepancies between Ward's and k-means groupings because 17 observations appeared in different clusters. The k-means method was started at the grouping resulting from Ward's method because it achieved the lowest value of the within clusters sum of squares, compared with the other two possible methods. The single linkage and centroid methods produce very skewed trees, possibly caused by the correlations among the genes and, as a result, there are many small clusters and high discrepancies with the other methods.

Table 10.1 Table of Discrepancies for Four Clustering Procedures Applied to a Subset of 100 Genes

	K-MEANS	WARD	AVERAGE	SINGLE	CENTROID
WARD	17				
AVERAGE	39	39			
COMPLETE	27	23	30		
SINGLE	79	78	64	73	
CENTROID	80	77	64	72	8

10.2.5 Model-Based Clustering

Model-based clustering is a partitioning method in which a probability framework is posited for the clusters. The model states that (i) the genes fall into k clusters; (ii) a proportion, p_r (where $\sum_{r=1}^{k} p_r = 1$), of the genes belong to the rth cluster; (iii) the genes that belong to the rth cluster were all generated from a distribution, $f(x; \theta_r)$; and (iv) the parameter, θ_r, is different from cluster to cluster. This, then, implies that any observation x is a realization from the *mixture model*:

$$f(x) = \sum_{r=1}^{k} p_r f(x; \theta_r).$$

Usually, $f(x; \theta_r)$ is taken to be a p-variate Gaussian distribution. In this case, θ_r has two components: $\theta_r = (\mu_r, \Sigma_r)$, where μ_r is the mean and Σ_r is the variance-covariance matrix for the Gaussian distribution in the rth cluster. Banfield and Raftery (1993) point out that a geometrical structure can be imposed on the clusters by specifying a format for the variance-covariance matrices, Σ_r. This has the advantage of reducing the otherwise large number of parameters that have to be estimated. Four structures worth considering for Σ_r are (i) $\Sigma_r = \lambda I$ (where I is the identity matrix), which forces spherical clusters of equal volume; (ii) $\Sigma_r = \lambda_r I$, which forces spherical clusters of possibly unequal volume; (iii) $\Sigma_r = \lambda DAD'$, where A is a diagonal matrix and D is an orthogonal matrix, which forces elliptical clusters having equal volume, shape, and orientation across the clusters; and (iv) not imposing any structure on Σ_r. The unconstrained model (iv) is, of course, the most general, but it requires a large number of observations per cluster in order to be fitted adequately. The model (i) appears to be closely related to k-means clustering.

Given a value for the desired number of clusters, k, the parameters, θ_r, of the individual clusters, and the mixing proportions, p_r, are estimated using the EM algorithm. The EM algorithm involves alternating through a series of expectation (E) and maximization (M) steps. In the E step, the probability of each observation belonging to the each cluster is estimated conditionally on the current values of θ_r, In the M step, the values for θ_r are estimated based on the current cluster membership probabilities. Once the algorithm ultimately converges, each observation becomes a member of the cluster in which it has the largest conditional probability. Banfield and Raftery (1993) and Fraley and Raftery (1998) provide additional details of the procedure.

One advantage of model-based clustering is that instead of having to heuristically judge which clustering result seems best, as has to be done with most other clustering procedures, with model-based clustering, one has recourse to a probabilistic framework that can be used to compare across competing clustering results. Thus, in practice, one would fit the model with different values of k and different structures of Σ_r, and, then, for each model fitted, a criterion function that judges how well the model fits the data, without overfitting, can be used to pick the best model and, thereby, the best clustering result. The two criteria that are generally used are the *Akaike information criterion (AIC)*:

$$\mathrm{AIC}_m = 2\log p(X|\hat{\theta}_m, M_m) - 2\nu_m$$

and the *Bayesian information criterion (BIC)*:

$$\mathrm{BIC}_m = 2\log p(X|\hat{\theta}_m, M_m) - \nu_m \log(G)$$

Here, M_m refers to the mth model, ν_m is the number of parameters in θ_m, and $\hat{\theta}_m$ is the maximum likelihood estimator of θ_m. Large values indicate better models. Model-based clustering will find spherical or elliptical clusters, depending on how Σ_r is specified, but will not find nonconvex structures. Model-based clustering has been applied to microarray data by McLachlan, Bean and Peel (2002), Pan et al. (2002), and Yeung et al. (2001). Somewhat similar approaches are described by Holmes and Bruno (2000) and Barash and Friedman (2002).

10.2.6 Chinese Restaurant Clustering

Chinese restaurant clustering, proposed by Lo et al. (2000), is a Bayesian approach to model-based clustering. The idea is to construct a Dirichlet prior distribution over the space of partitions and build a likelihood using the mixture model given in Section 10.2.5. Bayes' theorem is then applied to determine the posterior distribution and its mode over the space of partitions is calculated.

In practice, this involves the construction of a Gibbs sampler that produces a sequence of partitions. The iteration is continued until the mode partition of the posterior distribution is clearly identified. This algorithm has the drawback that it is computationally highly intensive, that is, it may take a long time to produce the desired partition. However, it is a very interesting approach because it does not separate the selection of the number of clusters from the assignment of the genes to the clusters. In that sense, it is more natural than many of the more conventional clustering algorithms. The "Chinese restaurant" label comes from the practice of some Chinese restaurants of sitting the entering customers at a vacant or new table according to a decision of the restaurant host. This phenomenon resembles the initial steps of the algorithm, where the genes are assigned to their respective initial clusters.

10.2.7 Ensemble Methods for Clustering Samples

The methods mentioned in the previous sections for clustering genes can also be used to cluster samples. To cluster the p samples, the G genes would be treated as predictors, the p samples as cases, and a cluster analysis algorithm would be applied. However, when clustering samples, all these methods often exhibit high error rates because of the huge excess of predictors (genes).

The usual resolution attempted has been to filter the genes based on variance or coefficient of variation. This has been found to reduce the error rates somewhat. On the other hand, Amaratunga, Cabrera, and Kovtun (2008) show that the error rates can be even more drastically reduced by filtering the genes repeatedly in parallel and applying an ensemble technique they call ABC.

The procedure is as follows.

1. Rank the variances of the genes from 1 (most variable) to G. The premise behind the ABC technique is that the higher variance (and thus lower ranked) genes are the ones most likely to be useful for separating the samples into meaningful clusters. The ranks can be used to determine weights for the genes: $W_g=1/(R_g+c)$, where c is chosen so that the 1% of genes with the highest variance have a combined probability of 20% of being selected.
2. Using these weights, draw a weighted random sample of $\sqrt{G}$ genes without replacement. The weighting with weights inversely proportional to the ranks guarantees that this random sample of genes contains an overabundance of the high variance genes that are the predictors most likely to be useful for separating the samples into meaningful clusters.
3. Draw a random sample of p samples with replacement, discarding any replicates.
4. Run Ward's clustering procedure on the resulting subset of the data to cluster the samples into $\sqrt{p}$ clusters.
5. Repeat steps 2, 3, and 4 many times (say 1000 times).
6. Collate the results: Let P_{ij} denote the proportion of runs in which the ith and jth samples cluster together.
7. Let $D_{ij} = 1 - P_{ij}$ and use P_{ij} as a dissimilarity measure in a standard clustering procedure (such as Ward's method described in Section 10.2.3).

The basis of the method is that a large value of P_{ij} implies that the ith and jth samples clustered together often and therefore can be inferred to be close to each other, whereas a small value of P_{ij} implies that the ith and jth samples are relatively distant from each other. Thus, P_{ij} is a measure of sample similarity, which can be converted into a measure of sample dissimilarity by setting D_{ij}= 1-P_{ij}. The D_{ij} are called *ABC-dissimilarities* as they are based on aggregating bundles of clusters.

Example.

1. For the full Golub data, which has three clusters, Ward's method with 1-correlation as the distance measure had an error rate of 23.6%, whereas ABC with 1000 runs had an error rate of 18.1%.
2. For the Sialin Day 18 data, which has two clearly differentiated groups of samples (wild type and knockout), both Ward's method with 1- correlation as the distance measure and ABC have error rates of 0%.
3. For the Sialin Day 0 data, which has two not-well-differentiated groups of samples (wild type and knockout), Ward's method with 1- correlation as the distance measure has an error rate of 25%, whereas ABC has an error rate of only 8.3%.

10.2.8 Discussion

It is highly unlikely that gene expression data can be clearly and unambiguously separated into a set of well-defined clusters. Consequently, different clustering algorithms will generally produce different, even conflicting, results. Loosely, a good clustering method will produce clusters whose within-cluster similarity is high and between-cluster similarity is low. However, the kinds of clusters found will vary according to the clustering method used and they may not be directly comparable. The best method, if one even existed, would be data dependent. Yeung et al., (2001) applied a leave-out-one procedure to assess the performance of clustering procedure. In general, it is impossible to assert that any one clustering method, or, for that matter, any one of the seemingly endless variations on the basic algorithms, is uniformly better than any other method. Hence, in practice, it is best to run more than one clustering method on any given data set.

10.3 SEEKING PATTERNS VISUALLY

Clusters and other patterns in multivariate data can also be captured by representing the data visually. To discuss this, we will treat the G genes as G variables and the samples as cases. Of course, the dimensionality of microarray data (i.e., the number of variables (genes) in microarray data) precludes displaying the data as is. Instead, the data must be *projected* onto a lower (say k) dimensional space (usually $k = 2$, maybe $k = 3$) and plotted in this latter space. Projecting G-dimensional observations into k-dimensional observations essentially involves fashioning k new variables out of the G original ones. The process of projecting the data this way is called *dimension reduction.*

There are a number of ways to reduce the dimensionality of a data set. For many of the simpler methods, such as principal component analysis (PCA) and factor analysis (FA), the k new variables are k linear combinations of the G original variables; these methods are called *linear reduction techniques*. On the other hand, methods such as multidimensional scaling are *nonlinear reduction techniques.*

Another method, projection pursuit (PP), was proposed by Friedman and Tukey (1974) as a way to explicitly "pursue" projections that have interesting structure.

10.3.1 Principal Components Analysis

We begin with PCA), a method of classical multivariate analysis that is the most commonly used technique for dimension reduction. Several data analysts have used PCA for working with microarray data (see, e.g., Raychaudhuri et al. (2000) and Yeung and Ruzzo (2001), who discuss PCA for analyzing a temporal microarray data set).

PCA is particularly useful in situations where we are dealing with many correlated, and therefore redundant, variables and we want to reduce them to a few new uncorrelated variables, constructed as *projections*, linear combinations of the original variables, without losing too much information. The first new variable, that is, the first principal component, is the linear combination of expression patterns that explains the greatest amount of variability in the data. The second principal component is the linear combination of expression patterns that explains the greatest amount of variability remaining in the data after accounting for the first principal component. Each succeeding principal component is similarly obtained.

Projecting the data into the dimensions spanned by the leading principal components will reveal data structures, such as clusters, which stretch the data point cloud out. This is why PCA is often used as a way of examining the data for clusters. When there are a few well-separated clusters, it is likely that PCA will find projections that separate the clusters. However, in other cases, it may not work so well: for instance, when there are a large number of noisy variables that do not contribute much information regarding the clusters or when the clusters themselves are located in such a way that they do not stretch the point cloud out, a rather extreme example of which occurs when the clusters are centered at the corners of a simplex.

Example. We now return to the top 100 gene data described in Section 10.1. Figure 10.7 shows a two-dimensional view of this 100-dimensional data. The two dimensions plotted are the first two principal components, denoted PC1 and PC2 (each is a linear combination of the 100 "variables"), obtained by PCA. In this view, it can easily be perceived that the data have two groups. Note, however, that this structure would not have been evident from a one-dimensional view in the PC1 direction.

The projection of X in the direction l is Xl, the variance of which is $l'Sl$. Thus, the first principal component is the projection l that maximizes $l'Sl$. Generally, principal components are calculated directly from the eigenvalues and eigenvectors of either the variance-covariance matrix of X or the correlation matrix of X. However, because, in microarray experiments, these matrices are of a very high dimension, $G \times G$, it is computationally much more efficient to use the singular value decomposition, in which the largest matrix that needs to be computed is of size $G \times p$, where p is considerably smaller than G.

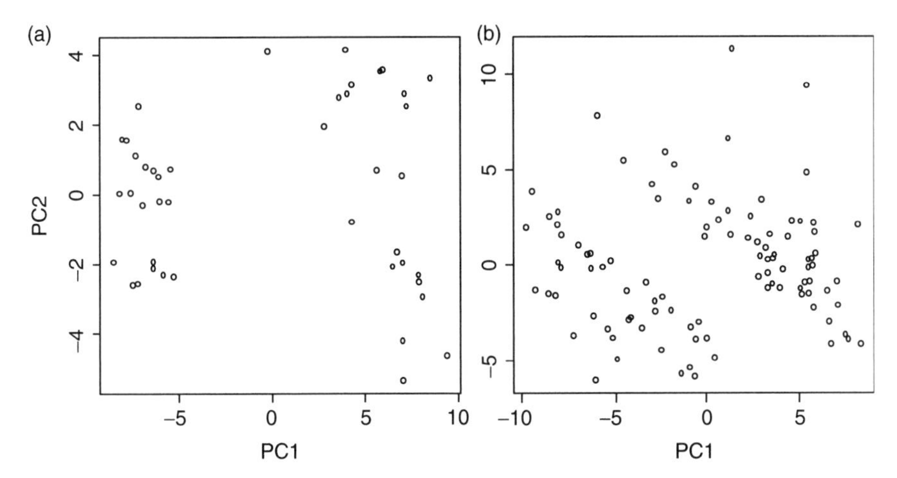

Figure 10.7 Principal components of the top 100 genes: PC2 versus PC1. (a) Cells are observations and genes are variables, (b) Cells are variables and genes are observations.

Suppose that the rows of X are centered, that is, the average of x_g is zero for all g. The singular value decomposition (SVD) of X is defined as

$$X = UDV^T,$$

where U is a $G \times p$ orthogonal matrix ($U^tU = I_r$) that projects the G-dimensional samples into p-dimensional samples, V is a $p \times p$ orthogonal matrix ($V^tV = I_r$), which projects the p-dimensional genes into other p-dimensional genes and D is a $p \times p$ diagonal matrix whose diagonal elements, s_h, are called *singular values*. We shall assume that $s_1 \leq s_2 \leq \cdots \leq s_p$. Alter et al. (2000) describe an analysis of microarray data using SVD.

From the SVD, it follows that the sample variance-covariance matrix of X with the genes as variables is

$$D^2 = \begin{pmatrix} s_1^2 ... 0 \\ ... \\ 0 ... s_p^2 \end{pmatrix}, U = (u_1, \ldots, u_p)$$

Denote the eigenvalues of S as $\lambda_1 = {s_1}^2, \ldots, \lambda_p = {s_p}^2$.

We can also obtain the eigenvalues and eigenvectors of the sample correlation matrix, R, using the same procedure if we standardize the vector x_g by subtracting the mean and dividing by the standard deviation.

As we mentioned in Section 10.1, our notation in this section differs from the standard SVD notation in classical multivariate analysis because, in microarray data, the multivariate observations are the columns and the variables (i.e., the genes) are the rows of the data matrix. In classical multivariate notation, the reverse is true, the observations are the rows and the variables are the columns of the data matrix.

For this reason, our formulas for the singular value decomposition and principal components are slightly different than the ones found in any classical multivariate analysis text.

The objective now is to select a subset of k principal components containing most of the information in the original data. There are several ways to select k. The proportion of the variance explained by the k components is $p_k = (\lambda_1 + \cdots + \lambda_k)/(\lambda_1 + \cdots + \lambda_p)$. The number of principal components could be selected by one of the following criteria:

1. k components explain some fixed percentage of the variance (70%, 80%).
2. k eigenvalues are greater than the average of the eigenvalues (for the correlation matrix the average is 1).
3. *Scree plot.* Graph the eigenvalues and look for the last sharp decline and choose k as the number of points above the cutoff.
4. Test the null hypothesis that the last m eigenvalues are equal (which is tantamount to testing that they are all essentially close to zero), using as test statistic:

$$u = (G - (2m + 11)/6)\left(m \times \log \overline{\lambda} - \sum_{i=p-m+1}^{p} \log \lambda_i\right),$$

where $\overline{\lambda} = \sum_{i=p-m+1}^{p} \frac{\lambda_i}{m}$. The null distribution of the test statistic, u, is approximately a chi-squared distribution with $(m - 1)(m + 2)/2$ degrees of freedom. In many microarray experiments, this method will eliminate only a few components because asymptotic results do not hold for cases with large number of variables and relatively few cases. However, this result is also true if we concentrate only in a range of components, say the first m, as long as certain assumptions about the multiplicity of eigenvalues are true.

Example. Returning to the example in Section 10.1, Table 10.2 shows the summary of the 43 principal components of the 100 genes. This table is used to decide how many components are needed when following the above methods for principal components selection.

1. Using criterion 1, it is appropriate to choose k between 2 and 12 because they determine the range of 70 – 90% variability. More than 12 components would mean very small increments in the variance.
2. The average of the eigenvalues is 1.24, which suggests that we should keep no more than five components.
3. The Scree plot is shown in Figure 10.8 suggesting that the number of components would be either 2 or 6 or 9.

Table 10.2 Principal Components Summary for All the 43 Principal Components

Component	Var	Cumulative Variance	Percent	Cumulative Percent
Comp.1	26.845	26.845	50.38	50.378
Comp.2	11.732	38.577	22.07	72.394
Comp.3	1.846	40.422	3.463	75.858
Comp.4	1.534	41.957	2.880	78.737
Comp.5	1.227	43.184	2.303	81.040
Comp.6	1.047	44.231	1.965	83.005
Comp.7	0.892	45.123	1.674	84.679
Comp.8	0.803	45.926	1.508	86.187
Comp.9	0.763	46.689	1.431	87.618
Comp.10	0.615	47.304	1.155	88.773
Comp.11	0.539	47.843	1.011	89.784
Comp.12	0.471	48.314	0.884	90.668
Comp.13	0.434	48.748	0.814	91.482
Comp.14	0.395	49.143	0.742	92.223
Comp.15	0.343	49.486	0.644	92.867
Comp.16	0.333	49.819	0.624	93.491
Comp.17	0.308	50.127	0.579	94.070
Comp.18	0.303	50.430	0.568	94.638
Comp.19	0.277	50.707	0.519	95.158
Comp.20	0.261	50.967	0.489	95.647
Comp.21	0.216	51.184	0.406	96.053
Comp.22	0.209	51.392	0.392	96.445
Comp.23	0.190	51.582	0.357	96.801
Comp.24	0.181	51.763	0.339	97.141
Comp.25	0.171	51.934	0.321	97.462
Comp.26	0.146	52.080	0.274	97.735
Comp.27	0.138	52.218	0.260	97.995
Comp.28	0.123	52.342	0.231	98.226
Comp.29	0.116	52.457	0.217	98.443
Comp.30	0.110	52.567	0.206	98.649
Comp.31	0.106	52.674	0.199	98.849
Comp.32	0.098	52.771	0.183	99.032
Comp.33	0.081	52.852	0.151	99.183
Comp.34	0.075	52.927	0.141	99.324
Comp.35	0.068	52.994	0.127	99.451
Comp.36	0.061	53.056	0.115	99.566
Comp.37	0.054	53.110	0.101	99.667
Comp.38	0.048	53.157	0.090	99.757
Comp.39	0.039	53.197	0.074	99.831
Comp.40	0.036	53.233	0.068	99.899
Comp.41	0.030	53.263	0.057	99.956
Comp.42	0.022	53.286	0.042	99.998
Comp.43	0.001	53.287	0.002	100.00

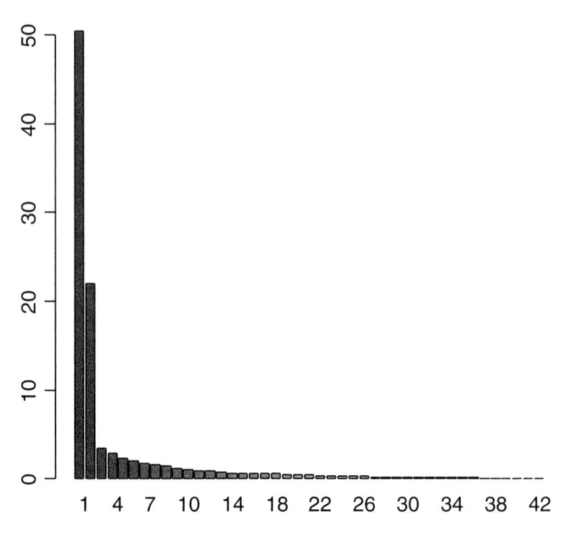

Figure 10.8 Scree plot.

4. There is a group of very small eigenvalues that we are going to discard or otherwise the method produces negligible results. We concentrate on the last 25 principal components. Then the test becomes significant for six components or less and it becomes very significant for two or less.

In conclusion, it appears that two is the best number of PCs because it satisfies criteria 1 through 3 and we saw in Figure 10.7 that the two-dimensional view in the plane spanned by the first two PCs does indeed show the primary structure in the data, which is the separation of the samples into two groups. If 72% of the variability is not regarded as high enough, either six or nine principal components could be chosen.

$p - m$	24	20	15	9	8	7	6	5	4	3	2	1
U	0.1	5	32	146	182	222	279	340	425	554	1632	3260
c^2	9.2	37	94	195	215	237	259	282	307	332	358	386

10.3.2 Factor Analysis

FA assumes the existence of a few latent variables that define the phenomena under study. The observations are functions of these unknown latent variables, or more specifically are linear combinations of the latent variables.

The objective of FA is to estimate the latent variables and to try to express them in a form as related as possible to the original observations. The statistical model for FA is

$$x = \Lambda f + \varepsilon,$$

where x is a column vector of G components and it is assumed that the vector f has k components and $E(f) = 0$, $\text{cov}(f) = I$. The matrix $\Lambda = \{\lambda_{ij}\}$ is a $G \times k$ matrix of the coefficients of the linear combinations of the factors that compose the observed variables. The error term, ε , is a G-dimensional vector satisfying $E(\varepsilon) = 0$ and $\text{cov}(\varepsilon) = \psi = \text{diag}(\psi_1, \ldots, \psi_G)$. In addition, f and e are assumed independent of each other in the sense that $cov(f, \varepsilon) = 0$. Next, we enumerate some of the important elements of the factor model as follows:

1. *Covariance Matrix.* The factor model expresses the $G \times (G - 1)/2$ covariances among the G coordinates of x in terms of $G \times k$ loadings $\{\lambda_{ij}\}$ and G variances $\{\psi_i\}$:

$$\Sigma = \text{cov}(f + \varepsilon) = \text{cov}(\Lambda f) + \text{cov}(\varepsilon) = \Lambda \text{cov}(f)\Lambda' + \psi = \Lambda\Lambda' + \psi.$$

2. *Factor Loadings.* The factor loadings λ_{ij} represent the covariances of the variables with the factors. For example, the loading of variable x_1 on factor f_2 is

$$\text{cov}(x_1, f_2) = \text{cov}(\lambda_{12} f_2, f_2) = \lambda_{12}\text{var}(f_2) = \lambda_{12}.$$

3. *Communality.* We break down the variance of a variable between a component because of the common factors and a variable-specific component.

$$\sigma_{ii} = \text{var}(x_i) = ({\lambda_{i1}}^2 + \cdots + {\lambda_{im}}^2) + \psi_i {h_i}^2 + \psi_i.$$

The communality component is h_i^2 and the component specific to the variable is y_i.

4. *Nonuniqueness.* The factors are identifiable only up to an orthogonal transformation. Let T be an orthogonal transformation, that is, $TT' = I$. Then,

$$\Lambda f + \varepsilon = \Lambda TT' f + \varepsilon = \Lambda^* f^* + \varepsilon,$$

where $\Lambda^* = \Lambda T$ and $f^* = T' f$. In addition, the properties of f are preserved by f^*. $E(f^*) = 0$, $\text{cov}(f^*) = I$, and $\text{cov}(f^*, \varepsilon) = 0$. In terms of the decomposition of the covariance matrix $S = \Lambda^* \Lambda^{*\prime} + y = \Lambda\Lambda' + y$, the communalities do not change because $h_i^{*2} = h_i^2$.

Estimation. We assume the factor model with m factors. There are two basic methods for estimating the factors.

1. *Principal Components Method.* $S = CDC' \cong C_1 D_1 {C_1}' + \hat{\Psi} = \hat{\Lambda}\hat{\Lambda}' + \hat{\Psi}$, where $\hat{\Psi}_i = s_{ii} - \sum_1^m \hat{\lambda}_{ij}^2$. This decomposition is iterated a few times.
2. *Maximum Likelihood Method.* Assume that the observations are $N(\mu,\Sigma)$ and obtain the maximum likelihood estimators of Λ and ψ.

Choosing the Number of Factors. The ideas parallel those of PCA.

1. m factors explain some fix percentage of the variance (70% or 80%).
2. m eigenvalues are greater than the average of the eigenvalues (for the correlation matrix the average is 1).
3. *Scree plot.* Graph the eigenvalues and look for the last sharp decline and choose m as the number of points above the cutoff.
4. *Test the null hypothesis that there are m factors.* The test statistic is

$$u = (G - (2p + 4m + 11)/6) \ln \left(\frac{|\hat{\Lambda}\hat{\Lambda}' + \hat{\Psi}|}{|S|} \right).$$

   The null distribution of the test statistic, u, is, approximately, a chi-squared distribution with $((p - m)2''p - m)/2$ degrees of freedom.

Rotations. As factors are identifiable only up to an orthogonal transformation, it is convenient to choose the orthogonal transformation or rotation that produces a set of factors that are the easiest to interpret. As it is likely that the number of factors m is much smaller than the number of variables G, the rotation is to be chosen so each variable contributes mainly to one or few factors. In some cases, rotations produce a grouping of G variables into m subgroups represented by the factors. There are several methods for obtaining the appropriate rotation.

1. *Graphical approach.* When m is 2 or 3, it is easier to just do a graph and find the best rotation by eye. Software such as Ggobi or JMP provide tools for performing the rotation with the aid of a mouse.
2. *Varimax.* This method computes the rotation that maximizes the variance of the square loadings in each column of $\hat{\Lambda}$.
3. *Quartimax.* Maximizes the variance of the square loadings of each row of $\hat{\Lambda}$.
4. *Promax.* Power transformation plus rotation, so it is a transformation.
5. *Procustes.* Rotation to match a canonical configuration.
6. *General Oblique.* $\hat{\Lambda}$ is now not necessarily orthogonal but it is a nonsingular matrix.

FA is sometimes criticized because the assumptions of the underlying factors may be unrealistic. Many phenomena are very complex in nature and may not fit into the FA framework. In addition, the application of a rotation may produce overoptimistic results just by chance. For these two reasons, we recommend that FA be used only as an exploratory data analysis technique that is helpful for summarizing the variables in problems, such as the microarray data analysis, where the number of variables (genes) requires simplification, and, hopefully, meaningful simplification.

Example. FA seems to suggest that nine factors or two are a good number. This is similar to the PCA conclusions in the sense of the dimensionality of the data. In Table 10.3, we give a table obtained from the `R` software with the factor loadings and it shows that the most substantial changes indicate that we should select either two or nine factors.

Table 10.3 Factor Analysis Results Using 10 Factors

	Fact1	Fact2	Fact3	Fact4	Fact5	Fact6	Fact7	Fact8	Fact9	Fact10
Ssloadings	17.73	11.42	1.187	1.055	1.015	0.891	0.822	0.632	0.56	0.317
Proportional variance	0.412	0.266	0.028	0.025	0.024	0.021	0.019	0.015	0.013	0.007
Cumulative variance	0.412	0.678	0.706	0.73	0.754	0.775	0.794	0.809	0.822	0.829

10.3.3 Biplots

The biplot (Gabriel, 1971; Gabriel and Odoroff, 1990) is a graphical display of X in which two sets of markers are plotted simultaneously. One set of markers $a_1, \ldots, a_G$ represents the rows of X and the other set of markers, $b_1, \ldots, b_p$, represents the columns of X. The basis of the biplot is that any matrix, X, can be approximated by a rank-two matrix, X_2, of the same size as X and that this latter matrix, X_2, can be factored as $X_2 = AB'$, where A is a $G \times 2$ matrix, whose ith row is a_i, and B is a $p \times 2$ matrix, whose jth row is b_j, so that $X \approx AB'$.

Such an approximation can be obtained in several ways. For example, in the SVD, $X = UDV'$, if only the two largest singular values, s_1 and s_2 are retained, a rank-two decomposition $X_2 = U_2D_2V_2^t$ can be obtained and factored as $A = U_2D_2^a$ and $B = U_2D_2^b$ with $a + b = 1$, for example, (a,b)=(0,1) or (a,b)=(1,0) or (a,b)=(0.5,0.5). Chapman et al. (2002) use biplots for visually exploring microarray data from plant pathology experiments.

Example. Figure 10.9a and b shows the two biplots, the first one is for the first two principal components. The points represent the 100 genes and they display a pattern of two clear clusters. The reason for these two clusters is that these 100 genes were selected for having a highly significant t-statistic for differentiating between two types of tumors. Hence, there are two types of genes: (i) those that are differentially upregulated for the first tumor group and (ii) those that are differentially upregulated for the second group. The PCA and FA methods capture this fact automatically and it shows as clusters in the biplot. In addition, the biplot shows that the cases are split into two groups that also correspond to the two groups of tumors. The biplot graph for the FA is better for this separation because it does a varimax rotation in the factor space.

10.3.4 Spectral Map Analysis

Wouters et al. (2003) found the spectral map, an extension of the SVD-based biplot originally developed by Lewi (1976) for displaying activity spectra of chemical compounds, useful as a means of uncovering patterns in microarray data (this concept has its basis in correspondence analysis, which has also been used for visualizing microarray data as described by Fellenberg et al., 2001).

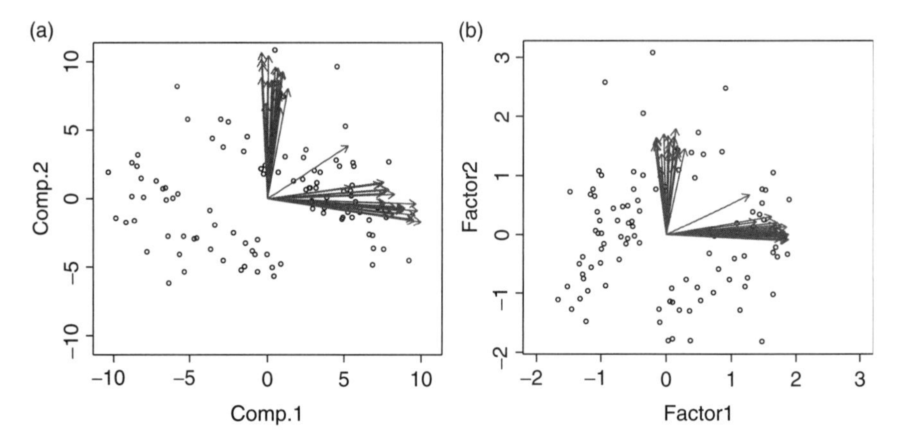

Figure 10.9 Biplot for the data. (a) Biplot of the first two principal components, (b) Biplot of the first two factors after Varimax rotation.

Spectral map analysis proceeds as follows. First, the data are transformed into relative values such that they sum to unity along the rows and along the columns. The row weighting has the effect such that genes that have lower, and therefore generally unreliable, intensity measurements get lower weights than the genes with higher intensity measurements. If x_{i+} is the ith row sum, x_{+j} is the jth column sum, and x_{++} is the overall total, this operation is

$$x_{ij} \rightarrow x_{ij}x_{++}/x_{i+}x_{+j}.$$

Next, the transformed data are doubly centered. This removes the "size" effect, leaving only contrasts between the different rows and contrasts between the different columns. If $\overline{x}_{i+}$ is the ith row mean, $\overline{x}_{+j}$ is the jth column mean, and $\overline{x}_{++}$ is the overall total, this operation is

$$x_{ij} \rightarrow x_{ij} - \overline{x}_{i+} - \overline{x}_{+j} + \overline{x}_{++}.$$

Next, the centered data are globally standardized. If $W_n = \text{diag}_n(1/n)$, $W_p = \text{diag}_p(1/p)$, and $d = 1_n W_n Y^2 W_p I_p$, this operation is

$$x_{ij} \rightarrow \frac{x_{ij}}{d}.$$

Let the resulting matrix be denoted Z. A generalized version of the singular value decomposition is used in spectral map analysis:

$$W_n^{1/2} Z W_p^{1/2} = UDV^T,$$

where again U and V are orthogonal matrices and D is a diagonal matrix of singular values.

The factor scores, $S = W_n^{-1/2} U D^{\alpha}$, and the factor loadings, $L = W_p^{-1/2} V D^{\beta}$, are plotted on a biplot for the first few singular values. Different values for α and β produce biplots with different characteristics. In drawing spectral maps, both are generally set to 0.5, which produces a distortion of the interpoint distances.

10.3.5 Multidimensional Scaling

In section 10.2, we described the methods for constructing similarity or dissimilarity measures among observations and how to use them for obtaining clusters. The reverse problem is also interesting. Suppose that we have obtained a measure of similarity or dissimilarity between a set of objects, can we produce a set of points that represent the objects in some low-dimensional Euclidean space?

In some microarray experiments, we may want to assign more importance to certain genes, truncate some low values, and in essence define a complicated measure of dissimilarity or similarity. In these cases, it may be useful to be able to represent the data in a low-dimensional space based on the dissimilarity or similarity measure.

One method of doing this is multidimensional scaling. We begin with a matrix of dissimilarities $D = (d_{ij})$ among n objects (objects could be subjects, genes, or any other). If the information available consists of a similarity matrix S then we proceed to obtain D as shown in Section 10.2.

Let $A = (a_{ij}) = (-1/2d_{ij})$ and let the matrix $B = (I - G^{-1}11')A(I - G^{-1}11')$, where I is the $G \times G$ identity matrix and 1 is a vector of length G with all its values equal to 1. Then, if B is positive semidefinite, let Y denote the first k eigenvectors of B, standardized so their length squared is the corresponding eigenvalue. The matrix Y gives a configuration of points in the k-dimensional real space with a distance matrix that is closest to D. The representation may not always be adequate if the dimension k is not sufficiently large for our data.

10.3.6 Projection Pursuit

Data of three or more dimensions are difficult to visualize. On the other hand, two-dimensional, or even three-dimensional, views (i.e., two- or three-dimensional projections) of the data are easy to visualize. In a two-dimensional graph, it is not hard to make out clusters or any other data structures. In a three-dimensional graph, we can use rotation software that enables us to visualize the data. However, as the dimension gets higher, visualization becomes difficult at best.

One solution is to look at low-dimensional projections of high-dimensional data but, again, we encounter a problem because, as the dimension gets higher, the number of views becomes far too large. The motivation behind PP methodology (Friedman and Tukey (1974); further developed by Friedman (1987); see also Barnett, 1981) is to find a few low-dimensional views of the data that describe the structure of the high-dimensional data set, such as clusters, outliers, or subspaces containing the data, as they may provide interesting information about the scientific questions motivating the data analysis.

A projection is considered interesting if it shows a nonrandom or nonnormally distributed point cloud. Projections showing a pattern of clusters or showing outliers are considered "interesting" because they differ markedly from a normal distribution. However, projections chosen at random are likely to be close to a normal distribution. This is a consequence of the central limit theorem because projections are linear combinations of variables.

The method of PP finds the projections that optimize a criterion called the *projection pursuit index* that measures how interesting a structure is within a view. The most common indices are the Legendre index and the Hermite index.

Let $Y = PX$ be a one-dimensional projection of our data. The Hermite index measures the distance from the empirical distribution of Y to a normal distribution. It was proposed by Hall (1989); Cook et al. (1993) and Cook et al. (1995) recommended using just two of the Hermite polynomial expansions of this distance resulting in a very simple expression that it is easily computable and hence not difficult to optimize. The two-term Hermite index is

$$I_H = a_1^2 - 2^{1/2}\pi^{-1/4}a_0 + \frac{1}{2}\pi^{-1/2},$$

where

$$a_0 = \text{ave}\left(\pi^{-1/4}e^{Y^2/2}\right) \text{ and } a_1 = \text{ave}\left(\pi^{-1/4}e^{Y^2/2} \times Y\right).$$

The function ave represents the average of the expression over the sample points.

In order to define the Legendre index, we transform the projection Y into a variable U in the interval $[-1, 1]$ by the function $U = 2\Phi(Y) - 1$, where $\Phi(t)$ is the normal distribution function. The Legendre index measures the L_2 distance between the distribution of U and a uniform distribution on the interval $[-1, 1]$. This index was proposed by Friedman (1987). Again, we use a two-term approximation based on Legendre polynomial expansion:

$$I_H(P) = a_1^2 - 2^{\frac{1}{2}}\pi^{-\frac{1}{4}}a_0 + \frac{1}{2}\pi^{-\frac{1}{2}},$$

where $a_0 = \text{ave}(\pi^{-\frac{1}{4}}e^{-\frac{Y^2}{2}})$ and $a_1 = \text{ave}(\pi^{-\frac{1}{4}}e^{-\frac{Y^2}{2}} \times Y)$. The function ave represents the average of the expression over the sample points.

In order to define the Legendre index, we transform the projection Y into a variable U in the interval $[-1, 1]$ by the function $U = 2\Phi(Y) - 1$, where $\Phi(t)$ is the normal distribution function. The Legendre index measures the L_2 distance between the distribution of U and a uniform distribution on the interval $[-1, 1]$. This index was proposed by Friedman (1987). Again, we use a two-term approximation based on Legendre polynomial expansion:

$$I_L(P) = a_1^2 + a_2^2,$$

where $a_1 = \sqrt{\frac{3}{2}}\text{ave}(U)$ and $a_2 = \sqrt{\frac{5}{8}}\text{ave}(3U^2 - 1)$.

The method of PP consists of selecting projections that optimize a projection pursuit index and examining these projections graphically for interesting structures. Cook et al. (1993, 1995) provide a detailed assessment of these and other indices.

10.3.7 Data Visualization with the Grand Tour and Projection Pursuit

Cook et al. (1993, 1995) describe Xgobi/Ggobi, a fascinating computer implementation of these ideas that combines the idea of a Grand Tour (essentially, a movie of data projections, a continuous sequence of two-dimensional projections of multidimensional data) (Asimov, 1985) with that of PP.

Example. Figure 10.10 shows a screen of the software Ggobi in action. The data set is the same tumor data except that now 63 patients are included, corresponding to four types of tumors. The PP method succeeds in identifying four clusters corresponding to the four types of tumors without using the tumor information. The main panel in Figure 10.10 shows a two-dimensional projection selected by the PP index with the four clusters in different colors and glyphs. The top left panel shows the main controls and the left bottom panel displays the controls and

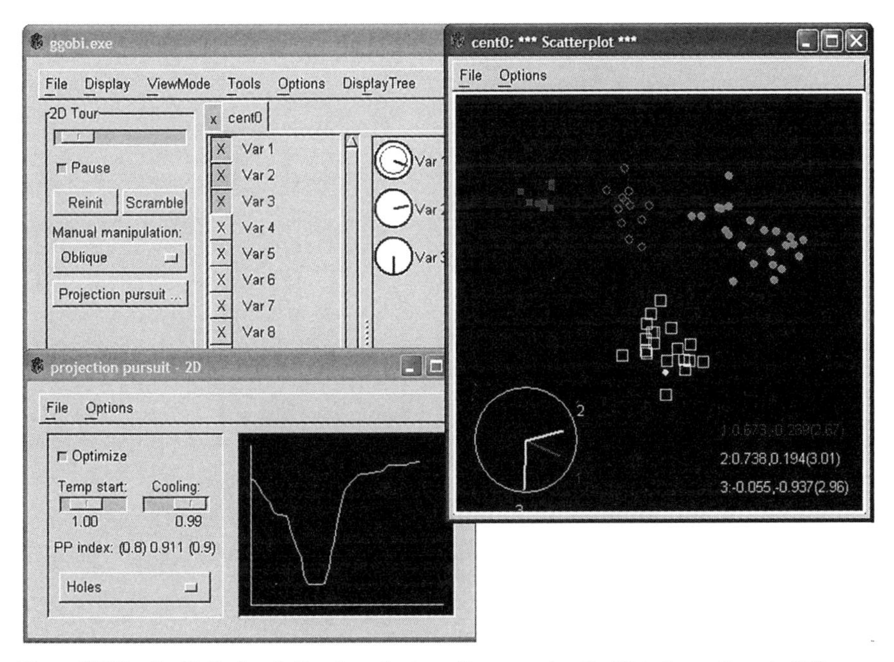

Figure 10.10 Ggobi display finding four clusters of tumors using the PP index on the set of 63 cases. The main panel shows the two-dimensional projection selected by the PP index with the four clusters in different colors and glyphs. The top left panel shows the main controls and the left bottom panel displays the controls and the graph of the PP index that has been optimized. The graph shows the index value for a sequence of projection ending at the current one.

the graph of the PP index that is being optimized. The graph shows a deep valley at whose bottom the optimization algorithm was turned on. The index value corresponds to a sequence of projections, ending at the current one, which is the optimum reached by the algorithm. This is the projection shown in the central panel.

10.4 BICLUSTERING

Section 10.2 dealt with methods for clustering genes (these same algorithms can also be applied to cluster samples), while Section 10.3 dealt with methods for spotting clustering samples (these same methods can also be applied to spot genes that cluster together). In fact, it makes sense to consider *two-way clustering*, or *biclustering* in which both genes and samples (i.e., both the rows and the columns of the expression matrix) are clustered simultaneously (Madeira and Oliveira, 2004). The goal of such an analysis is to identify groups of genes that participate in a biological activity taking place in only a subset of the samples and form a submatrix in the expression matrix. Such a submatrix is called a *bicluster*. An illustrative example of a bicluster is shown in Figure 10.11. Note how the genes that belong

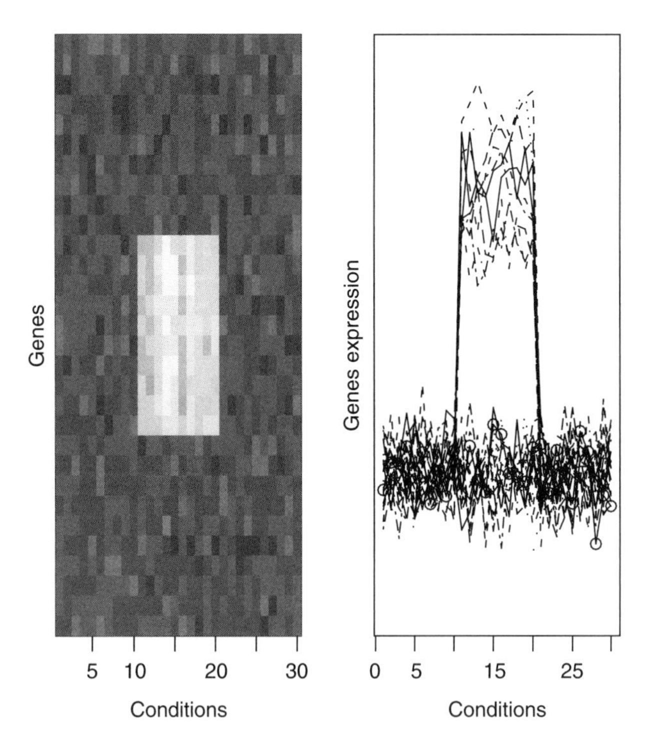

Figure 10.11 Illustrative example of a bicluster.

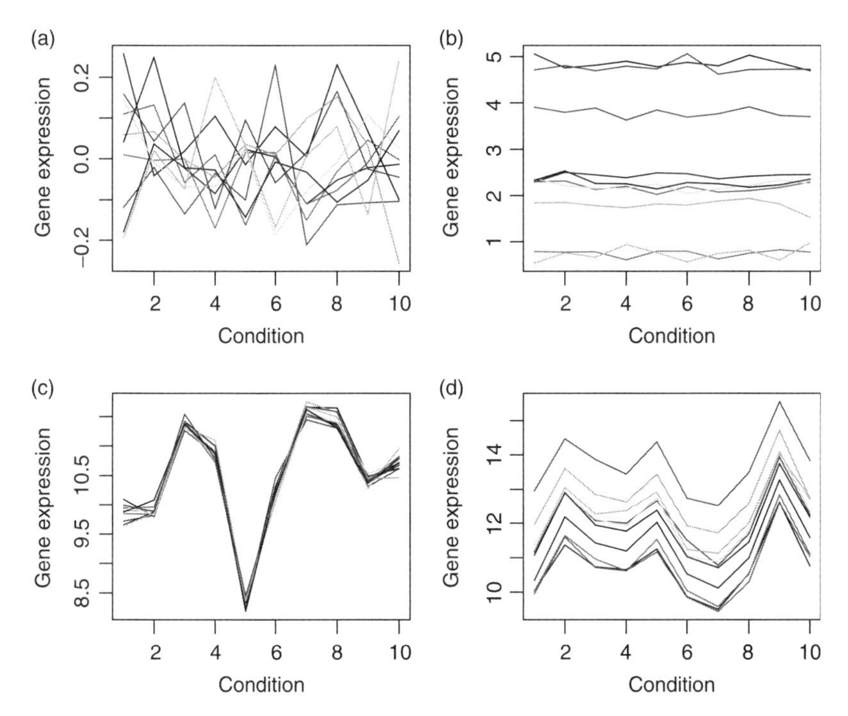

Figure 10.12 Types of bicluters. (a) Example of random noise. (b) A bicluster with constant values. (c) A bicluster with constant columns values. (d) A bicluster with both gene and samples effects.

to the bicluster have higher expression levels, across the conditions belonging to the bicluster compared to those that do not belong to the bicluster.

Madeira and Oliveira (2004) discussed several structures of biclusters: (i) bicluster with constant value, (ii) constant values by rows, (iii) constant values by columns, and (iv) coherent values/evolution of expression levels across the conditions. Examples of the different types of biclusters are shown in Figure 10.12.

Two-way clustering is somewhat more challenging than one-way clustering and new tools have been developed for this purpose. A straightforward approach, however, is to apply one-way clustering procedures separately to the rows and the columns and then to reorder the rows and the columns in such a way as to produce a two-way clustering.

10.4.1 Block Clustering

Block clustering (Hartigan, 1972; used by Tibshirani et al. (2000) for gene expression data) reorders the rows and columns of X to produce a matrix with homogeneous blocks of gene expression. The algorithm is started off with all the data in one block. At the next and each subsequent stage, the row or the column split of all existing blocks that reduces total within-block variance the most is used to create new blocks. If an existing row or column split intersects a block, the block has to be split accordingly. Otherwise, all split points are tried. The process is continued until a large number of blocks are obtained. Then some blocks are recombined until an optimum number of blocks are obtained.

A form of block clustering called *coupled two clustering* was applied to colon cancer data by Alon et al. (1999) and colon cancer and leukemia data by Getz et al. (2000).

10.4.2 Gene Shaving

Gene shaving (Hastie et al., 2000) is a two-way clustering procedure that finds possibly overlapping clusters.

Initially, each row of the gene expression matrix, X, is centered to have zero mean. Then, a linear combination of rows (i.e., genes) having maximal variation in the column space is found. This is the first principal component of the rows of X. A specified proportion (typically, 10%) of the genes having the lowest correlation with this linear combination is removed ("shaved") from the data. This process is repeated until only a single gene remains. This process generates a nested sequence of gene blocks, one of which is selected as the first cluster by optimizing a criterion, usually the gap statistic (Tibshirani et al., 2001; also see Section 10.2.3).

At the next and each subsequent step, the rows of the gene expression matrix are orthogonalized with respect to the average gene in the cluster and the above steps are repeated with the orthogonalized data to find more clusters.

10.4.3 The Plaid Model

Many biclustering methods exist and are discussed by Madeira and Oliveira (2004). In this section, we focus on the *plaid model* proposed by Lazzeroni and Owen (2002) as a method for identifying K, possibly overlapping, clusters of genes in which similarity within a cluster may extend across only a subset of the p samples.

The rough idea is that each cluster has its own mean expression level. Thus, the genes belonging to the kth cluster have mean $\mu_0 + \mu_k$ across the samples in that cluster, where μ_0 refers to a background expression level and μ_k refers to the average expression level unique to the kth cluster. This is equivalent to writing

$$X_{ij} = \mu_0 + \sum_{k=1}^{K} \mu_k \rho_{ik} \kappa_{jk} + \varepsilon_{ij},$$

where $\rho_{ik} = 1$ if and only if the ith gene belongs to the kth cluster and is zero otherwise, $\kappa_{jk} = 1$ if and only if the jth sample belongs to the kth cluster and is zero otherwise and ε_{ij} is a zero-mean error term.

The formulation can be set to be highly flexible. The constraint $\sum_{k=1}^{K} \rho_{ik} = 1$ that insists that a gene belongs to one and only one cluster is not imposed. Instead, some genes may appear in more than one cluster, so that $\sum_{k=1}^{K} \rho_{ik} \geq 2$ for those genes, and some genes may not appear in any of the clusters, so that $\sum_{k=1}^{K} \rho_{ik} = 0$

for those genes. The constraint $\sum_{k=1}^{K} \kappa_{jk} = 1$ that insists that a sample belongs to only one cluster is also not imposed. Instead, some samples may appear in more than one cluster, so that $\sum_{k=1}^{K} \kappa_{jk} \geq 2$ for those samples, and some samples may not appear in any of the clusters, so that $\sum_{k=1}^{K} \kappa_{jk} = 0$ for those samples.

It is useful to add more structure to this basic model by extending it to allow for a distinct regulatory effect for each gene and each sample within a cluster:

$$X_{ij} = \mu_0 + \sum_{k=1}^{K} (\mu_k + \alpha_{ik} + \beta_{jk}) \rho_{ik} \kappa_{jk} + \varepsilon_{ij}.$$

Observe that this model is essentially a superposition of K two-way ANOVA models. The constraints

$$\sum_{k=1}^{K} \rho_{ik} \alpha_{ik} = 0 \text{ and } \sum_{k=1}^{K} \kappa_{jk} \beta_{jk} = 0$$

are imposed to avoid over parameterization of the model. Somewhat more generality is obtained by rewriting the model as

$$X_{ij} = \sum_{k=0}^{K} \theta_{ijk} \rho_{ik} \kappa_{jk} + \varepsilon_{ij}.$$

Note that the type of the bicluster is defined by the model which is used for θ_{ijk}

$$\theta_{ijk} = \begin{cases} \mu_k, \\ \mu_k + \alpha_{ik}, \\ \mu_k + \beta_{jk}, \\ \mu_k + \alpha_{ik} + \beta_{jk}. \end{cases}$$

The case for which $\theta_{ijk} = \mu_k$ implies a constant bicluster, while $\theta_{ijk} = \mu_k + \alpha_{ik}$ and $\theta_{ijk} = \mu_k + \beta_{jk}$ imply biclusters with constant rows and constant columns, respectively. Finally, $\theta_{ijk} = \mu_k + \alpha_{ik} + \beta_{jk}$ implies a bicluster with coherent values across the genes and condition in the bicluster.

The algorithm developed by Lazzeroni and Owen (2002) is implemented in the R package `biclust`.

Example. Figure 10.13a shows an illustrative example of a 100-gene expression matrix with two biclusters. Figure 10.13b shows the first bicluster identified by the plaid model. Note that the genes belonging to the first bicluster are downregulated across the condition associated with the bicluster compared to their expression levels outside the bicluster. Figure 10.13c shows the profile plot of the genes that belong to the second bicluster across all conditions. We notice that the second bicluster is a constant bicluster for which the expression levels of the genes in the bicluster are upregulated.

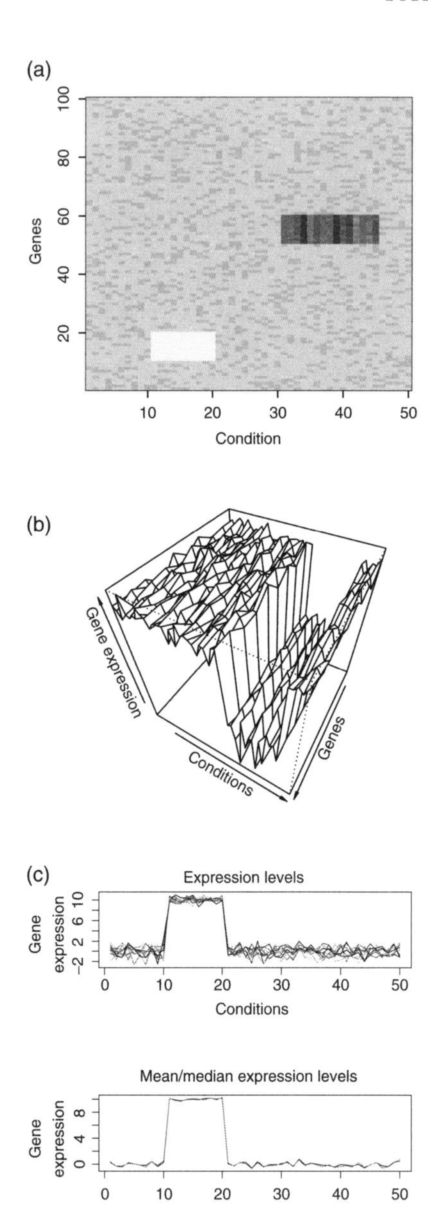

Figure 10.13 Solution of the Plaid model. (a) Illustrative example of an expression matrix with 100 genes and 50 samples with two biclusters. (b) Bicluster 1. (c) Bicluster 2.

SUPPLEMENTARY READING

There has been such an extensive body of work on the subject of cluster analysis that there are entire books devoted just to this topic, including Aldenderfer and Blashfield (1984), Everitt (1993), Gordon (1999), Hartigan (1972), and Kaufman and Rousseeuw (1990). The latter emphasizes outlier-resistant techniques. Surveys are provided by Cormack (1971) and Gnanadesikan and Kettenring (1989). A number of multivariate analysis textbooks also provide detailed accounts of clustering techniques, including Gnanadesikan (1997), Krzanowski (2000), Mardia, Kent, and Bibby (1979), and Seber (1984). The books by Hastie, Tibshirani, and Friedman (2009) and Ripley (1996) lie at the interface of statistics and data mining.

SOFTWARE NOTES

`DNAMR 2.0`

This package implements the basic methods for multivariate analysis adapted for microarray analysis that are included in this chapter. In particular it contains (i) PCA (ii) Biplot (iii) Microarray Clustering (iv) ABC clustering and (v) microarray plot `www.rci.rutgers.edu/~cabrera/DNAMR`.

`Clustering`

Functions for conventional cluster analysis methods are available in R. These include hclust (for hierarchical clustering, as described in Section 10.2.3) and kmeans (for k means clustering, as described in Section 10.2.4). The function cluster.stats in the R package fpc can be used to compare the similarity of two cluster solutions.

`ABC`

The R function ABC, which implements the ABC clustering algorithm (described in Section 10.2.7), is available in DNAMR or via the authors' websites.

`Biplots and spectral maps`

The R function biplot implements the biplot (described in Section 10.3.3) and the R library mpm implements spectral map analysis (described in Section 10.3.4).

`GGobi`

The GGobi visualization program (described in Section 10.3.7) is available at the website `http://www.ggobi.org`. It can be used for exploring high-dimensional data, both via modern dynamic and interactive graphics, as well as via more conventional visualizations.

`biclust`

The R package `biclust` available from CRAN and can be used for biclustering analysis. Several algorithms to find biclusters in two-dimensional data are implemented: Cheng and Church, Spectral, plaid model, Xmotifs, and Bimax.

`fabia`

FABIA, factor analysis for bicluster acquisition, is a biclustering method based on the FA model. The method is implemented in the bioconductor R package `fabia`.

`isa2`

The iterative signature algorithm (ISA) is a biclustering algorithm that classifies simultaneously the rows and columns of an input matrix into biclusters. The algorithm is implemented in the R package `isa2`.

`Bcdiag`

The R package `BcDiag` is available from CRAN and can be used for diagnosis of biclustering output.

`GGobi and RGobi`

This is a stand alone software for data visualization that runs on Unix and on Windows. There is also an R package called RGgobi which interfaces GGobi with R. `www.ggobi.org`

`cluster`

The R package cluster is available form CRAN and implements the k-medioids clustering algorith. It also includes a visaulisation tool called silhouette plot.

EXERCISES

10.1. Verify that D_{E}, D_{M}, D_{∞}, D_{CAN} satisfy the dissimilarity axioms (i)–(v).

10.2. Use the full Khan et al. (2001) data set of 88 samples that is included in the DNAMR package.

- **(a)** Use principal components analysis to reduce the dimension of the gene expression matrix.
- **(b)** Select the number of principal components that appears to represent the entire data set using the four criteria that are given for this purpose.
- **(c)** Graph the principal components using the (i) biplot and (ii) spectral map analysis and try to identify the clusters.

10.3. Continue with the full Khan et al. (2001) data set of 88 samples that is included in the DNAMR package.

- **(a)** Perform factor analysis (FA) using the varimax rotation procedure.

(b) Select the number of factors that appears to represent the entire data set using the four criteria that are given for this purpose.

(c) Graph the main factors using the biplot and try to interpret the factors in the graph and try to identify clusters.

(d) Compare the results with those of Problem 3.

10.4. Continue with the full Khan et al. (2001) data set of 88 samples that is included in the DNAMR package. Use a few principal components selected in Problem 2 or otherwise use the principal components data set provided in the web page of this book.

(a) Perform a cluster analysis to search for patterns among the genes using single linkage hierarchical clustering.

(b) Compare the result from part (a) with other methods such as Ward's method and average linkage.

(c) Use the results of the previous part (b) as the initial configuration for the k-means clustering procedure and compare the results.

(d) repeat part (c) using the robust k-medioids algorithm (pam) from the cluster package and compare the results with part (c).

(e) Graph the results from (a), (b), and (c) using the microarray plot in DNAMR.

10.5. Prove that when $n <=$ than p the ranks of the correlation and covariance matrices (R and S, respectively) are both at most $p-1$.

10.6. Use the R package `biclust` in order to discover biclusters in the Golub data, discussed in Chapter 1, using the Plaid model. What is the difference between the biclustering analysis in this question and the clustering methods discussed in Section 10.2?

10.7. Read the paper "FABIA: factor analysis for bicluster acquisition" by Hochreiter et al. (2010) and use the R package `fabia` in order to discover biclusters in the Golub data discussed in Chapter 1. Compare between the biclusters discovered using FABIA to the biclusters discovered using the Plaid model (implemented in the R package `biclust`).

10.8. Use the R package `bcdiag` in order to visualize one of the biclusters discover in questions 10.7 and 10.8.

CHAPTER 11

Class Prediction

Microarray experiments can be used to classify mRNA samples on the basis of the type of mRNA that is present in them. For example, suppose that mRNA samples are available from several tumors. The tumors are known to be of various different classes, but for this set of tumors, we know to which class each tumor belongs. Now, it is likely that different genes are expressed in the cells of different tumor classes. Therefore, it can be conjectured that it ought to be possible to differentiate among the tumor classes by studying and contrasting their gene expression profiles; that is, by studying how the types and amounts of mRNA present in them vary from class to class and applying *class prediction* or *supervised classification* techniques to develop a classification rule to discriminate them. The knowledge gleaned from this exercise can be used not only to gather valuable information regarding the gene expression pattern of the underlying disease process but also to predict the class of a new tumor of unknown class based on its gene expression profile.

This paradigm has tremendous potential as it is sometimes difficult to distinguish among certain tumor/cancer subtypes by clinical and histopathological means, as is current practice, but yet it is possible to discriminate among them by studying their gene expression data. The seminal paper in this regard was by Golub et al. (1999), who demonstrated its feasibility by separating out two different but clinically indistinguishable types of leukemia, ALL and AML, based on gene expression information. Incidentally, this data has been subsequently reanalyzed many times using various different methods (the book by Lin and Johnson, 2002, has several reanalyses).

Since then, many applications of this idea have been reported. For instance, Hedenfalk et al. (2001) compared gene expression profiles for two types of hereditary breast cancer (breast cancer with BRCA1 mutation and BRCA2 mutation) and found that distinctly different groups of genes are expressed by the two types, suggesting that a heritable mutation affects the gene expression profile of the cancer. Yeang et al. (2001) performed multi-class classification of 14 tumor classes by running and combining multiple binary classifiers.

Exploration and Analysis of DNA Microarray and Other High-Dimensional Data, Second Edition.
Dhammika Amaratunga, Javier Cabrera, Ziv Shkedy.

In addition, quite a few applications have used cluster analysis to analyze microarray data even when class information was available. The better the resulting clusters matched the known classes, the better the clustering was deemed to be performing and the more informative the data structures that produced those clusters. This, however, is an indirect and thereby a highly inefficient approach to the problem of classification.

We will use the Khan and Sialin data sets (see Chapter 1) to illustrate the methods of this chapter.

11.1 INITIAL CONSIDERATIONS

As in Chapter 10, the data in this chapter will be set up as a *gene expression matrix*, a $G \times p$ matrix, $X = \{x_{ij}\}$, whose G rows and p columns represent, respectively, the G genes and p samples. Depending on the experiment, the p samples may correspond to p tissues, cell lines, tumors, or something else. The p samples belong to k different classes. It is known a priori to which class each sample belongs and there are n_j samples from the jth class, $\Sigma_{j=1}^{J} n_j = p$. The p-vector, $\mathbf{y} = \{y_j\}$, indicates to which class each sample belongs: thus $y_j = s$ if the jth sample belongs to the sth class.

The values x_{ij} that make up the gene expression matrix could be either the measured gene expression level for the ith gene in the jth sample, suitably transformed and normalized, or, particularly in two-channel experiments, the log of the ratio of the normalized gene expression level for the ith gene in the jth sample relative to its corresponding value in a reference sample. A generic G-vector, $\mathbf{x} = (x_1, \ldots, x_G)$ will denote a gene expression profile, a vector of gene expression data for the G genes.

The gene expression matrix, X, functions as a *training set* (also called a *learning set* or *design set*) for classification as it is a set of samples for which the classes are known and gene expression data are available. The objective of supervised classification is to use the training set data for "training" purposes, that is, to develop a *classification rule*. The idea is that given a new sample with gene expression profile x, the classification rule can be used to predict, as accurately as possible, the true class of the new sample (assuming that its true class is one of the k classes) based on its gene expression profile, x. Generally, the classification rule will be based on a classifier that partitions the space of all possible x's into k disjoint subsets, $A_1, \ldots, A_k$, such that, if x falls into A_s, then x is predicted to belong to class s.

11.1.1 Misclassification Rates

If a classification rule predicts that x belongs to class s when the truth is that x belongs to some other class $t (t \neq s)$, then a misclassification is deemed to have occurred. The proportion of misclassifications in the training set, called the *misclassification rate*, is the most natural measure for evaluating the performance of a classification procedure.

However, because the classification rule would have been optimized, in some sense, for the training set, this raw misclassification rate tends to seriously underestimate the true error rate of the procedure.

One way to circumvent this problem is *test set cross-validation*, which consists of setting aside a portion of the samples as a *validation set* or *test set*, then constructing the classification rule based on the training set, which is now all the samples other than the test set, and using the proportion of misclassifications in the validation set as an assessment of the performance of the procedure.

Another strategy that is on the same lines, but is less wasteful use of resources, is *leave-out-one cross-validation* (LOOCV). In LOOCV, each sample in turn is set aside as a one-sample validation set and its class is predicted by constructing the classification rule based on the rest of the samples as the training set. The proportion of misclassifications is an indication of the performance of the classification procedure. A variant of this strategy is *leave-out-k cross-validation* or *V-fold cross-validation*, in which the number of samples set aside as the validation set at each step is k (where $p = kV$) rather than 1.

Bootstrap methodology (Efron and Tibshirani (1993) is a good general reference) can be used to improve the behavior of the raw misclassification rate, E_{obs}, as a measure of the true misclassification rate, E, of a classification procedure. A set of p samples, chosen at random with replacement from the original p samples, is used as the training set (called the *bootstrap training set*), with which a classification rule is constructed. The original p samples are used as the validation set, from which a misclassification rate can be determined. This is repeated several times and the average misclassification rate, E^*, is determined. The misclassification rate of the procedure is taken to be $E_{\text{boot}} = E_{\text{obs}} + (E^* - E_{\text{obs}}) = E^*$. A slightly modified version of this, called the .632 bootstrap, that has been shown to be an improvement is $E_{0.632} = 0.368E_{\text{obs}} + 0.632E^{**}$, where E^{**} is the average bootstrap misclassification rate for those samples that are not included in the bootstrap training set.

11.1.2 Reducing the Number of Classifiers

The idea is to use either the genes or certain combinations of the genes as classifiers for classifying the samples into classes. As the number of genes generally greatly exceeds the number of samples, if we were to treat all the genes as classifiers, there will a great deal more classifiers than samples. By retaining such a large number of classifiers, it is incredibly easy for a classification rule to overfit and "discover" good-looking but irreproducible and meaningless separations. This will result in a spuriously low misclassification rate in the training set, but a high misclassification rate in a test set.

There is an intuitive geometrical argument that illustrates this fact. Suppose that we have a data set of three samples and two genes, where the three samples are members of two classes. If we represent the three samples as three points in the two-dimensional plane, it is easy to see that, if the points are not aligned, there is always a line in the plane that splits the three samples into the two classes.

The same is true if we have four samples and three genes in three dimensions divided into two classes, as there is a two-dimensional plane that produces the correct classification. The argument generalizes to a data set with $p+1$ samples and p genes that spans the p-dimensional space and the samples are members of two classes. Then, there is a $(p-1)$-dimensional plane that produces the correct classification. The good behavior of this linear classification is just a geometrical artifact and should not be taken to imply that the genes in the data set are good classifiers. However, when the number of samples is much greater than the number of genes, the geometrical artifact disappears and any good classification will be a consequence of the relationship between the gene expression levels and the classes. This means that in order to demonstrate that a set of genes are genuinely good classifiers, we need to have many more samples than classifiers.

Besides this issue, biological considerations make it highly likely that, among the thousands of genes printed on an array, only a handful are really useful as classifiers in any situation, with the retention of the rest merely contributing noise and obfuscating the separation between classes. Thus, the performance of a classification procedure would be vastly improved by reducing this number beforehand to a much smaller number of relevant genes, a process known as *gene filtering*. It is best that this reduction be carried out independently of the classification rule as, otherwise, there will be a risk of overfitting, but this is rarely possible.

Besides the use of prior knowledge, the simplest strategy to reduce the number of genes is to argue that the genes that are likely to be the best classifiers will express differentially across the different classes. If this is the case, they can be identified using the tests for differential expression (e.g., the t-test, SAM, CT, or F-test, with a sufficiently low FDR) that were discussed in Chapters 7 and 8. On the other hand, Bourgon et al. (2010) argue that filtering should be done using a criterion that is independent of the separation, such as variance.

While it makes sense to eliminate as a potential classifier any gene that expresses at about the same level in all the samples, there are some problems with this approach: (i) filtering out too many genes may lead to loss of most of the classification information, particularly with the risk that some of those genes are just false discoveries, while retaining too few genes may not reduce enough noise; (ii) there may exist a set of genes that together acts as a classifier, but each individual gene in the set does not; (iii) there could be a redundancy of information as many genes may be picking up the same pattern of differential expression; and (iv) because, in microarray experiments, the gene pool is very large, there will be individual genes that, just by chance, may appear to be good classifiers in the data set at hand but this result may not be reproducible. In fact, it is possible that some of the extraordinarily good-looking results that were reported in the early days of microarray research but that subsequently failed to reproduce could be due to this phenomenon.

Another way to filter genes that overcomes many of the previous objections is to consider multiple genes simultaneously. Bo and Jonassen (2002) show that a pair of genes in combination separates two classes better than doing the filtering gene by gene. Gene pairs (or other multiples) can be selected using Hotelling's t-test (see, e.g., Mardia et al., 1979), the multivariate form of the t-test. Another effective approach to gene filtering is a by-product of the FA-based FARMS approach to summarization (described in Chapter 6.10). The percentage of variance explained by the FA generates a measure referred to as the "Informative/NonInformative call" (or "I/NI call") that captures the degree of separation information contained in a gene (Talloen et al., 2007; see also Talloen et al., 2010). This measure can be used to classify genes as potentially informative or noninformative.

Multiple genes can also be considered simultaneously by constructing linear combinations of genes. This can be done using dimension reduction methods, such as PCA or FA, which were introduced in Section 11.3. By dropping all but the most important linear combinations, these methods will produce a small set of classifiers made up of features, linear combinations of the genes, in such a way that they preserve, in some sense, almost all the information contained in the original genes. The classifiers are then *features* rather than individual genes.

Khan et al. (2001) use PCA to generate features for class prediction with microarray data. However, one nagging concern with using PCA this way is that the information we are most interested in, that is, information related to class differences, could be overwhelmed by other aspects of the data that are irrelevant to the class prediction problem. Preceding PCA or FA by a gene filtering step should mitigate this concern somewhat.

Partial least squares (PLS) is another method for defining features. PCA sequentially constructs orthogonal linear combinations, Xl, of the G genes that maximize the variance, $\text{var}(Xl)$, without paying any heed to the response or group variable, y, whereas PLS sequentially constructs orthogonal linear combinations, Xl, of the G genes that maximize the covariance, $\text{cov}(Xl, y)$ between Xl and the classes, y. This seems to address the concern with PCA mentioned above, but, if PLS was preceded by a gene filtering step, it is unlikely to produce results that are substantially different from PCA. However, Nguyen and Rocke (2002) do report an improvement in classification by using PLS rather than PCA for feature selection in a microarray context. Similar to PCA, we could obtain the PLS components using the singular value decomposition. However, the following algorithm is generalizable to the case of binary or categorical response by replacing linear regression by logistic regression.

1. Normalize all predictor variables (genes) to have mean 0 and variance 1.
2. Perform individual regression (or logistic regression) for each predictor variable x_i with the response y and get slope estimate b_i. The first PLS component is

$$X_1 = \frac{\sum_{i=1}^{G} b_i x_i}{\sqrt{\sum_{i=1}^{G} b_i^2}}.$$

3. Orthogonalize each x_i with respect to the first PLS component X_1 by

$$x_i^{\text{new}} = \frac{x_i - (x_i^T X_1)X_1}{\|x_i - (x_i^T X_1)X_1\|}.$$

4. Repeat steps 2 and 3 k times as needed, replacing x_i by x_i^{new} to obtain X_2, $X_3, \ldots, X_k$. k must be less or equal the minimum of n and G.

This algorithm does not need to modify y during the iterations and the model in step 2 could be a linear model or a logistic model or any other suitable model to predict y, so it is very general. Examples of this algorithm are shown with the enriched methods in Section 11.7.

An alternative is to run a PCA as above and then rank the principal components in the order suggested by the ratio of between-class variance to within-class variance. This strategy was originally proposed by Krzanowski (1992) for a chemometrics problem and then was implemented and extended by Landgrebe et al. (2002) and Coombes (2002) for classifying microarray data. An alternative that may be able to do this more directly is projection pursuit regression (Friedman and Stuetzle, 1981), which tries to find smooth functions of the linear combinations Xl that correlate with the response, y.

Yet another way to reduce the effective number of classifiers is to run a clustering procedure over the set of genes or a large interesting subset of them and form features that are the averages of the clusters or, alternatively, one or two principal components.

Many researchers have recognized the importance of classifier selection for microarray classification problems. Golub et al. (1999), Dudoit et al. (2002) and Bourgon, Gentleman, and Huber (2010) discuss individual gene selection, and the latter two, in particular, demonstrate how the performance of many classification rules can be improved by reducing the number of classifiers. Several papers in the book edited by Lin and Johnson (2002) also discuss the general issue.

For simplicity, in the remainder of this chapter, we refer to G classifiers even though the actual number of classifiers may have been reduced to a smaller number.

Example. We illustrate some of the proposed dimension reduction techniques with the Khan data set example of the four types of SRBCT.

Method 1. Take the first 10 principal components for the entire set of 2308 genes. As the sample covariance matrix is a 2308×2308 singular matrix of rank 62, we use the singular value decomposition described in Chapter 9. Figure 11.1 shows the scatterplot of the 63 training samples and the 25 test samples in the coordinates of the first two principal components (i.e., the first two PCA basis). The training samples are represented by small filled symbols, while the testing samples are the unfilled larger symbols. The test set symbols in the graph show a nearly random pattern indicating that two principal components are not enough to produce a good classification rule.

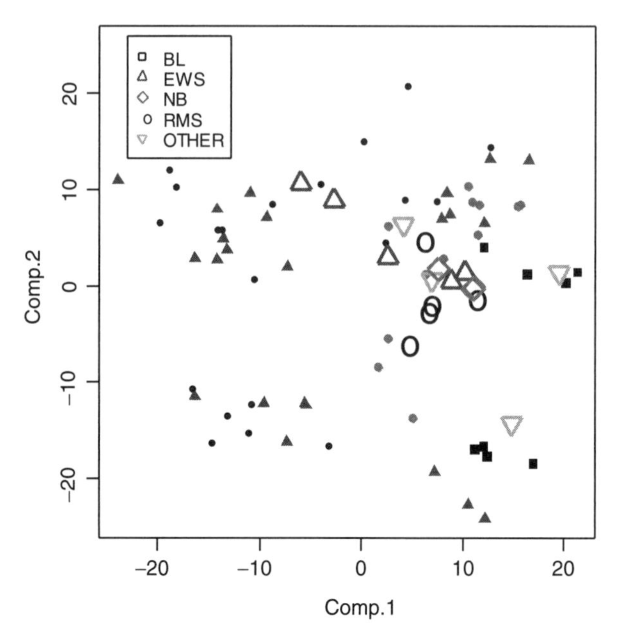

Figure 11.1 This graph shows the 63 training samples and the 25 test samples in the coordinates of the first two PCA basis. The training samples are represented by small filled symbols, while the testing samples are the unfilled larger symbols. The data shows a nearly random pattern that illustrates the poor performance of this classification rule.

Method 2. Select the genes that have a significant F-statistic at $\alpha = 0.001$ the level and take the top 10 principal components. This subset contains a total of 450 significant genes. As in the previous case, the sample covariance matrix is high dimensional and highly singular and hence the principal components are calculated with the singular value decomposition method. Figure 11.2 shows the scatterplot of the 63 training samples and the 25 test samples in the two first PCA basis with the same style as Figure 11.1. The data shows a clear separation between the four classes for both training and testing sets that suggest that this dimension reduction method will produce good classification rules.

Method 3a. Select the 50 most significant genes for the F-statistic and cluster the genes into 10 clusters. Take the average of the genes in each cluster to produce a set of 10 classification variables. The variables can be sorted in order of significance using the values of the F-statistic. Figure 11.3 shows the scatterplot of the 63 training samples and the 25 test samples in the two first PCA basis with the same style as Figures 11.1 and 11.2. The data shows a clear separation between the four classes for both training and testing sets that is almost as good as the one in Figure 11.2. This suggests that this dimension reduction method will produce good classification rules.

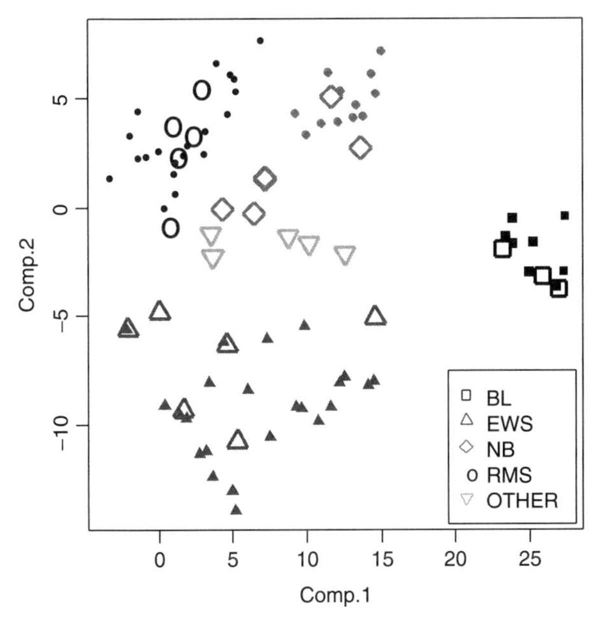

Figure 11.2 Principal components for 450 significant genes. This graph shows the 63 training samples and the 25 test samples in the two first PCA basis. The data shows a strong clustering pattern that explains the excellent performance of the classification rules. The solid symbols represent the training set points and the hollow symbols represent the testing set.

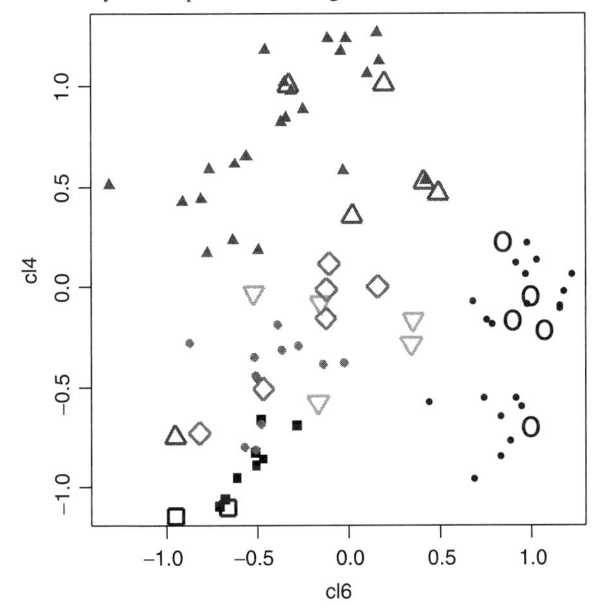

Figure 11.3 Two cluster means of 50 significant genes. This graph shows the 63 training samples and the 25 test samples in the two first PCA basis. The data shows a strong clustering pattern that explains the excellent performance of the classification rules. The solid symbols represent the training set points and the hollow symbols represent the testing set.

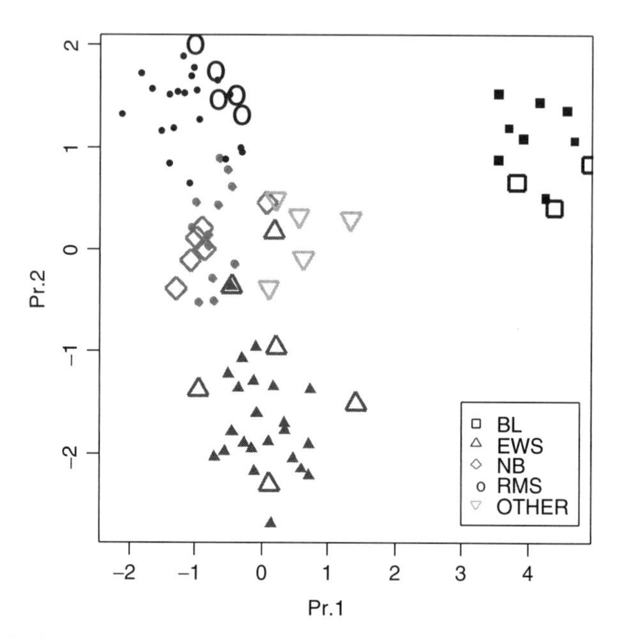

Figure 11.4 The first two principal components for the means of 10 clusters obtained from a subset of the top 50 significant genes. This graph shows the 63 training samples and the 25 test samples in the two first PCA basis. The graph shows that for the EWS tumors two observations in the testing and one in the training are in the boundary with the group of NB tumors.

Method 3b. This is a variant of the previous method. Take the 10 classifiers in method 3a and calculate the 10 principal components. The 10 principal components will produce the same classification rule similar to that of the previous 10 cluster mean variables but there maybe subsets of principal components that perform better than equal size sets of cluster means. Figure 11.4 shows a clear separation between the four classes for both training and testing sets that is as good as the one in Figure 11.1. This suggests that this dimension reduction method will produce good classification rules.

Method 4. Select the 30 most significant genes for the F-statistic and take the top 10 principal components. Figure 11.5 shows the scatterplot of the 63 training samples and the 25 test samples in the two first PCA basis. The data shows a clear separation between the four classes for both training and testing sets that suggest that this dimension reduction method will produce good classification rules.

11.2 LINEAR DISCRIMINANT ANALYSIS

The oldest and one of the simplest methods of supervised classification, *linear discriminant analysis* (LDA; Fisher, 1936), endures to this day as one of most

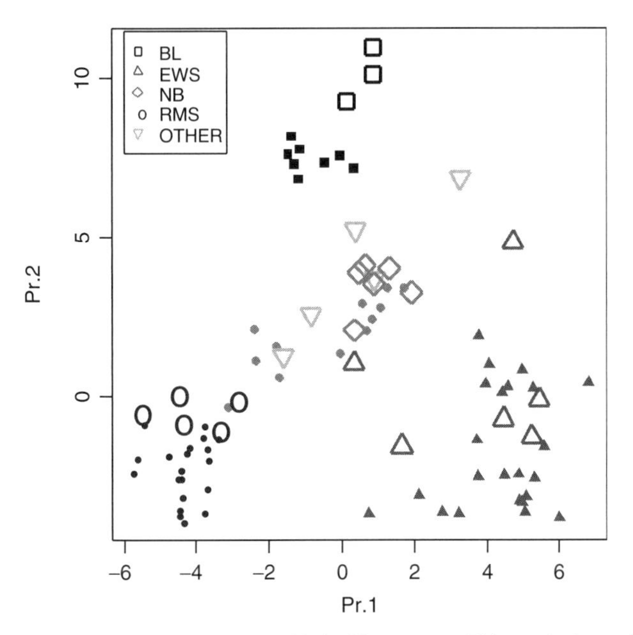

Figure 11.5 Principal components for the top 30 significant genes. This graph shows the 63 training samples and the 25 test samples in the two first PCA basis. The data shows a strong clustering pattern that explains the excellent performance of the classification rules.

popular classification techniques. It is based on finding the linear projections (views) of the data that most effectively separates out the k-classes.

The most common situation is the case $k = 2$, that is, when there are just two classes of samples. In this case, classification can be based on the projection $w'x$, where the projection is made in the direction w where the classes are most widely separated in the training set. Letting n_s, the G-vector $\overline{x}_s$, and the $G \times G$ matrix S_s denote, respectively, the sample size, the mean, and the variance-covariance matrix of the sth class in the training set, and letting $S = (n_1 - 1)S_1 + (n_2 - 1)S_2/(n_1 + n_2 - 2)$ denote the pooled variance-covariance matrix, a standardized measure of the separation between the two samples in the training set in the direction w is given by

$$\lambda = \frac{(w'\overline{x}_1 - w'\overline{x}_2)^2}{w'Sw}.$$

The direction w that maximizes λ is

$$w = S^{-}(\overline{x}_1 - \overline{x}_2),$$

where S^{-} denotes the generalized inverse of S, because, with microarray data, S will almost always be singular. The classification rule is then based on the *linear classifier*:

$$w'x = (\overline{x}_1 - \overline{x}_2)'S^{-}x.$$

The classification rule is

If $w'x > w'(\overline{x}_1 - \overline{x}_2)'/2$ then x is classified as belonging to Class 1. Otherwise x is classified as belonging to Class 2.

While no distributional assumptions were made in the above derivation, this rule can also be obtained under the assumption that the data are normally distributed with the same variance-covariance matrix, in which case the rule can also be shown to possess various optimality properties.

This method can be readily generalized to the case of more than two classifiers (Rao, 1948). Again let n_s, the G-vector, and the $G \times G$ matrix S_s denote, respectively, the sample size, the mean, and the variance-covariance matrix of the sth class in the training set. Let

$$\overline{x}\frac{\Sigma_{s=1}^{k} n_s \overline{x}_s}{\Sigma_{s=1}^{k} n_s} \text{ and } S = \frac{\Sigma_{s=1}^{k}(n_s - 1)S_s}{\Sigma_{s=1}^{k}(n_s - 1)},$$

denote the overall mean and pooled variance-covariance matrix. Then, a standardized measure of the separation between the k sample means in the training set in the direction w is given by

$$\lambda = \frac{w'Bw}{w'Sw},$$

where $B = \Sigma_{s=1}^{k}(\overline{x}_s - \overline{x})(\overline{x}_s - \overline{x})'$ is the between-class matrix.

The extreme values of λ correspond to the eigenvalues, $\lambda_1, \ldots, \lambda_t$, and eigenvectors, $w_1, \ldots, w_t$ of $S^{-}B$, where S^{-} denote the generalized inverse of S. There are at most $t = \min(k-1, G)$ distinct eigenvalues. The eigenvector that corresponds to the largest of these eigenvalues is the direction in which the classes are maximally separated in the training set and provides the view of most interest. On the other hand, the eigenvectors corresponding to the smallest eigenvalues tend to obscure the separation of the samples into classes.

Let $D_h(x) = \Sigma_{s=1}^{i}[(x - \overline{x}_h)'w_s]^2$ denote the squared distance (in terms of the t eigenvectors) of x from the hth class mean. Then, x is predicted to belong to the class whose mean is closest to x, that is, to the class, h, which has the smallest value of $D_h(x)$. This is equivalent to using the linear discriminant function:

$$L_h(x) = \overline{x}_h' S^{-} x - \frac{1}{2}\overline{x}_h' S^{-} \overline{x}_h$$

and assigning x to the class with the largest $L_h(x)$.

It has been found that LDA with no initial gene filtering does not perform well. Indeed, in the comparison study of Dudoit et al. (2002), it was one of the worst performers. Besides the issues discussed in Section 11.1.2, the difficulty of estimating S efficiently with a very small p, a common problem in microarray studies where replication is limited, is at least partly responsible for this phenomenon. In fact, the performance of LDA improves significantly with aggressive gene filtering.

Example. In order to illustrate the use of the LDA method and the improvement garnered by gene filtering, we apply it to the four variable reduction methods in Section 11.2. Since each reduction method produces 10 classifiers in a given order, we apply LDA to a few subsets in the given order. The results are shown in Table 11.1. The message is very clear, because procedures 2, 3, and 4 did reasonably well and much better than 1. In particular, procedures 3 and 4 used very few genes. Procedure 3 with four classifiers used only 20 genes, which was the lowest in terms of number of genes.

11.3 EXTENSIONS OF FISHER'S LDA

Fisher's basic method has, over the years, been extended in various ways.

- *Quadratic Discriminant Analysis (QDA).* Dropping LDA's assumption that the true variance covariance matrices of the classes are the same produces the QDA classification rule: assign x to the class with the largest value of

$$Q_h(x) = (x - \overline{x})S_h^{-}(x - \overline{x}_h)' + \log(s_h).$$

Example. We repeated the LDA analysis using the QDA method. As each reduction method produces 10 classifiers in a given order, we apply LDA to a few subsets in the given order. The results are shown in Table 11.2 are more or less the same as Table 11.1, perhaps slightly worse in the sense that they vary a bit more among the last three variable reduction procedures. The explanation is that some of the class sizes are very small (8 is the smallest one, so we may use a maximum of seven classifiers), and in such cases, using a QDA rule means increasing the numbers of parameters in the model to a point that it may produce a worse fit. In any case, the differences between QDA and LDA are small.

- *Diagonal Linear Discriminant Analysis (DLDA).* A special case of QDA occurs when S_h is set to be a diagonal matrix that is the same for every class. Thus, correlations between genes and variance differences between

Table 11.1 Results of Fisher LDA for the Four Rules for Selecting Classifiers Giving the Number of Misclassifications for Both Training and Testing Samples

	10 PC of 2308 Genes		10 PC of 450 Genes		10 Cluster Means of 50 Genes		10 PC of 30 Genes	
	Training	Testing	Training	Testing	Training	Testing	Training	Testing
2 Classifiers	35	13	0	2	4	2	3	2
3 Classifiers	5	5	0	0	0	1	1	1
4 Classifiers	0	3	0	0	0	0	0	0
10 Classifiers	0	3	0	0	0	0	0	0

Table 11.2 Results of QDA for the Four Rules for Selecting Classifiers Giving the Number of Misclassifications for Both Training and Testing Samples

	10 PC of 2308 Genes		10 PC of 450 Genes		10 Cluster Means of 50 Genes		10 PC of 30 Genes	
	Training	Testing	Training	Testing	Training	Testing	Training	Testing
2 Classifiers	26	14	0	2	3	2	4	6
3 Classifiers	0	6	0	1	1	1	0	5
4 Classifiers	0	6	0	1	0	0	0	0
7 Classifiers	0	3	0	0	0	0	0	0

samples are ignored. It turns out that similar to LDA, DLDA is a linear classification rule. Dudoit et al. (2002) found that DLDA to be one of the strongest performers in their comparison study.

- *Diagonal Quadratic Discriminant Analysis (DQDA).* Another special case of QDA is when S_h is set to be a diagonal matrix that is different across classes. This is a quadratic classification rule.
- *Regularized Discriminant Analysis (RDA).* When the sample sizes in the training set are small, as is typically the case with microarray data, it is likely to be difficult to estimate S_h efficiently. Consequently, the performance of QDA may not offer an improvement over LDA, even though the covariance matrices of the classes are moderately different (as we saw in the above example). A compromise is to use a weighted average of S_h and S,

$$S_h^* = \frac{(\alpha - 1)S_h + \alpha S}{(\alpha - 1)n_h + \alpha n},$$

as an estimate of the covariance matrix of the hth class. QDA is then applied as above with $S*_h$ in place of S_h, with the value of α estimated to maximize performance via cross-validation. This compromise was reached by shrinking S_h toward a common value, S, along the lines of the concept of regularization, which suggests shrinking a highly parametrized model towards one that is less highly parametrized. It has been demonstrated that regularization improves certain properties of the estimation, at the cost, however, of a slightly biased fit. Another mode of regularization is to shrink S toward a diagonal matrix. It has being argued (see, e.g., Friedman, 1989) that one advantage of this double regularization for the classification problem is that it can be used to reduce the emphasis of the smaller eigenvalues.
- *Prediction Analysis for Microarrays (PAM).* The plan behind this method proposed by Tibshirani et al. (2002) is to use a simple centroid distance classification rule but to regularize by shrinking the centroids in a similar way as was done in the SAM method described in Section 7.3. Define the G-dimensional vector, $d_j = (\overline{x}_j - \overline{x})/[m_j(s + s_0)]$, where $m_j = \sqrt{1/n_j + 1/n}$, s is a vector of length G containing the within-class standard deviations for

each of the G genes and s_0 is a fixed constant equal to the median of the components of s. We define the new shrunken centroids as

$$\overline{x}_j = \overline{x} + m_j(s + s_0)d'_j,$$

where $d'_j = \text{sign}(d_j)(|d_j| - \Delta)_+$ and Δ is a fixed scalar. The sign function gives a vector of the signs of the components of d_j, that is, it returns a vector of $+1$'s, -1's, and 0's for positive, negative, and zero components, respectively. The value of Δ is chosen according to the method of cross-validation described in Section 11.5. The procedure has an in-built gene selection mechanism as the vector d'_j may have some zero components, which would imply that those genes are automatically excluded as classifiers.

- *Flexible Discriminant Analysis (FDA).* This method consists of two steps. First, a nonlinear model is fitted to the data using a binary numeric representation of the response. For this step, any nonlinear nonparametric regression estimator, such as generalized additive models, lowess, projection pursuit regression, or MARS, can be used. Second, a linear discriminant classification rule is applied to the fitted values from the first step as predictor variable and the same response variable. Hastie et al. (1994) provide further details.
- *Bayes Rule.* In the event that prior probabilities $(\pi_1, \ldots, \pi_k)$ can be assigned to the k classes, classification by Bayes' rule is to assign x to the class with the largest value of

$$L_h^B(x) = \overline{x}'_h S^- x + \frac{1}{2}\overline{x}'_h S^- \overline{x}_h + \log(\pi_h).$$

Other regularization methods for discriminant analysis are described in the Section 11.4.

11.4 PENALIZED METHODS

One of the most popular general ideas for gene selection is to estimate a model such as a linear or logistic model by adding a constraint to the criterion that is being minimized.

For least squares regression, the criterion being minimized becomes

$$\tilde{\beta} = \text{argmin}_\beta \sum_{i=1}^{n} \left(y_i - \beta_0 - \sum_{j=1}^{G} x_{ij}\beta_j \right)^2 + \lambda \sum_{j=1}^{G} |\beta_j|^k \qquad (11.1)$$

When k=1, the resulting method is called the *LASSO* (Tibshirani, 1996). When k=2, the resulting method corresponds to ridge regression. The case when k=0 corresponds to variable selection. The idea is to estimate β along the values of λ creating a "solution path," which is a regularization path of estimates of the β_i's given a sequence of λ's. LARS (Efron et al., 2004; Rosset and Zhu, 2007) is an algorithm for efficiently computing the solution path for the LASSO.

Once the solution path is computed, we find the optimal λ and the corresponding β_i's that optimizes some performance criteria such as the cross-validated mean square error (MSE) along the solution path.

One interesting feature of the LASSO is that along the solution path many β_i's may become zero, thus performing gene selection automatically. Hence, the LASSO may be used for gene selection by selecting those genes with non-zero coefficients.

One variant of the LASSO is elastic net (Zou and Hastie, 2005) that combines both LASSO and ridge penalties by minimizing

$$\tilde{\beta} = \text{argmin}_\beta \sum_{i=1}^{n} \left(y_i - \beta_0 - \sum_{j=1}^{G} x_{ij}\beta_j \right)^2 + \lambda \left(\sum_{j=1}^{G} \alpha|\beta_j| + \frac{1-\alpha}{2}|\beta_j|^2 \right)$$

For $\alpha = 0$, the elastic net constraint corresponds to ridge regression, and for $\alpha = 1$, it is the same as the LASSO.

The elastic net solution path is computed by a step of data augmentation followed by the LASSO algorithm. It has the advantage of providing more stable solutions that are less affected by colinearities because of the effect of the ridge part of the penalty.

And, similar to the LASSO, it also performs gene selection, although the final fit will not be as sparse as with LASSO (i.e., more genes are retained with non-zero coefficients).

However, the computational burden is increased by the data augmentation step.

A faster algorithm but follows a different regularization path is GLMNET (Friedman et al., 2010). GLMNET uses cyclical coordinate descent, and it is computationally faster and more suitable for microarray data.

One reasonable procedure to use the GLMNET algorithm is to start with $\alpha = 0.99$ (i.e., a bit below $\alpha = 1$) because it stabilizes the LASSO in cases where there are strong colinearities. Then, proceed by lowering the value of α and compare the performance of the different models estimated for different α's.

We will show examples of these methods in Section 11.11 with the enriched methods.

11.5 NEAREST NEIGHBORS

Nearest-neighbor methods for classification (first proposed by Fix and Hodges, 1951) are among the oldest and more successful classification methods.

Following the notation in Section 11.1, let x_j represent the jth sample and y_j give the class number of the jth sample. Let x be the candidate sample for classification, and let $S_{k,x}$ be the set of the k-nearest neighbors (kNNs) of x in the training set. The simplest kNN method consists of estimating the probability that

x belongs to the ith class $p(i|x)$ by the proportion of the kNNs that belong to the ith class

$$p(i|x) = \frac{\#\{g_j = i|x_j \in S_k, x\}}{k}$$

The classification rule is based on a "majority vote": x is assigned to the ith class if i maximizes the probability $\hat{p}(i|x)$.

This method assumes that $p(i|x)$ is approximately constant in the region containing the kNNs of x, for all i. In practice, this means that the number, p, of samples should be large and the number, G, of genes should be small compared to p, which is a typical of microarray experiments. As this is never the case, a few of the principal components or factors should be taken as classifiers as explained in Section 11.1.1.

Dudoit et al. (2002) found that, along with DLDA, kNN had very good performance in their comparison study, particularly when it was preceded by gene filtering. Pomeroy et al. (2002) analyzed microarray data from 99 patients using kNN after gene filtering and demonstrated that medulloblastomas, the most common malignant brain tumors of childhood, were molecularly distinct from other brain tumors.

More sophisticated implementations of the kNN method are readily available, for example,

1. The decision rule can be rendered more complex by introducing the idea of a loss function. Let l_{ij} represent the loss that is sustained by stating that x belongs to the ith class when, in reality, x belongs to the jth class. Then, we calculate the risks as

$$r_i = \Sigma_{j=1}^{p} l_{ij} \hat{p}(j|x).$$

   The decision rule will assign x to the class that gives the minimum of the risks r_i.
2. By rescaling the variables by dividing them by their corresponding standard deviations before computing the kNNs, the distance between the samples will be scale independent.
3. Friedman (1994) introduced a combination of nearest neighbors and recursive partitioning that is very successful.

Example. We redo the classification using the kNN method. The results are shown in Table 11.3 are more or less the same as Table 11.1, perhaps slightly worse in the sense that only procedure 3 achieves zero misclassifications.

11.6 RECURSIVE PARTITIONING

A classification rule induces a partition in the space of all possible samples that assigns each possible sample to a class. The best partition is usually selected by optimizing a classification criterion. In reality, the number of possible partitions

Table 11.3 Results of ANN for the Four Rules for Selecting Classifiers Giving the Number of Misclassifications for the Testing Samples

	10 PC of 2308 Genes		10 PC of 450 Genes		10 Cluster Means of 50 Genes		10 PC of 30 Genes	
	Training	Testing	Training	Testing	Training	Testing	Training	Testing
2 Classifiers	18	14	0	2	0.5	1.5	0	3.5
3 Classifiers	8	14	0	1	0	0.5	0	1.5
4 Classifiers	0	3	0	0.5	0	0.5	0	1.5
10 Classifiers	0	8	0	0.5	0	0.5	0	1.5

produced by a method depends only on the configuration of the observed samples, and as a result, the number of possible partitions grows exponentially with the number of samples in our data set. In most practical cases, it is not possible to find the globally optimal partition and we resort to methods that produce nearly optimal partitions. One such method is recursive partitioning that is used to generate classification trees.

Trees are the obvious method for displaying the results of recursive partitioning and, consequently, statisticians have been growing them at least since Sonquist and Morgan (1964). Many methods for growing classification trees have been proposed by statisticians [e.g., CHAID (Hartigan, 1975), FIRM (Hawkins and Kass, 1982), CART (Breiman et al., 1984), SPlus TREE (Clark and Pregibon, 1992)] and computer scientists [e.g., C4.5 (Quinlan, 1993)]. These conventional recursive partitioning methods generate partitions of the samples with the goal of reaching a partition that generates a good prediction rule. Zhang et al. (2001) apply recursive partitioning to classify tumors using microarray data.

In Figure 11.6a, we show a simple classification function of two variables $f(X, Y)$, which is expressed in the form of a tree rule in Figure 11.6b. The way to read the tree is "If $X \geq 2$ then class 1, if $X < 2$ and $Y \geq 2$ then class 2," and so on. One of the nice properties of such trees is that they produce classification rules that have a wide appeal because they resemble decision rules that are easier to understand compared to most other competitive methods.

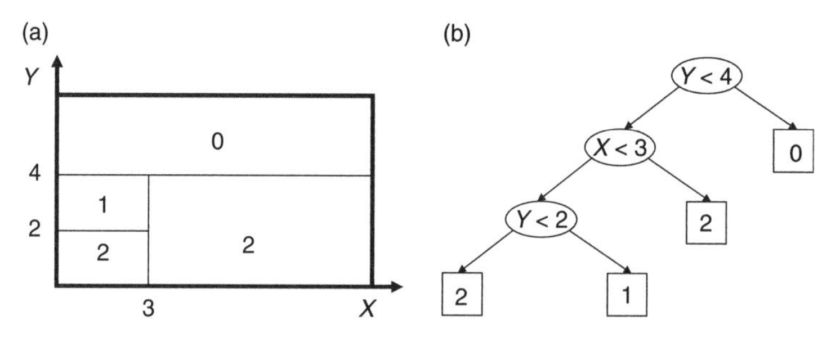

Figure 11.6 Classification tree for a function $f(X, Y)$. (a) Function $f(x, y)$ and (b) tree form of $f(x, y)$.

11.6.1 Classification Trees

A *classification tree* is an easily understandable way of graphically displaying the results of a recursive partitioning procedure. For gene expression data, the inputs to a classifier are gene expressions, ratios of gene expressions, or linear combinations thereof, obtained from PCA or FA. The example in Figure 11.7 shows a classification tree. The process of building a classification tree has two stages (i) building the tree and (ii) pruning the tree.

Building the Tree. A binary tree begins at a root node where the data is split into two buckets using one of the classification variables from the set. The split is performed by optimizing one of the criteria below over all possible partitions generated by some logical condition in any of the classification variables. The conditions are of the form: $x_i > c$ goes to the right bucket and $x_i \leq c$ goes to the left bucket. This produces two new nodes, right and left (R, L), which are split into two buckets each by the same process that took place at the root node. If the size of a node is less than a predetermined constant m then the node is labeled a terminal node, and it is not split. The process continues until all nodes have either been split or are terminal nodes. The result is a binary tree that produces a partition (made up of terminal nodes).

In some microarray data analysis classification problems, we may use categorical classifiers; for example, instead of using the spot intensity X as a classifier variable, we find that the spot intensities have been categorized into variables Z reflecting that a group of one or more genes are all highly expressed $(Z = 1)$, or not all

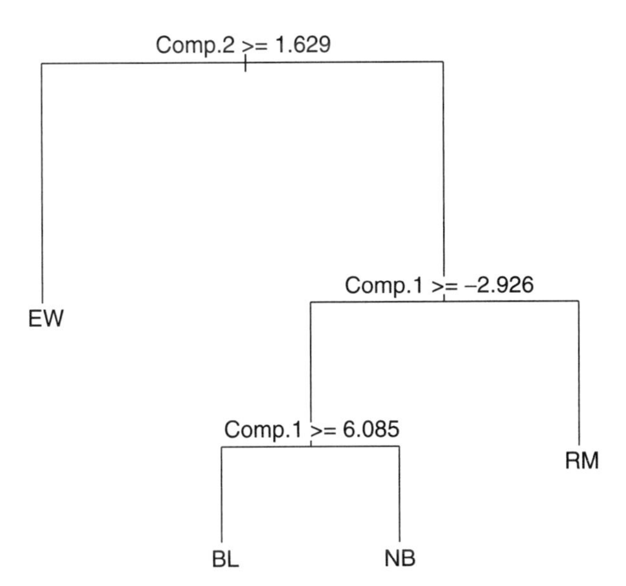

Figure 11.7 Classification tree for the cancer groups using 10 principal components of the top 100 cancer genes. The classification rule produces zero mistakes in the training set and five mistakes in the testing set.

highly expressed ($Z = 0$). These classifiers may generate categorical splits where the categories of Z are split into two groups such that the splitting criterion is minimized.

Let us consider the case when the objective is to classify the samples into only two classes, class 0 and class 1. The objective of the tree method is to produce a partition of terminal nodes that are relatively pure in the sense that almost all the observations at a terminal node belong to only one class. The most popular criteria that have been proposed to achieve this goal are as follows:

- *Gini Index.* This is the criterion used in the original version of *classification and regression tree* (CART) methodology by Breiman et al. (1984). The objective function is
$$C_g = qq_R P_R + pq_L P_L,$$
where p and q are the proportions of observations going to the left and right buckets, p_L and q_L are the proportions of 0's and 1's in the left side bucket and p_R and q_R are the proportion of 0's and 1's in the right side bucket, respectively.
- *Entropy.* This criterion is used by the C4.5/C5 algorithms by Quinlan (1993) that is very widely used in computer science applications:
$$C_e = q(-q_R) \log q_R - p_R \log p_R) + p(-q_L \log q_L - P_L \log P_L).$$
- *Tree.* A deviance-based criterion proposed by Clark and Pregibon (1992) has been implemented in statistical software such as `SPLUS` and `R`:
$$C_t = q \min(p_L, p_R).$$

A less well-known, but interesting, criterion is Buja and Lee's (2001) data mining criterion,
$$C_{LB} = \frac{n_L \hat{\sigma}^2 L + n_R \hat{\sigma}^2 R}{n_R + n_L}.$$

Many criteria described above are widely used by practitioners and the choice of the "best" criterion remains an open question.

The tree method can also be applied for regression analysis, that is, when there is a continuous response variable that is analyzed by a tree model. The splitting criterion is
$$C_r = \frac{n_L \hat{\sigma}^2 L + n_R \hat{\sigma}^2 R}{n_R + n_L},$$
where $n_R, \hat{\sigma}_R^2$ and $n_L, \hat{\sigma}_L^2$ are the number of observations and sample variance in the right and left buckets, respectively.

Pruning the Tree. The tree-building step is likely to experience two kinds of problems:

1. An overfitted tree, with small buckets at the terminal nodes.
2. An oversized tree that is hard for the practitioner to interpret.

A way to correct these problems is by pruning the tree. As step 1 of the tree-building procedure produces an ordered sequence of trees, the question becomes where to stop.

One procedure to do this is *test set cross-validation*, which consists of separating a portion of the data (25–50%) that we will call testing set and leave the remaining part of the data set for training (as described in Section 11.1.1). The tree is built using the training set alone and results in an ordered sequence of trees. For each tree in the sequence, a misclassification rate is estimated using the testing set alone, and the tree with the lowest misclassification rate is chosen. This procedure requires a large initial data set and, even then, it seems unnatural to discard a part of the data set for training because it will reduce the performance of the method. An alternative technique that improves on this is called *V-fold cross-validation* details, which can be found in Breiman et al. (1984).

One weakness of classification trees is that some nodes may have few observations, making the predictions at those nodes unreliable. Techniques have been proposed to improve the predictive ability at those nodes and therefore of the tree, in general. Two such procedures are bootstrap aggregating or bagging (Breiman, 1996) and boosting (Freund and Schapire, 1997). The idea behind both these methods is to produce slightly perturbed classifiers from the training data by resampling. Bagging generates replicate training sets by sampling with replacement from the training set. Boosting retains all the samples, but weights each sample differently and generates different classifiers by adjusting the weights. Each method generates multiple classifiers that are combined by voting to form a composite classifier. In bagging, each component classifier has the same vote, while in boosting, each component classifier has a different vote based on the assessment of its accuracy. Dudoit et al. (2002) found that boosting and bagging improves the performance of CART-like procedures with microarray data.

Example. In Figure 11.7, we show a tree graph generated using the tree method with the four-tumor data example. The input classifiers are the two top principal components of the best 100 genes and the node splitting criterion used was the Gini index. The method produced a tree with three splits and four terminal nodes that fits the training data perfectly and has five misclassification errors in the 20 testing samples. This performance is typical of trees with small training sets.

11.6.2 Activity Region Finding

The activity region finding (ARF) method for growing classification trees was proposed by Amaratunga and Cabrera (2003a). ARF trees are trees that exclude large parts of the data where no information is available and concentrate only in subsets that contain the important information. The advantage of ARF over recursive partitioning (RP) methods is that it produces simpler more condensed trees in cases where RP methods give very complex and elaborate trees that are hard to interpret.

Building the ARF Tree. The ARF tree is a ternary tree, that is, each node is split into three groups. The splits are of the form $c_1 < x_i < c_2$, so there are three subgroups.

The basis of the ARF approach is the H criterion. For data of the form $D = \{(Y_i, x_i)\}$, where $i = 1, \ldots, N$, Y_i is a Bernoulli variable, which is either 0 ("failure") or 1 ("success"), and $x_i = (x_{1i}, \ldots, x_{ri})'$ is an r-vector of predictor variables. The objective is to discover *high activity regions* (HARs) ranges of values of x (i.e., subsets of the form $S = \Pi I_k$, as described above) associated with high values of $\text{Prob}(Y = 1|S)$ (i.e., with high success probabilities).

It is natural to consider that, for the kth predictor variable, x_k, an "interesting" interval, $I_k = \{a_k \leq x_k \leq b_k\}$, is one that has a substantially higher proportion of successes compared to D, that is, one such that $p(I_k) = \text{Prob}(Y = 1|I_k)$ is substantially larger than $p(D) = \text{Prob}(Y = 1|D)$. In order to compare $p(I_k)$ across subsets, I_k, of different sizes on an equal footing, we need a statistic that is not much dependent on $n(I_k)$, the number of observations in I_k. Such a statistic is

$$z(I_k; D) = \frac{p(I_k) - p(D)}{\sigma_p},$$

where $\sigma_p^2 = P(D)(1 - P(D))/n(I_k)$, as $z(I_k; D)$ is approximately N(0, 1), irrespective of sample size, except for very small samples, for a random binary series of length N with success probability $p(D)$. The larger the value of $z(I_k; D)$, the more interesting is I_k.

11.7 ENSEMBLE METHODS

The idea underlying ensemble methodology is to generate multiple model fits from a single training set with the intention of combining them so as to produce a single classification for each test sample that is more accurate and reliable than a prediction based on any single model fit. It is akin to seeking several opinions before making a crucial decision, weighing the individual opinions, and then combining them to reach a final decision.

Generally, ensembles are collections of model fits that are minor variants of the same basic model fit. The variation in these ensembles is generated via random perturbations of the fitting procedure. Hybrids in which the variants are not from the same model family have also been proposed. In either case, the basic general criteria for the variants is the same: each constituent fit should be reasonably accurate and also reasonably diverse. If most of the fits were not accurate, then it is unlikely that a combination would be either. If the fits were not diverse, then generating multiple model fits would not be necessary, one should suffice. Ultimately, the expectation is that, if the model fits were indeed generally accurate and diverse, then even if a few of the fits were erroneous, there is a chance that the other fits would be correct and, as a result, the consensus decision should also be correct.

Ensemble methods have been found to be among the most successful methods for classifying high-dimensional data.

11.7.1 Random Forest

We begin with a description of the most popular ensemble method: random forest (Breiman (2001); Breiman and Cutler (2003) provide further details).

In a random forest, a tree, rather than being trained on the entirety of the training set, is trained only on a sample of p' samples drawn at random with replacement from the complete set of p samples (where $p' < p$). These are called the *in-bag samples*; the rest are set aside as *out-of-bag samples*. In addition, when determining which gene to split on at each node, only a subset of g of the G genes (usually $g = G^{1/2}$) are considered eligible; this subset is drawn at random without replacement independently at each node from the complete set of G genes.

A random forest is an ensemble (i.e., a collection) of some number R of such trees, where each tree is called a *base classifier*. Classes are assigned to test samples by majority vote: when given a test sample, each tree assigns it a class according to its classifier; this information is collated, and overall, the forest assigns it the most frequent class.

The out-of-bag samples in any tree can be regarded as test samples for that tree as they were not used to build it and thus they can be used as an independent test set in any run to assess the performance of the forest as a whole; this is done via the out-of-bag error rate, which is the proportion of times an out-of-bag sample is misclassified.

Most classification procedures when dealing with a situation in which there are a large number of predictor variables to choose from tend to overfit. However, a major advantage of random forests is that they are able to keep the likelihood of overfitting low by using different subsets of the training data and different subsets of genes for training the different base classifiers. Thus, only patterns consistently present in the data would be detected reliably by a majority of the base classifiers and the majority votes turn out to be good indicators of class.

As for as ensemble methods in general, for the random forest classifier to be effective, each base classifier must have reasonably good classification performance and the trees must be diverse and only weakly correlated. The first of these, individual performance, is obtained by using strong performing tree classifiers and the second, diversity, is obtained by randomly choosing samples on which to train each tree and by randomly choosing attributes at each node of each tree.

Example. Table 11.5 shows the results of running random forest on the three Sialin data sets. The method works well on the Day 18 data where there is a clear separation between the knockout and wild-type mice. However, on Day 10 and Day 0, where the separation is less clear, the overabundance of noninformative genes tends to overwhelm the procedure and the performance is less stellar.

Boosting is another ensemble procedure. The difference in boosting is that instead of the model fits being generated via random-independent perturbations as in random forest, in boosting methods, models are fitted sequentially with the training of each fit tilted towards samples that were found by the preceding model fits to be the most difficult to classify.

11.7.2 Enriched Random Forest

When the number of possible genes is huge and the percentage of truly informative genes is small, it is possible that the performance of the base classifiers could degrade. This is because, if simple random sampling is used for selecting the subset of g eligible genes at each node, almost all these subsets are likely to contain a preponderance of noninformative genes. Consider a situation with G genes of which only H are informative. Then, if at any node g genes are selected by resampling randomly with equal weights, the probability distribution of the number of informative genes selected is binomial with g trials and probability $p = H/G$, so that the mean number of informative genes selected at each iteration is $m = pg$. As p is typically tiny, so will be m. For example, if $H = 100$, $G =$ 10,000, and $g = G^{1/2} = 100$, the resulting m is only one informative gene per node. The base classifiers built using such nodes will have low accuracies, and overall, the performance of the ensemble will suffer.

This can be remedied by using weighted random sampling instead of simple random sampling (an analogous issue arising in unsupervised classification is addressed similarly by Amaratunga et al., 2008). By tilting the random sampling of genes so that less informative genes are less likely to get selected, the odds of trees containing the more informative genes being included in the forest increases. Consequently, the resultant random forest will be composed of a higher proportion of better base classifiers, resulting in a better fit. Owing to the enormous choice of genes available, the diversity of the ensemble is not compromised and can be controlled to be more diverse than prefiltering. The value of doing the weighting is amply demonstrated in the performance improvement over both nonfiltering and prefiltering reported in Section 11.3.

Weighting can be done by scoring each gene based on its ability to separate the groups, for example, via a t-test, and using these scores to assign weights, w_i, so that the genes that most separate the groups are the only ones assigned high weights. Once the weights have been determined, the algorithm as described in Section 11.7.1 is run with the only modification being that when, at any node, the subset of g eligible genes is selected, it is selected from the G genes using weighted random sampling with weights w_i, rather than simple random sampling.

The key to the modified algorithm is to score each gene based on how well it separates the two groups. Such a score can be generated by testing each gene for a group effect using a standard two-sample t-test and calculating the p-value, small p-values indicating greater separation and large p-values indicating less. In general if Y is not binary but categorical or continuos the t-test maybe replaced by any goodness of fit or any other test derived from the modeling of Y given X. The p-value of this later test is used in place of the t-test p-value. However, to weigh using the p-values themselves would be inappropriate because of two factors: (i) the multiplicity of tests being performed and (ii) the small sample size that is typical of microarray experiments.

To adjust for (i), we instead look at FDR-adjusted p-values (Benjamini and Yekutieli, 2001; Storey and Tibshirani, 2003) or q-values. Genes are then assigned weights, w, where either $w = 1/q$ or $w = -\log(q)$. Thus, genes with less separability (which will have high p-values) will receive almost zero weight and genes with high separability (which will have low p-values) will receive large weights. It is important to carry out the testing and weighting within the loop (rather than as a preprocessing step) to avoid the problem of selection bias in feature selection described by Ambroise and McLachlan (2002).

There are two small modifications to these potential weights. First, to prevent a large fraction of genes getting essentially zero weight and reducing too much the diversity of genes across the eligible subsets, we threshold the lower weights to a_{min}. Second, to prevent a small number of genes with very small p-values from receiving very large weights, which could also drastically reduce the diversity of the ensemble, we threshold the high weights to a_{max}. Thus, the weights assigned are $w(k) = median(a_{\text{min}}, w(k), a_{\text{max}})$.

To adjust for (ii), even though the t-test is the simplest way to assess separation for a gene, microarray experiments typically have small sample sizes and thus the t-tests have low power and thus low discriminatory ability. Therefore, an analysis method that borrows strength across genes, such as conditional t (see Chapter 7), is likely to generate a better ranking of genes.

Example. Table 11.5 shows that enriched random forest (ERF) has zero misclassification errors with the Sialin data, thus illustrating the importance of the enrichment by weighting.

11.8 ENRICHED ENSEMBLE CLASSIFIERS

Even though ERF outperforms random forest in situations where there are a large number of genes, it inherits some of the pitfalls of random forest. For example, random forest will likely miss a structure that is hidden in the dimensionality and that is oblique to a coordinate-wise grid. It turns out that it is beneficial to also replace classification trees with more stable classifiers such as LDA. These new ensembles attain superior performance compared to random forest and even ERF. These are described in Section 11.11.

11.9 NEURAL NETWORKS

Inspired by the way the brain supposedly processes information, neural networks are a class of highly flexible nonlinear models for studying complex patterns in data and for predicting new observations from existing ones. Use of these models is very popular in data mining, machine learning, and other application areas related to computer science, although they are significantly less favored by statisticians. One reason is that neural networks intentionally tend to be heavily overparametrized, which goes totally against conventional statistical wisdom that identifies overparametrization with overfitting.

However, in many modern classification problems, this overparametrization may not be a serious concern because the data may have the following characteristics: there is no overlap between the classes, the surface that separates the classes is highly nonlinear, and there are massive amounts of data so that the separation can be identified by the procedure. For problems with such characteristics, the risk of overfitting is less of a concern than the ability to capture highly nonlinear separations.

A basic model for neural networks appears under the name *feed forward single hidden layer neural nets*, which consist of an input layer, an output layer, and a hidden layer in between. Figure 11.8 gives a visual scheme of the structure of such neural nets. Each node has one or more inputs and one output. The neural net model is structured as follows:

1. The input layer (or first layer) consists of as many nodes as classifiers are available for the fit. The output of each node is the corresponding value of the classifiers assigned to it (Fig. 11.8).
2. Each node inputs the outputs of the nodes of the prior layer and it outputs a fixed function of the linear combination. The function, sometimes called a *transfer function*, is usually a logistic function or any other sigmoidal-shaped function for classification problems and the identity function for regression problems. The sigmoidal function is

$$h(x, y) = \tanh(\alpha_0 + \alpha_1 (x'y)^2)$$

3. The output layer (or last layer) has as many nodes as responses are available for the fit.

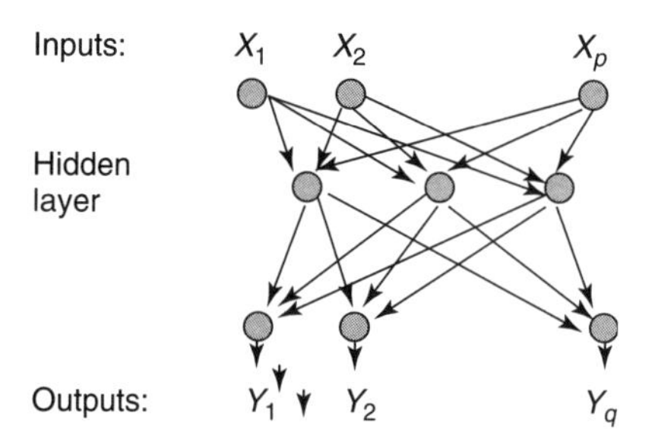

Figure 11.8 Graph of an ANN with one hidden layer.

The process of estimating the parameters of the neural net ("learning") uses a very complicated "backfitting" algorithm that does not always find the optimal parameter values. However, a nice feature of the neural net model is that it can be implemented in computer hardware. It would be a mistake for statisticians to ignore neural net methodology because it does produce excellent results in many applications. The difficulties mentioned above will likely be overcome with new research and greater computational resources.

Example. We redo the classification using the `ann` (which stands for *artificial neural network*) function in the `R` software. We used one hidden layer with $K = 0, \ldots, 20$ nodes and found that the number of nodes made little effect. We allowed direct links between the input layer and the output layer. The results are shown in Table 11.4 are more or less the same as Table 11.3. The 0.5 in the table means that different trainings produced different results in the classification because of the differences in the initial conditions. The ANN was trained 1000 times and the results are reported as 0.5 when about half of the time we get 0 misclassifications and the other times we have one or more misclassifications. It appears that procedures 2 and 3 performed slightly better than procedure 4.

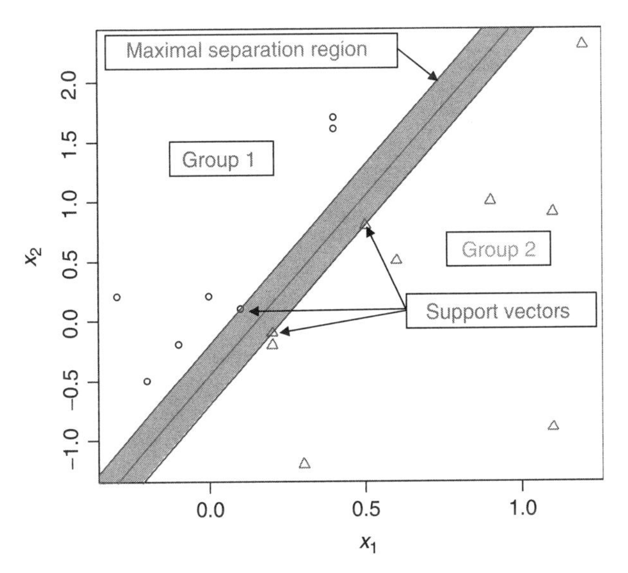

Figure 11.9 SVM example with two groups of points. The shaded area represents the separation region. The arrows indicate the location of the support vectors.

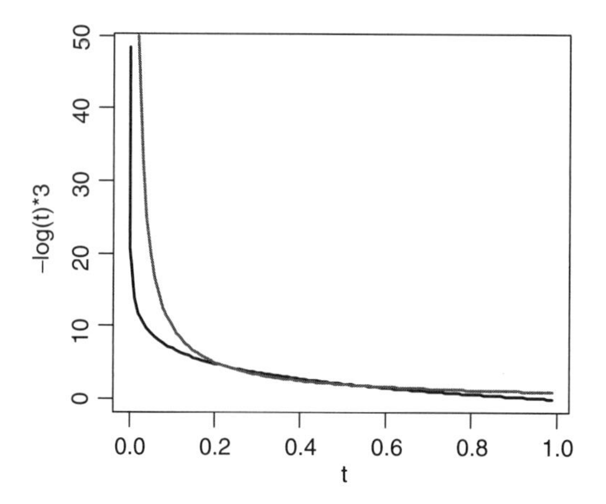

Figure 11.10 A comparison between $1/t$ and $-\log(t)$. $1/t$ gives higher weight near zero than $-3\log(t)$.

11.10 SUPPORT VECTOR MACHINES

Support vector machines (SVM) are generalizations of the linear classifier methods (such as LDA) that have become very popular in the machine-learning literature (Fig. 11.9).

Suppose that the training set is classified into two classes $\{+1, -1\}$, then the SVM classification rule is of the form $r(x) = \text{sign}(\beta' x - \beta_0)$. This function defines a separation hyperplane between the two classes. Some of the features that make SVM popular are as follows:

1. The criterion for estimating the hyperplane is to maximize the margin of separation between the classes, as shown in Figure 11.10, by the shaded region in the graph. This is an interesting idea, but it is not affine invariant and it may not be optimal in situations when the scales of the different classifiers may not be very similar.
2. The linear classifiers can be extended to nonlinear ones by augmenting the set of classifiers to the sometimes-called "feature" space, which includes the classifiers plus nonlinear functions of them. The form of the nonlinear classifier is

$$r(x) = \text{sign}\left(\sum_{i=1}^{p} \beta_i h(x_i, x) - \beta_0\right),$$

where the most popular forms for h are

(a) *Radial basis functions:*

$$h(x, y) = \exp\left(\frac{-(\|x - y\|)^2}{2\sigma^2}\right).$$

(b) *Sigmoidal functions:*

$$h(x, y) = \tanh(\alpha_0 + \alpha_1 (x'y)^2).$$

3. The estimation of the classifier rule parameters is performed using a quadratic programming algorithm. The solution can be expressed as a function of a few of the samples that are called *support vectors* that gives the name to the method. Figure 11.10 shows a graph of an example of SVM in two dimensions indicating the support vectors and the maximal separation region.

SVMs have been used for analyzing microarray data. For example, Brown et al. (2000) use SVMs to predict functional roles for uncharacterized yeast ORFs.

A good general introduction to SVM can be found in a collection of four papers by Hearst (1998), where the authors give high praise to the theoretical simplicity of SVM compared to neural nets, and is the reason why SVM is becoming very popular in the area of machine learning. On the other hand, they point out that there are still no applications where these methods have been shown to be significantly superior to other nonlinear classification techniques. Our intuition of SVMs is that they are different from other methods in the sense that they pay special attention to the boundary of separation between the regions corresponding to each class and this may yield small improvements of the classification prediction rate.

Incidentally, computer-intensive nonlinear classification methods are becoming more and more popular because of the widespread availability of very fast computers and there are many implementations of them in modern software. See Burges (1998) for a tutorial.

11.11 GENERALIZED ENRICHED METHODS

The methodology of ERF described in Section 11.7.2 can be extended to other methods using two different paradigms.

On one hand, we could describe ERF as an ensemble of trees in which variables (i.e., genes) are assigned weights. Therefore, one extension of ERF to other methods is by producing enriched ensembles that are just like regular ensembles except that the variables are selected with probabilities given by the enriched weights.

A general algorithm consists of the following steps:

1. Assign the enriched weights to the set of predictors.
2. Choose the ensemble subsets by weighted random sampling of variables using the enrichment weights and split the subset into training and testing set.
3. Apply the generic method to the training subset and observe the results on the testing subset.
4. Iterate steps 2 and 3 for as many simulations as necessary and collect and summarize the results from all the testing sets.

This algorithm is very general and can be applied to any generic method. It should work in almost all situations.

A second generalization of *ERF* is ignoring the ensemble part and incorporating the weights directly to the generic method.

This modification could be applied to most of the existing classification and prediction methods but perhaps not all.

For example, enriched weights could be easily added to the following methods: PCA, PLS, Lasso, ridge regression, elastic net, SVM, nearest neighbors, and many others.

All these methods are not scale invariant, and therefore, the weights could be incorporated by scaling the variables by the weights.

This will not work with unconstrained linear regression because the scale will absorb the weights and produce the same predictive model.

One question now is how to define the weight function.

In principle, the weight function can be any generic monotonic function that gives high weights to "important" genes, where the measure of "importance" is based on the statistical evidence that a gene is predictive of a response.

The statistic that reflects this importance measure is the p-value from some test that assesses the significance of the gene prediction or correlation according to some model.

The weight functions that we consider are the minus log, $y = -\log(p)$ and the reciprocal $y = 1/p$. In Figure 11.10, we compare $1/t$ with $-3\log(t)$ over the interval (0, 1) in order to show that $1/t$ gives more weight to the region near zero.

To avoid overfitting, the p-values are corrected for multiplicity by converting them into FDR corrected p-values (Benjamini and Hochberg, 1995; Benjamini and Yekutieli, 2001), which have been coined q-values (Storey, 2001). To obtain q-values, we divide each p-value by $Q_{(i)}(\alpha)$, the αth quantile of the null distribution of the order statistic corresponding to the p-value. Then, $q_{(i)} = p_{(i)}/Q_{(i)}(\alpha)$. Usually, as the null distribution we use the Uniform(0, 1) distribution and we set $\alpha = 5\%$, and under this null, the distribution of the order statistic is $p_{(i)} \sim \text{Beta}(i, G - i)$, where G is the number of genes.

If the null distribution of tp-values is not uniform but has a different null distribution F that is known, then using the same argument as above the new q-values become $q_{(i)} = p_{(i)}/F^{-1}(Q_{(i)}(\alpha))$.

This derivation assumes that the p-values are independent. Sometimes there might be evidence to the contrary. The correlations among the p-values is a direct effect of the correlations among genes but usually the sample size is too small to be able to estimate it.

As stated earlier, there are at least two different enrichment weight functions that may be used. The reciprocal weights (Amaratunga et al., 2012) are $w_i = 1/q_i$, with a threshold from above when q_i is zero or near zero. Another function is the negative of logarithm of the q-values, $w_i = -\log(q_i)$, which is motivated by the weights of the first PLS component of a linear fit because $\hat{\beta}_{\text{PLS}} \approx -\log(p\text{-value})$ (see Cherkas, 2012).

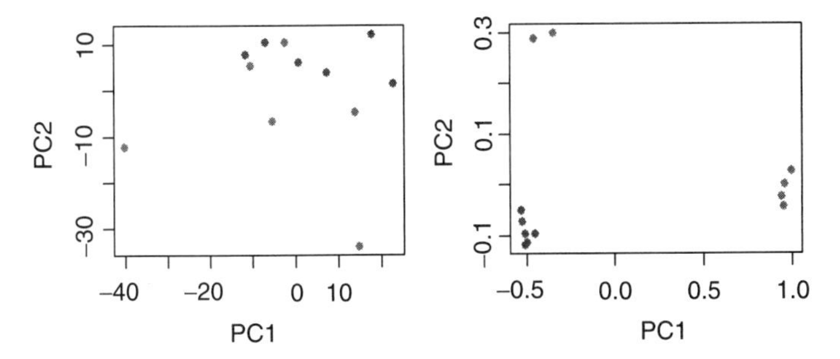

Figure 11.11 Plot of the first principal components for the Sialin 0 data. (a) The standard PCA graph and (b) the enriched PCA graph. The black dots indicate the knockout mice and the grey dots indicate the wild type mice.

11.11.1 Enriched Principal Components Analysis and Biplots

In Section 11.3.1, we introduced one of the fundamental methods for analysis of multivariate data: PCA. We noted that for high-dimensional data, we need to transpose the X data matrix and get to a new centered data matrix Z of dimension $G \times p$.

Then, the singular value decomposition of $Z = UDV^T$ will yield the p principal components of X, namely, the matrix U.

To produce an enriched version of PCA, we first calculate the weights $w_1, \ldots, w_G$ and put them into a diagonal matrix $W = \text{diag}(w_1,\ldots,w_G)$.

Then we just modify Z to create a new matrix $Z^* = WZ$. Then we perform the singular value decomposition on $Z^* = U^*D^*V^{*T}$ and obtain the new enriched principal components U^*.

In Figure 11.11, we display the results of performing PCA on the Sialin Day 0 data (Sialin 0) with and without enrichment.

The left panel shows the graph of the first two principal components from the standard PCA analysis. There is clearly no separation between the knockout group and the wild-type group. The second graph on the right shows the same graph for the output of the enriched PCA and this time the separation is perfect.

This shows clearly the value of enriching.

The same ideas lead to the formulation of enriched biplots, enriched FA, and enriched spectral maps that were described in Sections 11.3.2 through 11.3.4. All the corresponding results are achieved by just applying the standard methods to the matrix Z^*.

For example, in Figure 11.12, we have the enriched biplot of the Sialin Day 0 data. It shows the same pattern for the observations as the enriched PCA graph in Figure 11.11, but in addition, it also shows two clearly defined groups of variables that contributed to the principal components. The first component is dominated by genes 1417210_at, 1426438_at, 1427262_at, and 1436936_s_at, whereas the second principal component is dominated by genes 1429116_a, 1435559_at, 1437522_x_at, and 1454905_at.

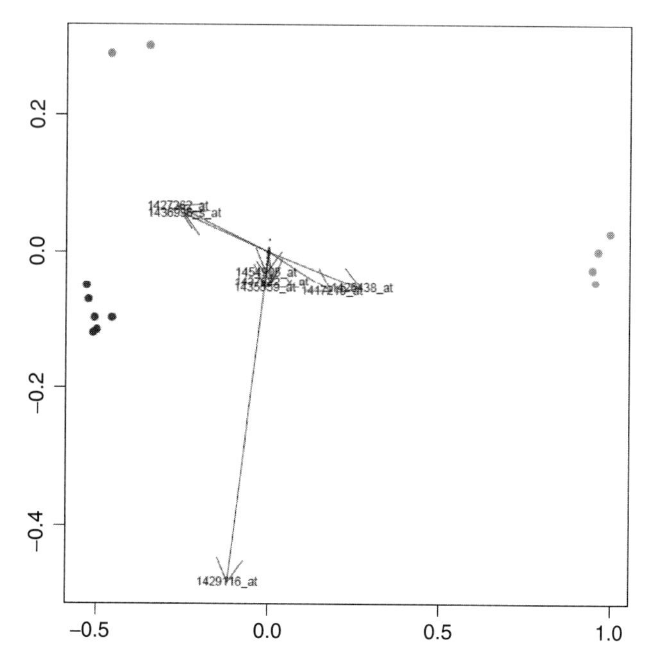

Figure 11.12 Plot of the first principal components for the Sialin Day 0 data. (a) The standard PCA graph and (b) the enriched PCA graph

In Table 11.4, we give a description of the annotations for each of the genes that contributes to the first and second principal components. It appears that the first principal component is loaded with genes that are part of the X and Y chromosomes and, therefore, the first component corresponds to gender. This is what we call a nonspecific signal. The fact that the two groups are not balanced with respect to the response implies that gender genes are differentially expressed and contribute to the signal.

However, the second component is specific and contains the Sialin gene plus other genes whose annotations indicate their contribution to growth pathways. This is in fact the type of signal that we are after and is specific and helps us learn which pathways are affected by the knocked out gene at the embryo phase of mouse development.

This example helps us understand the three types of signals that appear in microarray data:

- The signal found in the second principal component is specific and is the primary signal of interest.
- The signal found in the first principal component is a nonspecific signal that is attributable to a secondary effect in the data.
- The spurious signal of standard principal components analysis is shown in Figure 11.10.

Table 11.4 Gene Annotations for the Two Components of the Enriched PCA of the Sialin Day 0 Data

Genes in the Second PCA	Annotation
1429116_a	SLC gene that was knocked out in treatment group.
1435559_at	Myo6, Growth.
1437522_x_at	Gh growth hormone.
1454905_at	Inhibitor of Bruton agammaglobulinemia tyrosine kinase.
Genes in the first PCA	**Annotation**
1417210_at	Eukaryotic translation initiation factor 2, subunit 3, structural gene Y-linked Eif-2gy, Spy, Tfy
1426438_at	Box polypeptide 3, Y-linked 8030469F12Rik, D1Pas1-rs1, Dby
1427262_at	Inactive X-specific transcripts A430022B11, AI314753. Exper Embryonic brain development.
436936_s_at	Inactive X-specific transcripts A430022B11, AI314753 Experiment embryonic brain development.

The enriched method was able to avoid the spurious signal but detected the other two. Then it is up to the scientist or analyst to separate the specific signals from the rest. Usually this will have to be done using biological knowledge associated with the genes which are most contributing to the principal component of interest.

11.11.2 Enriched Penalized Methods: Lasso, SVM, P-SVM

Penalized methods may achieve the same result as enriched methods for a moderate number of predictors, but for a typical microarray experiment where the number of predictors is very large and much larger than the number of genes, we may also improve the prediction by enriching. We introduce the enriched weights in the LASSO penalty, which results in the following modification to Equation 11.1.

$$\tilde{\beta} = \text{argmin}_{\beta} \sum_{i=1}^{n} (y_i - \beta_0 - \sum_{j=1}^{G} x_{ij}\beta_j)^2 + \lambda \sum_{j=1}^{G} w_j^{-1}|\beta_j| \tag{11.2}$$

Note that if we apply the transformation $\beta_j = w_j \beta_j^*$ then Equation 11.2 becomes

$$\tilde{\beta} = \text{argmin}_{\beta} \sum_{i=1}^{n} (y_i - \beta_0 - \sum_{j=1}^{G} w_j x_{ij}\beta_j^*)^2 + \lambda \sum_{j=1}^{G} |\beta_j^*| \tag{11.3}$$

Therefore, to compute the enriched LASSO, we only need to replace X with $X^* = WX$ as we did in the enriched PCA method.

The same idea could be used to extend the enriched methodology to SVM and penalized-SVM (Becker et al., 2009). The case for enriched SVM is quite strong for $G >> n$. SVM finds a linear subspace that separates the data into two groups.

Table 11.5 Comparing Cross-Validated Prediction Error Rates for the Sialin Day 0, Day 10, and Day 18 Data

Method	Day 0 Prediction Error	Day 10 Prediction Error	Day 18 Prediction Error
Enriched PCA	0%(0)	0%(0)	0%(0)
Enrich forest (W=-log)	0%(0)	0%(0)	0%(0)
Random forest (500)	41%–75%(5–9)	16%–50%(2–6)	(0%–25%)0–3
Random forest (1000000)	41%(5)	16%(2)	(8%)1
GLMnet	0%(0)	0%(0)	0%(0)
SVM (e1071)	50%(6)	50%(6)	50%(6)
Enriched (1/t) SVM (e1071)	0%(0)	0%(0)	0%(0)
Enriched(-log) SVM (e1071)	50%(6)	0%(0)	0%(0)
Proximal SVM	50%(6)	50%(6)	50%(6)
Penalized SVM (LASSO)	0%(0)	50%(6)	50%(6)
Penalized SVM (SCAD)	0%(0)	50%(6)	50%(6)

In two dimensions, this corresponds to a line that separates the data into two groups. Suppose that there are many lines that do that, then SVM chooses the line corresponding to the widest gap between the two groups which we call the "margin."

Suppose that we have a very large number G of variables where a small number of them contain the signal and the rest are noise.

Then for each subset of p variables in the noise part, there will be a hyperplane that separates the p observations into two groups correctly and there will be a margin associated with this hyperplane. As the number of noisy variables grows, the maximum margin among all subsets of p variables will also grow and could easily surpass the margin obtained from a small or moderate signal.

Table 11.6 Comparing Prediction Error Rates for the Sialin Data, Training with Day 0, Testing on Day 18 and Vice-Versa

Method	Day 0 to Day 18 Prediction Error	Day 18 to Day 0 Prediction Error
Enriched PCA	0%(0)	0%(0)
Enrich forest (W=-log)	0%(0)	0%(0)
Random forest (500)	41%–75%(5–9)	16%–50%(2–6)
Random forest (1000000)	41%(5)	16%(2)
GLMnet	0%(0)	0%(0)
SVM (e1071)	50%(6)	50%(6)
Enriched (1/t) SVM (e1071)	0%(0)	0%(0)
Enriched(-log) SVM (e1071)	50%(6)	0%(0)
Proximal SVM	50%(6)	50%(6)
Penalized SVM (LASSO)	0%(0)	50%(6)
Penalized SVM (SCAD)	0%(0)	50%(6)

Enrichment would reduce the effect of the spurious signal and that will improve the performance of SVM.

Table 11.5 gives a performance evaluation of the previous methods for the three Sialin data sets corresponding to Day 0, Day 10, and Day 18. It shows that enriched methods and glmnet outperform other nonenriched methods in these three data sets. In particular, we observe poor performance for random forest and all forms of SVM (proximal and penalized), which is significantly improved by the enrichment.

The results of Table 11.5 were obtained using cross-validation. It is a concern that there are many different ways to evaluate performance, and they often do not yield similar results; therefore there is always the question of the validity of comparisons like those reported in Table 11.5.

In the Sialin example, we have a unique opportunity because the three data sets are different but they share a common signal; that is, the differential expression of growth-related genes induced by the knockout of the Sialin gene. So one question that arises here is whether we could predict the Day 18 classification from the Day 0 classification and vice-versa.

We evaluated these methods using one data set as training and another as testing. Table 11.6 shows this.

11.11.3 Enriched Partial Least Squares (PLS)

In Section 11.1.2, we provided an algorithm for PLS for continuous response and for binary response using linear and logistic regression, respectively.

There is a clear connection between this algorithm and the algorithm for enriched PCA.

The first component of PLS can be written as $X_1 = c\sum_{i=1}^{G} \hat{\beta}_i z_i$, where the $\hat{\beta}_i$ come from individual linear regression of z_i on y and z_i are the z-scores associated with the initial variable x_i.

Cherkas (2010) showed that this is approximately equal to $X1 = c\sum_{i=1}^{G} -\log(p_i)z_i$. Therefore, enriched PLS could easily follow by replacing the $-\log(p_i)$ by the enriched weights $X_{1_{\text{enriched}}} = c\sum_{i=1}^{G} W_i z_i$.

This formula is applied to the linear and logistic versions of PLS described in Section 11.1 and it also applies to not only the first component but also all the components of the PLS algorithm. In Figure 11.13a, we show a comparison of the exponential and t-distribution tails to show that, for not small degrees of freedom the approximation of the *minus log* weights is good. In Figure 11.13, we show that the actual weights are computed with the standardized *minus log* weights and the formula for our data example and are very close.

In Figure 11.14, we plot the two top PLS components for the Sialin Day 0 data and a second data set, which is the same Day 0 data with the response scrambled. When we use logistic PLS without enriching, the results show a good fit on both the good data and the scrambled data, which proves that PLS overfits when used with megavariate data. However, this is not the case for enriched PLS because it fits the good data very well but it does not fit the scrambled data well.

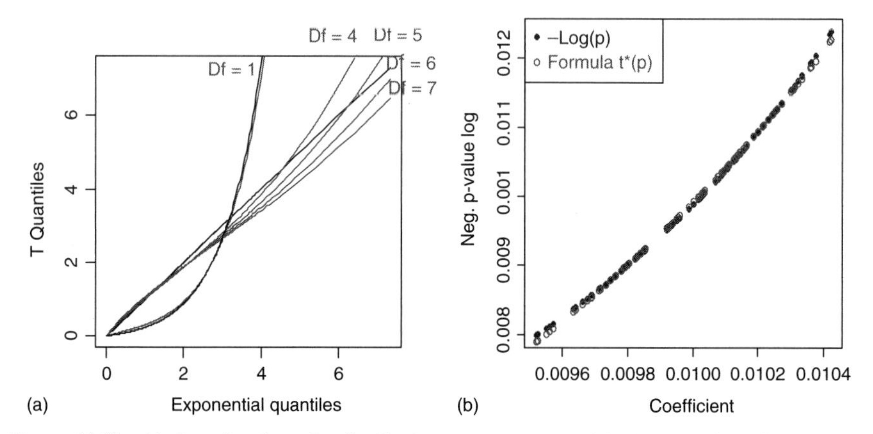

Figure 11.13 (a) Quantile plots of t-distributions versus exponential. (b) Plot of the Sialin Day 0 weights calculated with the minus log transformation.

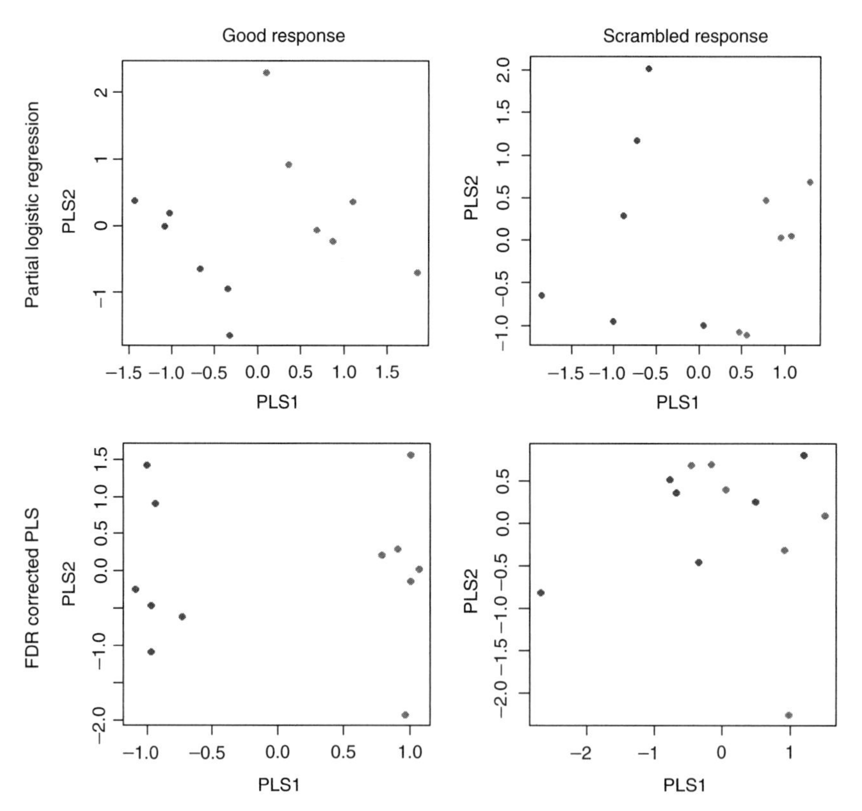

Figure 11.14 PLS results for the Sialin Day 0 data with PLS (first row) versus enriched PLS (second row). The columns correspond to the true response and the scrambled random response.

For the binary case, another way to calculate the weights for the PLS components is to compute two sample test p-values (from CT or Limma or two-sample t-test) and calculate the enriched weights from those p-values and use those weights to build $X1_{\text{enriched}}$. Then proceed the same way as the PLS algorithm and compute $X2_{\text{enriched}}, \ldots, Xk_{\text{enriched}}$. This algorithm is easy to implement and makes use of the moderated p-values that usually outperform the individual p-values (see Cherkas, 2010).

11.12 INTEGRATION OF GENOME INFORMATION

Gene expression information from microarray studies can be integrated with information from other sources, such as annotation, partial information regarding genetic pathways, and so on, to develop more complete views of biological processes. We outline briefly some efforts in this regard.

11.12.1 Integration of Gene Expression Data and Molecular Structure Data

Blower et al. (2002) describe a method called *SAT* analysis for systematically associating molecular features of compounds with gene expression patterns, with the objective of predicting which molecular substructures would be present in drugs that are active in cells whose genes are expressed according to a specific pattern. SAT analysis links together three databases of information on cells and chemical compounds. The three databases are A, a $k \times l$ "activity matrix" consisting of experimental measures of the inhibitory effect of each of the k compounds against each of l cell lines; T, a $G \times l$ "target matrix" of gene expression patterns measured by DNA microarrays for G genes in the l cell lines; and S, a $h\text{x}k$ "structure matrix" of 0′s and 1's that identifies which of a very large number, h, of molecular structural features are present in each of the k compounds.

If A and T are properly standardized, the $k \times G$ matrix AT^t consists of Pearson correlation coefficients and the $k \times G$ matrix SAT^t consists of association measures, the (i, j)th one of which measures the tendency of the ith structural feature to occur in cell lines in which the jth gene is expressed. Mining this latter matrix via a series of targeted subsetting strategies leads to insights regarding these associations.

11.12.2 Pathway Inference

The study of coexpression of genes across a series of experimental conditions, such as time, provides an assortment of clues from which it is hoped that the genetic pathways involved in a biological process could be reconstructed. The simplest way of assessing these clues is by determining the functional classes to which coexpressing genes belong and using any knowledge gained from doing this to "fill in the blanks" whenever partial information about a biological pathway is available. More complicated assessments involve the use of Bayesian network models.

A Bayesian network model can be graphically represented as a directed graph. The nodes of the graph represent genes. Arrows connect those nodes where the expression of one gene regulates the expression of another, either directly or because of an external stimulus. The state of a daughter node conditional on the state of its parent nodes is modeled by a probability distribution. The whole model is fitted either by using a scoring function to evaluate how well the network matches the observed data or by performing tests for conditional independence on the observations. However, definitive conclusions are difficult to reach from fitting these models because of various reasons such as (i) the lack of availability of sufficient data to adequately and reliably fit the model and (ii) the nonuniqueness of the fit, indicating the statistical equivalence of totally different gene regulation pathways.

As functional genomics develops, research that involves integrating genomic data from diverse sources will lead to a better understanding of complex biological processes.

SUPPLEMENTARY READING

As with cluster analysis, the literature on class prediction is very broad. The book by Hand (1997) is a useful general reference. A number of multivariate analysis textbooks also provide detailed accounts of supervised classification methodologies, including Gnanadesikan (1997); Krzanowski (2000); Mardia, Kent, and Bibby (1979), and Seber (1984). The books by Hastie, Tibshirani, and Friedman (2009); McLachlan (1992), and Ripley (1996) lie at the interface of statistics and data mining.

SOFTWARE NOTES

Software for commonly used supervised classification techniques has been implemented in a number of different platforms and is available in all statistical packages. As with clustering algorithms, some implementations are better than others at handling large data sets and applications with large numbers of variables.

In `R` and `SPLUS` and its associated libraries, some relevant functions are `lda` for Fisher's linear discriminant analysis, `qda` for quadratic discriminant analysis, `knn` for the nearest neighbors method, `rpart` for classification trees, `randomForest` for random forest, and `nnet` for neural networks.

`DNAMR`
The library contains functions for ERF (Enriched Random Forest) and other enriched and ensemble techniques.

`CMA`
The bioconductor R package `CMA` contains many methods for class prediction of high-dimensional data. A complete description of package is given in Slawski, Daumer, and Boulesteix (2008)

`glmnet, lars`
The glmnet and lars R packages are available in CRAN

`e1071, penalizedSVM`
The e1071 and penalizedSVM R-package implement support vector machines and the penalized version of SVM. They are available from CRAN.

`ARF, ERF and ECLASS`
`R` software for the enriched methods and ARF are available online at
`www.rci.rutgers.edu/~cabrera/DM`.

`DNAMR 2.0`
This package implements the enriched methods that are included in this chapter which are (i) Enriched random forest (ERF) with continuous and categorical responses. (ii) Enriched PCA, (iii) Enriched Biplot, (iv) Enriched LASSO, (v) Enriched SVM, (vi) Enriched Discriminant Analysis, (vi) Enriched PLS.
`www.rci.rutgers.edu/~cabrera/DNAMR`.

EXERCISES

11.1. Golub et al. (1999) performed a supervised classification on oligonucleotide microarray data (the data is available online) related to two types of leukemia: AML and ALL. Read the article and answer the following questions:

(a) Briefly outline the authors' goals, the analysis they performed, and the conclusion that they reached.
(b) Summarize the data using PCA or FA on all the genes. Compare the summary produced by PCA with the outcome of Enriched PCA
(c) Perform a classification using (i) LDA, (ii) DLDA, (iii) QDA, and (iv) GLMNET, and (v) kNN using all the genes in the data. Report the misclassification rate in the training set and the test set.
(d) Repeat (b) and (c) using only the 50 genes identified in the paper as being the strongest classifiers. Report the misclassification rate in the training set and the test set.
(e) Compare the results of the various analyses that you performed and draw your conclusions.

11.2. Use the Khan et al. (2001) data that was covered in this chapter and from the training set, select the top five genes that produce the most significant F-statistic for comparing the mean expression between the four tumor classes.

(a) Use the LDA procedure to produce a classification rule for the four tumor classes and estimate the misclassification rate for the training and testing sets.

(b) Repeat the procedure for the top 10 genes, 15 genes, 20 genes, and 25 genes. Make a table showing the misclassification rates of the five classification rules and comment on the table.

(c) Repeat the procedure but for all the previous cases, but instead of using the raw gene data take the top two principal components and use them as classifiers. Make a new table of the performance of all the previous classifiers and try to summarize your findings.

11.3. For the Khan et al. (2001) data in the previous problem:

(a) Draw a biplot using the top 100 genes according to the F ratio criterion.

(b) Once this is done, draw a biplot of the training sets and try to find clusters by hand, that is, print the biplot graph and use a pencil and draw the regions corresponding to each class.

(c) Proceed by graphing the dots corresponding to the testing set and check the misclassification rate of your clusters.

11.4. Consider the data set MUS. The first 10 columns refer to samples from tissue type A, the second 10 columns refer to samples from tissue type B, and the third 10 columns refer to samples from tissue type C. Assume that the data set has been log transformed and adequately normalized (therefore, do not retransform or renormalize the data). In addition, unless otherwise stated, use MUS without the one outlying array discovered in Question 9.1 above.

(a) Carry out one-way ANOVA F tests to determine which genes are differentially expressed across the three tissue types. Let $I1$ denote the subset of genes that are significant at the 0.0001 level. Take MD_{gh} to denote the median of gene g in tissue group h, and suppose that R_g denotes the range (i.e., the maximum minus the minimum) of the MDgh values for gene g. Let $I2$ denote the subset of genes with the highest 5% R_g values. Let $I3$ denote the subset of genes common to both $I1$ and $I2$. What percentage of the 3000 genes are in $I3$?

(b) Run Fisher's LDA to classify the samples using only the genes in $I3$. What is the misclassification rate of the procedure? According to the LDA classifier, to which tissue type does the one outlying array belong?

(c) Cluster the genes in $I3$ into six groups, using Ward's hierarchical clustering method with Euclidean distance as dissimilarity metric. Let MC_{ch} denote the mean of the cth cluster in the hth sample. Plot MC_{ch} versus h (make separate plots for the different values of c). In words, characterize the six clusters (i.e., explain briefly what characteristics of the three tissue types are being picked up by each cluster).

11.5. Read the paper "CMA: a comprehensive Bioconductor package for supervised classification with high dimensional data" by Slawski, Daumer and

Boulesteix (2008). Use the R package `CMA` in order to classify subject to the ALL and AML groups in the Golub data discussed in Chapter 1. Note that the paper by Slawski , Daumer and Boulesteix (2008) is relevant for questions 11.5–11.7.
Choose few classification methods avilavle in the `CMA` package and compare the miss-classification error obtained from the different classification methods.

11.6. In this question use the `CMA` package in order to classify patients to the AML and ALL group using the LDA method discussed in Section 11.2.
Use different feature selection methods and compare the miss classification obtained from different feature selection methods. Do you select the same features (genes) for the signature when using different feature selection methods?

11.7. In this question use the `CMA` package in order to classified patients to the AML and ALL group using the LDA method discussed in Section 11.2.
Foe the classification procedure, use different proportion of data used in the test set in the cross validation: 50%, 33% and 25%. Do you see difference in the miss classification error when different proportion of the data is used for the test set?

11.8. Read the paper "Regularization and variable selection via the" by Hui Zou and Trevor Hastie (2005). The aim of this question is to predict the disease status (AML/ALL) in the Golub data using logistic regression. Use the R package `glmnet` to fit a regularized GLM to the data.
How many genes seems to be relevant with coefficient different from zero?

11.9. Repeat on the analysis in 11.8 using random forest. Do you select the same genes that were selected in 11.X. Explain why there is a difference between the two gene lists?

11.10. Consider the Sialin day 0 data

(a) Run the enriched PCA analysis and compare it with regular PCA analysis.

(b) Run the enriched PLS analysis and compare it with regular PLS analysis.

(c) Compare the enriched PCA analysis with the enriched PLS analysis.
Are they similar? Can you identify the specific and non-specific signals?

(d) Could you use the analyses in (c) for predicting the Sialin day 18 data and how does it compare with the penalized SVM and with GLMnet. Use the Silain day 18 data as the testing set and the Silaing day 0 dataset as training set.

CHAPTER 12

Protein Arrays

Protein array experiments display strong similarities to their DNA microarray counterparts. Protein arrays are rapidly becoming established as a powerful means to detect proteins, to monitor their expression levels, to ascertain their functions, and to investigate how they interact with each other and with external effects. Although the protein array field is still in its infancy, it is gaining momentum and is fast becoming one of the most promising areas of biomedical research.

12.1 INTRODUCTION

Proteins Proteins are the workhorses that regulate and perform the main functions of the cell (Chapter 2). They carry out all kinds of housekeeping activities, are catalysts of chemical reactions, act as channels and pumps, and perform motor functions. Some of the proteins involved in protein array experiments are as follows:

- *Antibodies.* They are the proteins produced by B-lymphocyte cells, which are a certain type of white blood cell. As part of the immune system, the function of an antibody is to bind with a specific protein (antigen) lying on the surface of a foreign cell. This protein-binding property plays an important role in the technology for the realization of protein array experiments. There are five classes of antibodies that are also called *immunoglobulins*: lgA, lgD, lgE, lgG, and lgM.
- *Antigens.* They are proteins that lie on the surface of foreign cells and that are detected by specific antibodies. Antibodies will bind with antigens in order to neutralize them and to help other parts of an organism's immune system to recognize foreign cells such as bacteria or viruses.

Exploration and Analysis of DNA Microarray and Other High-Dimensional Data, Second Edition.
Dhammika Amaratunga, Javier Cabrera, Ziv Shkedy.

- *Enzymes.* These are proteins that perform catalytic functions, that is, they accelerate a chemical reaction without being consumed by it. In particular, enzymes are involved in the synthesis of DNA and proteins. Enzymes are involved in the synthesis of proteins from RNA code by translation. The RNA code is subdivided into triplets of ordered nucleotides that are called *codons*. Proteins are formed of chains of amino acid molecules. There are 20 possible amino acids and each codon codes for one specific amino acid—but more than one codon may code for the same amino acid. The process of protein formation consists of translating the RNA code into a chain of amino acids bonded together to form the protein molecule. The enzyme's role in the protein formation is similar to the role of an assembly line in the making of a product. Although some of the basic concepts of protein arrays are covered in this chapter, some more complete general references in the genomics literature are Kodadek (2001); MacBeath (2002), and Angenendt et al. (2002).

12.2 PROTEIN ARRAY EXPERIMENTS

In principle, a protein array experiment can be fashioned to follow a path similar to a DNA microarray experiment. A protein sample is extracted from cells or whole tissues and labeled with dye, the labeled protein sample is incubated with a prefabricated array consisting of a large number of proteins printed in high density on a glass slide, any unbound labeled protein sample is removed via a filtration process, and the array is scanned to measure the amount of bound sample protein.

However, there are some crucial differences between a protein array experiment and a DNA microarray experiment. In addition to its amino acid sequence, the three-dimensional structure a protein folds into is an essential determinant of its function. Thus the protein on the array must be folded appropriately but in such a way that the recognition sites on the protein are not obscured. Clearly, proteins cannot simply be printed onto a two-dimensional glass surface to study function as is done with DNA. Thus, the technology of DNA microarrays described in Chapter 3 has to be modified considerably.

Several methods for fabricating protein arrays have been proposed. The basic idea is to bind the protein onto the glass slide with some agent and to label it with a fluorescent dye that can be detected by a scanner. The following are the three methods that have been proposed for constructing protein arrays.

1. *Sandwich Immunoassays.* The microarray spots are made of packed antibodies that will bind with specific proteins and then a second set of antibodies that have been labeled with a fluorescent dye will bind with the captured proteins. The scanner will read the fluorescence signal and assign a measure of protein abundance.
2. *Antibody Capture Immunoassays.* This method is similar to sandwich immunoassays except that the second antibody with the fluorescent tag is not used (Fig. 12.1b). Instead, it requires chemical labeling of the proteins

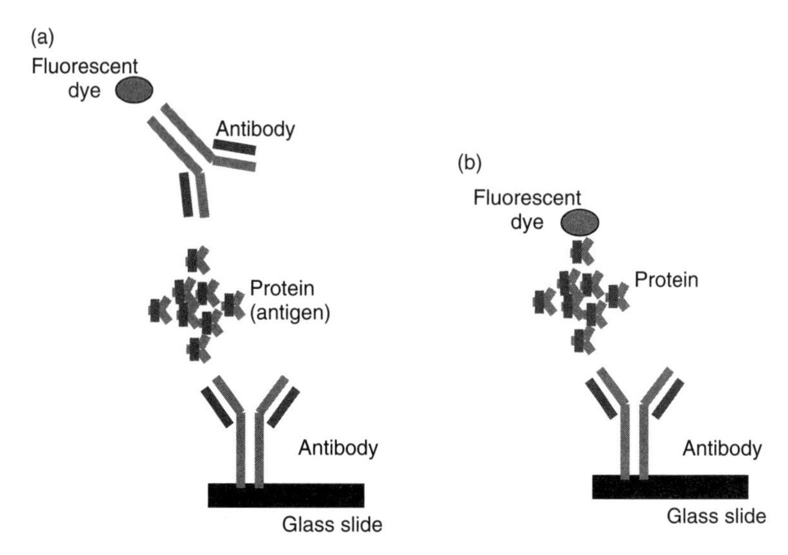

Figure 12.1 Protein array types: (a) Sandwich method (b) Antigen method.

(or, perhaps, some alternative method of measuring protein abundance on each spot).

3. *Antibody Capture Immunoassays.* This approach consists of immobilizing the protein molecules in the sample directly. An antibody labeled with fluorescent dye is used to detect any particular protein.
   When two dyes are used, dye-swap type designs may be used in case one dye binds more efficiently with certain proteins better than the second dye.

12.3 SPECIAL ISSUES WITH PROTEIN ARRAYS

Although there are many similarities between the images scanned from protein arrays and DNA microarrays, the processes that generated them (described in Section 12.2 and in Chapter 3) are quite different. Some of the issues that differentiate protein arrays from their DNA siblings that affect the data analysis are the following.

1. The objective of protein arrays is not only the detection of protein but also the measurement of protein abundance, whereas the objective of most DNA microarray experiments is focused on which genes are expressed or differentially expressed.
2. In DNA microarray experiments, there is a PCR step that amplifies the sample. In protein arrays, there is no such amplification step. For single-dye experiments, it is possible to amplify the signal by three orders of magnitude using

enzyme catalyzers (Knezevic et al., 2001), but, for two-dye experiments, this technology has not been developed as yet. Consequently, the detection level is an important issue because a protein that is present in the sample at a low concentration may not be detected by the protein array experiment.

3. Cross detection is also an issue because some antigens may bind to more than one protein.
4. The protein population is much more diverse than the gene population and involves many more interactions. For example, there are more than 2000 proteins in the human cell controlling gene expression only. Therefore, there is great potential for much larger microarrays and more complex experiments than for the DNA case. The technology for protein array spotting is advancing rapidly and will be a useful means of analyzing patterns of variation in hundreds of thousands of proteins.

Besides this application of protein detection, another role of protein arrays is to study the functions of proteins. The advantage of protein arrays for this purpose is that they are specially suited so the investigator can control the conditions of the experiment. A typical experiment consists of studying the interaction between two proteins. The aim is to be able to study the functionality of many proteins at once in one experiment.

12.4 ANALYSIS

Fluorescence data from protein arrays is analyzed using an analogous approach to that used with DNA microarray data. In the schematic display shown in Figure 12.2, we outline a series of steps that need to be followed for analyzing protein array data. Observe that, although Figure 12.2 is a modification of the DNA microarray analysis, schematic display shown in Figure 1.1, the data analysis part is essentially similar. We now review a few of the main steps here:

1. *Spotting of Microarray and Background Array.* The input data is the raw image produced by the scanner; the output data are the spotted intensities and spotted background.
2. *Log (or Similar) Transformation.* This is to remove, totally or partially, the heavy skewness of the spotted intensities.
3. *Quality Control.* The procedures described in Chapter 4 can be used to check the quality of the spotted arrays and the spots themselves.
4. *Normalization.* Global or intensity-dependent normalization among a group of arrays is applied to correct for any systematic biases in the measurement scales. With protein arrays, this step should be applied with caution because it could lower the signal of some high signal spots.
5. *Outliers among the Proteins.* These can be identified using the methods outlined in Chapter 5.

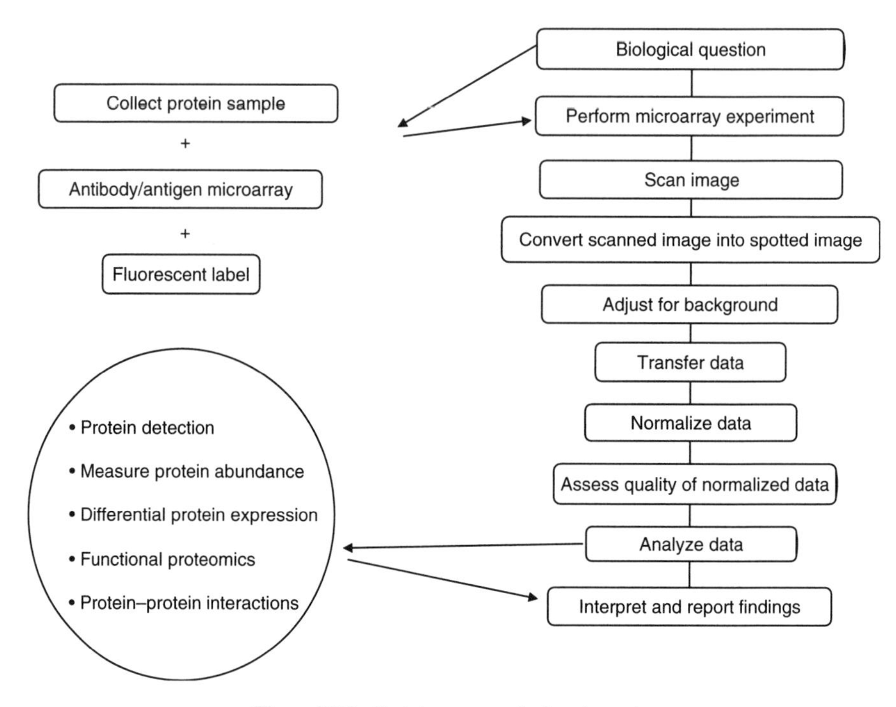

Figure 12.2 Protein array analysis schematic.

6. *Outliers among the Arrays.* These can be identified using concordance correlation coefficients and the other methods outlined in Chapter 5.
7. *Analysis of the Corresponding Biological Problem.* A consolidated approach to analyzing data from protein arrays is described by Lubomirski et al. (2007).

Please follow this steps when analyzing protein array data. It is often the case that the software that is attached to the protein array hardware comes with documentation suggesting that protein arrays are not as noisy as gene expression microarrays. Our experience suggests that this is not the case (Lubomirski et al. 2007).

12.5 USING ANTIBODY ANTIGEN ARRAYS TO MEASURE PROTEIN CONCENTRATIONS

In these early days of protein array experiments, some researchers are exploring groups of antibody/antigen pairs to show that it is possible to estimate protein concentrations using antibody/antigen microarrays. Haab et al. (2001) developed a method for protein array printing and used the arrays to measure the quantities of many specific proteins in complex solutions. They conducted a comparative fluorescence assay with two dyes, using 115 antibody/antigen pairs, with 6–12 replicates per pair, comprising a total of 1188 spots per microarray. In one group of six arrays, antibodies were employed to detect their corresponding antigen pair, and in another group of six microarrays, the reverse experiment was performed, that is, using antigens to detect antibodies. The researchers reported that 50% of the antigen array and 20% of the protein array allowed the detection of proteins at some of the antibody–antigen pairs and allowed the detection of proteins at concentrations of 1 ng/ml. Haab et al. (2001) indicated that these sensitivities are great enough for measuring many clinically important proteins in patient blood samples.

The method used to determine when a protein was detected relayed on using six arrays at six different concentrations of the sample. Recall that each individual array contains 6 replicate spots (except for a few with up to 12) of the same antibody/antigen so for each protein we observe a 6×6 array of logged ratios. A threshold value was assigned for each protein by calculating the mean of the six replicates at the lowest concentration plus twice their standard deviation. For each of the remaining five concentrations, if all the six spots gave ratios above the threshold value, then the protein was detected at that concentration. The results of the experiment showed a 50% detection rate of arrayed antigens and a 20% of detection of arrayed antibodies at the highest concentration and lesser values for the lower concentrations.

This method of calculating the threshold is highly variable. Suppose that, for simplicity, the ratios for the low-concentration sample for a particular protein has a normal distribution with 0 mean and standard deviation 1. Then the ideal threshold would be equal to 1.96 but, because we are calculating the threshold with only six values, the resulting threshold would range between 0.5 and 3.5, approximately 95% of the time.

An alternative way to check if a protein is detected by the microarray is to consider the concordance correlation between the observed values and the true protein concentration values. The concordance correlation coefficient (Section 5.6) measures the agreement between two sets of paired numbers.

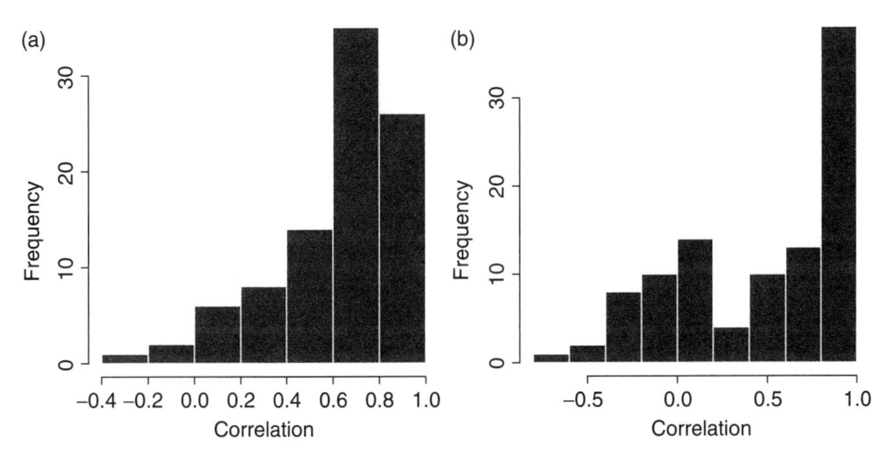

Figure 12.3 Histograms of the concordance correlations for antigen and antibody arrays.

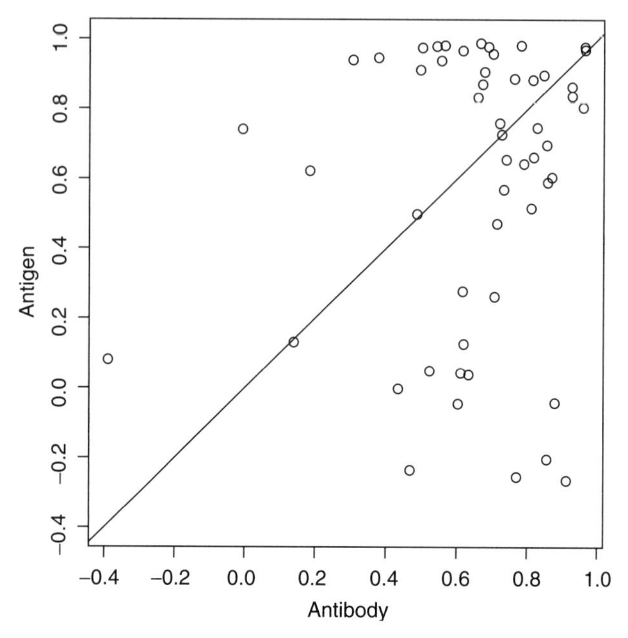

Figure 12.4 Concordance correlations for antigen arrays versus antibody arrays (with the identity line).

Figure 12.3 shows the histogram of the observed concordance correlation coefficient of the observed ratios and their corresponding ideal values for both sets of antibody and antigen microarrays. A simple way to compare these two sets of concordance correlation coefficients is by drawing their scatterplot as in Figure 12.4. In Figure 12.4, there appear to be two distinct groups of proteins on the top right corner, some are above the diagonal line indicting that the concordance correlation coefficients are higher for the arrayed antigens and some are below the line indicating that the concordance correlation coefficients are higher for the arrayed antibodies. In order to estimate a threshold for the concordance correlation, we permuted the samples and calculated a null distribution for the concordance correlation coefficients. It turned out that the 95th percentile of the null distribution corresponded to, approximately, a 0.75 concordance, although the values differ from protein to protein. The number of detected proteins with arrayed antibodies was 59, or approximately 50%, and the number of detected proteins with arrayed antigens was 31, which is approximately 27%. These numbers appear to be different enough to suggest that the detection rates for antibody arrays are slightly higher than that for the antigen arrays.

This kind of study is only the beginning in a new period of biological research. As advances in technology propel genomics and proteomics forward, novel technologies will emerge generating fresh challenges for the sophisticated data analyst.

EXERCISES

12.1. In the analysis in Section 12.4, in the third paragraph, it was suggested that, if the low-concentration sample for a particular protein has a normal distribution with 0 mean and standard deviation 1, the ideal threshold would be equal to 1.96, but, because we are calculating the threshold with only six values, the resulting threshold would range between 0.5 and 3.5, approximately 95% of the time.

(a) Perform a small simulation to verify this result.

(b) Repeat the procedure assuming that the distribution of the low concentration ratios is a chi-squared distribution with 2 degrees of freedom.

12.2. The data set E11 in the DNAMR library consists of 12 samples containing 1200 spots corresponding to 200 proteins with six replicates each. The first six samples are technical replicates at a concentration of 1 ng/ml. The second set of six samples are also technical replicates but spotted at a concentration of 10 ng/ml. The objective is to determine which proteins are detected in the sense of being differentially expressed between both groups. Carry out this analysis making sure that you follow the basic analysis steps and use the quantile normalization option.

References

Agresti A. *Categorical Data Analysis*. 2nd ed. New York: John Wiley & Sons; 2002.

Alberts B, Bray D, Lewis J, Raff M, Roberts K, Watson J. *Molecular Biology of the Cell*. New York: Addison-Wesley; 1994.

Aldenderfer MS, Blashfield RK. *Cluster Analysis*. London: Sage Publications; 1984.

Alizadeh AA, Eisen MB, Davis RE, Ma C, Lossos IS, Rosenwald A, Boldrick JC, Sabet H, Tran T, Yu X, Powell JI, Yang L, Marti GE, Moore T, Hudson J Jr., Lu L, Lewis DB, Tibshirani R, Sherock G, Chan WC, Greiner TC, Weisenburger DD, Armitage JO, Warnke R, Levy R, Wilson W, Grever MR, Byrd JC, Botstein D, Brown PO, Staudt LM. Distinct types of diffuse large B-cell lymphoma identified by gene expression profiling. *Nature* 2000;**403**:503–511.

Allison DB, Gadbury GL, Heo M, Fernndez JR, Lee CK, Prolla TA, Weindruch R. A mixture model approach for the analysis of microarray gene expression data. *Comput Stat Data Anal* 2002;**39**:1–20.

Alon U, Barkai N, Notterman DA, Gish K, Ybarra S, Mack D, Levine AJ. Broad patterns of gene expression revealed by clustering analysis of tumor and normal colon tissues probed by oligonucleotide arrays. *Proc Natl Acad Sci U S A* 1999;**96**:6745–6750.

Alter O, Brown PO, Botstein D. Singular value decomposition for genome-wide expression data processing and modeling. *Proc Natl Acad Sci U S A* 2000;**97**:10101d2-1010106.

Amaratunga D, Cabrera J. Statistical analysis of microchip data. Unpublished material presented at the Joint Statistical Meetings. Baltimore, MD; 1999.

Amaratunga D, Cabrera J. Outlier resistance, standardization and modeling issues for DNA microarray data. In: Fernholz LT, Morgenthaler S, Stahel W, editors. *Statistics and Genetics for the Environmental Sciences*. Basel, Switzerland: Birkhauser Verlag; 2001a.

Amaratunga D, Cabrera J. Statistical analysis of viral microchip data. *J Am Stat Assoc* 2001b;**96**:1161–1170.

Amaratunga D, Cabrera J. Mining data to find subsets of high activity. *J Stat Plann Infer* 2003a;**122**:23–41.

Amaratunga D, Cabrera J. Methods for assessing the quality of DNA microarrays; 2003b, Unpublished.

Exploration and Analysis of DNA Microarray and Other High-Dimensional Data, Second Edition.
Dhammika Amaratunga, Javier Cabrera, Ziv Shkedy.

Amaratunga D, Cabrera J. A robust Bayes analysis of DNA microarray data; 2003c, Unpublished.

Amaratunga D, Cabrera J. A conditional t suite of tests for identifying differentially expressed genes in a DNA microarray experiment with little replication. *Stat Biopharm Res* 2009;**1**:26–38.

Amaratunga D, Cabrera J, Kovtun V. Microarray learning with ABC. *Biostatistics* 2008;**9**:128–136.

Amaratunga D, Cabrera J, Cherkas Y, Lee YS. Ensemble classifiers. In: Fourdrinier D, Marchand E, Rukhin AL, editors. *Beachwood, Ohio, USA: IMS Collection Volume 8: Contemporary Developments in Bayesian Analysis and Statistical Decision Theory: A Festschrift for William E. Strawderman*; 2012.

Amaratunga D, Cabrera J, De Bondt A, Tryputsen V. Using Fisher's method to identify enriched gene sets. Unpublished; 2013.

Amaratunga D, Cabrera J, Lee YS. Enriched random forests. *Bioinformatics* 2008;**24**: 2010–2014.

Ambroise C, McLachlan GJ. Selection bias in gene extraction on basis of microarray gene expression data. *Proc Natl Acad Sci U S A* 2002;**99**:6562–6566.

Angenendt P, Glokler J, Murphy D, Lehrach H, Cahill DJ. Toward optimized antibody microarrays: a comparison of current microarray support materials. *Anal Biochem* 2002;**309**:253–260.

Anscombe F, Tukey JW. The examination and analysis of residuals. *Technometrics* 1963; **5**:141–160.

Asimov D. The grand tour: a tool for viewing multidimensional data. *SIAM J Sci Stat Comput* 1985;**6**:128–143.

Astrand M. Contrast normalization of oligonucleotide arrays. *J Comput Biol* 2003; **10**:95–102.

Baldi P, Long AD. A Bayesian framework for the analysis of microarray expression data: regularized t-test and statistical inferences of gene changes. *Bioinformatics* 2001;**7**:509–519.

Banfield JD, Raftery AE. Model-based Gaussian and non-Gaussian clustering. *Biometrics* 1993;**49**:803–821.

Barash Y, Friedman N. Context-specific Bayesian clustering for gene expression data. *J Comput Biol* 2002;**9**:169–191.

Barnett V, editor. *Interpreting Multivariate Data*. New York: John Wiley & Sons; 1981.

Barnett V, Lewis T. *Outliers in Statistical Data*. 3rd ed. New York: John Wiley & Sons; 1994.

Barlow RE, Bartholomew DJ, Bremner MJ, Brunk HD. *Statistical Inference Under Order Restriction*. New York: John Wiley & Sons; 1972.

Bassett DE, Eisen MB, Boguski MS. Gene expression informatics - it's all in your mine. *Nat Genet Suppl* 1999;**21**:51–55.

Ben-Hur A, Elisseeff A, Guyon I. A stability-based method for discovering structure in clustered data. *Pac Symp Biocomput* 2002;**7**:6–17.

Benjamini Y, Hochberg Y. Controlling the False Discovery Rate: a practical and powerful approach to multiple testing. *J R Stat Soc B* 1995;**57**:289–300.

Benjamini Y, Yekutieli D. The control of the false discovery rate in multiple testing under dependency. *Ann Stat* 2001;**29**(4):1165–1188.

Bittner M, Meltzer P, Chen Y, Jiang Y, Seftor E, Hendrix M, Radmacher M, Simon R, Yakhini Z, Ben-Dor A, Sampas N, Dougherty E, Wang E, Marincola F, Gooden C, Lueders J, Glatfelter A, Pollock P, Carpten J, Gillanders E, Leja D, Dietrich K, Beaudry C, Berens M, Alberts D, Sondak V, Hayward N, Trent J. Molecular classification of cutaneous malignant melanoma by gene expression profiling. *Nature* 2000;**406**:536–540.

Blower PE, Yang C, Fligner MA, Verducci JS, Yu L, Richman S, Weinstein JN. Pharmacogenomic analysis: correlating molecular substructure classes with microarray gene expression data. *Pharmacogenomics J* 2002;**2**:259–271.

Bo TH, Jonassen I. New feature subset selection procedures for classification of expression profiles. *Genome Biol* 2002;**3**:(research) 0017-1-0017-11.

Bolstad BM, Irizarry RA, Astrand M, Speed TP. A comparison of normalization methods for high density oligonucleotide array data based on variance and bias. *Bioinformatics* 2003;**19**:185–193.

Bourgon R, Gentleman R, Huber W. Independent filtering increases detection power for high-throughput experiments. *Proc Natl Acad Sci U S A* 2010;**107**(21):9546–9551.

Bouton CM, Pevsner J. DRAGON: database referencing of array genes online. *Bioinformatics* 2000;**16**:1038–1039.

Bouton C, Pevsner J. DRAGON view: information visualization for annotated microarray data. *Bioinformatics* 2002;**18**:323–324.

Brazma A, Vilo J. Gene expression data analysis. *FEBS Lett* 2000;**480**:17–24.

Breiman L. Bagging predictors. *Mach Learn* 1996;**26**:123–140.

Breiman L, Cutler A. Random Forests Manual (version 4.0), Technical Report of the University of California. Berkeley: Department of Statistics; 2003.

Breiman L. Random forests. *Mach Learn* 2001;**45**:5–32.

Breiman L, Friedman JH, Olshen RA, Stone CJ. *Classification and Regression Trees*. Monterey (CA): Wadsworth; 1984.

Brillinger DR, Fernholz LT, Morgenthaler S, editors. *The Practice of Data Analysis*. Princeton (NJ): Princeton University Press; 1997.

Broberg P. Ranking genes with respect to differential expression. *Genome Biol* 2002;**3**, preprint 0007.1-preprint 0007.23.

Brown CS, Goodwin PC, Sorger PK. Image metrics in the statistical analysis of DNA microarray data. *Proc Natl Acad Sci U S A* 2001;**98**:8944–8949.

Brown MP, Grundy WN, Lin D, Cristianini N, Sugnet CW, Furey TS, Ares M Jr., Haussler D. Knowledge-based analysis of microarray gene expression data by using support vector machines. *Proc Natl Acad Sci U S A* 2000;**97**:262–267.

Brown PO, Botstein D. Exploring the new world of the genome with DNA microarrays. *Nat Genet Suppl* 1999;**21**:33–37.

Buja A, Lee Y. S. Data mining criteria for tree-based regression and classification, KDD 2001: *Proceedings of the Seventh ACM SIGKDD International Conference on Knowledge Discovery and Data Mining*, 2001; 27–36.

Burges CJC. A tutorial on support vector machines for pattern recognition. *Data Mining Knowl Discov* 1998;**2**:121–167.

Cabrera J, Fernholz LT. Target estimation for bias and mean square reduction. *Ann Stat* 1999;**27**:1080–1104.

Cabrera J, McDougall A. *Statistical Consulting*. New York: Springer-Verlag; 2001.

Calinski T, Harabasz J. A dendrite method for cluster analysis. *Commun Stat* 1974;**3**:1–27.

Calza S, Raffelsberger W, Ploner A, Sahel J, Leveillard T, Pawitan Y. Filtering genes to improve sensitivity in oligonucleotide microarray data analysis. *Nucleic Acids Res* 2007;**35**(16).

Chambers J, Angulo A, Amaratunga D, Guo H, Jiang Y, Wan JS, Bittner A, Frueh K, Jackson MR, Peterson PA, Erlander MG, Ghazal P. DNA microarrays of the complex human cytomegalovirus genome: profiling kinetic class with drug sensitive viral gene expression. *J Virol* 1999;**73**:5757–5766.

Chambers JM, Cleveland WS, Kleiner B, Tukey PA. *Graphical Methods for Data Analysis*. Boston (MA): Duxbury Press; 1983.

Chapman S, Schenk P, Kazan K, Manners J. Using biplots to interpret gene expression patterns in plants. *Bioinformatics* 2002;**18**:202–204.

Chen Y, Dougherty ED, Bittner ML. Ratio-based decisions and the quantitative analysis of cDNA microarray images. *J Biomed Opt* 1997;**2**:364–374.

Cherkas Y. Classification and multiple testing for microarray data [PhD dissertation]. Newark (NJ): Rutgers University; 2010.

Chu S, DeRisi J, Eisen M, Mulholland J, Botstein D, Brown PO, Herskowitz I. The transcriptional program of sporulation in budding yeast. *Science* 1998;**282**:699–705.

Chu T-M, Weir B, Wolfinger R. A systematic statistical linear modeling approach to oligonucleotide array experiments. *Math Biosci* 2002;**176**:35–51.

Chu T-M, Weir B, Wolfinger R. Comparison of Li-Wong and loglinear mixed models for the statistical analysis of oligonucleotide arrays. *Bioinformatics* 2004;**20**:500–506.

Churchill GA. Fundamentals of experimental design for cDNA microarrays. *Nat Genet* 2002;**32**:490–495.

Churchill GA, Oliver B. Sex, flies, and microarrays. *Nat Genet* 2001;**29**:355–356.

Clark D, Russell L. *Molecular Biology Made Simple and Fun*. Vienna (IL): Cache River Press; 1997.

Clark LA, Pregibon D. Tree-based models. In: Chambers J, Hastie TJ, editors. *Statistical Models in S*. Wadsworth; 1992.

Clark PJ, Evans FC. Distance to nearest neighbor as a measure of spatial relationships in populations. *Ecology* 1954;**35**:445–453.

Cleveland WS. Robust locally weighted regression and smoothing scatterplots. *J Am Stat Assoc* 1979;**74**:829–836.

Cochran WG, Cox GM. *Experimental Designs*. New York: John Wiley & Sons; 1992.

Cochran WG. *Sampling Techniques*. New York: John Wiley & Sons; 1977.

Colantuoni C, Zeger S, Pevsner J. Local mean normalization of microarray element signal intensities across an array surface: quality control and correction of spatially systematic hybridization artifacts. *Biotechniques* 2002;**32**:1316–1320.

Cook D, Buja A, Cabrera J. Projection pursuit indices based on orthogonal function expansions. *J Comput Graph Stat* 1993;**2**:225–250.

Cook D, Buja A, Cabrera J, Hurley C. Grand tour and projection pursuit. *J Comput Graph Stat* 1995;**4**:155–172.

Coombes KR. PCANOVA: Combining principal components with analysis of variance to assess group structure; 2002, Unpublished.

Cormack RM. A review of classification. *J R Stat Soc [Ser A]* 1971;**134**:321–367.

Cox DR, Hinkley D. *Theoretical Statistics*. London: Chapman and Hall; 1974.

Cui X, Kerr MK, Churchill GA. Data transformation for cDNA microarray data; 2002, Unpublished.

Daniel C, Wood FS. *Fitting Equations to Data*. New York: John Wiley & Sons; 1971.

Debouck C, Goodfellow PN. DNA microarrays in drug discovery and development. *Nat Genet Suppl* 1999;**21**:48–50.

Dempster AP, Laird NM, Rubin DB. Maximum likelihood from incomplete data via the EM algorithm. *J R Stat Soc Ser B* 1977;**39**:1–38.

DeRisi JL, Iyer VR, Brown PO. Exploring the metabolic and genetic control of gene expression on a genomic scale. *Science* 1997;**278**:680–686.

Dudoit S, Fridlyand J. A prediction-based resampling method to estimate the number of clusters in a dataset. *Genome Biol* 2002;**3**: 0036-1-0036-21.

Dudoit S, Fridlyand J, Speed T. Comparison of discrimination methods for the classification of tumors using gene expression data. *J Am Stat Assoc* 2002;**97**:77–87.

Dudoit S, Yang YH, Callow MC, Speed TP. Statistical methods for identifying differentially expressed genes in replicated cDNA microarray experiments. *Stat Sin* 2002;**12**:111–140.

Durbin B, Hardin J, Hawkins D, Rocke DM. A variance-stabilizing transformation for gene expression microarray data. *Bioinformatics* 2002;**18**:S105-S110.

Efron B, Hastie T, Johnstone I, Tibshirani R. Least angle regression. *Ann Stat* 2004;**32**:407–451.

Efron B. Robbins, empirical Bayes, and microarrays. Technical Report of the Stanford University Department of Statistics; 2001.

Efron B, Tibshirani R. *An Introduction to the Bootstrap*. London: Chapman and Hall; 1993.

Efron B, Tibshirani R. Empirical Bayes methods and false discovery rates for microarrays. *Genet Epidemiol* 2002;**23**:70–86.

Efron B, Tibshirani R. On testing the significance of sets of genes. *Ann Appl Stat* 2007;**1**:107–129.

Efron B, Tibshirani R, Storey JD, Tusher V. Empirical Bayes analysis of a microarray experiment. *J Am Stat Assoc* 2001;**96**:1151–1160.

Efron B, Storey JD, Tibshirani R. Microarrays, empirical Bayes methods, and false discovery rates. Technical Report of the Stanford University Department of Statistics; 2001.

Eisen MB, Spellman PT, Brown PO, Botstein D. Cluster analysis and display of genome-wide expression patterns. *Proc Natl Acad Sci U S A* 1998;**95**:14863–14868.

Everitt BS. *Cluster Analysis*. 3rd ed. London: Halsted Press; 1993.

Ewens WJ, Grant GR. *Statistical Methods in Bioinformatics: An Introduction*. Secaucus (NJ): Springer-Verlag; 2001.

Friedman J, Hastie T, Tibshirani R. Regularization paths for generalized linear models via coordinate descent. *J Stat Softw* 2010;**33**:1–22.

Fayyad UM, Piatetsky-Shapiro G, Smyth P, editors. *Advances in Knowledge Discovery and Data Mining*. Menlo Park (CA): AAAI Press / MIT Press; 1996.

Fellenberg K, Hauser N, Brors B, Neutzner A, Hoheisel J, Vingron M. Correspondence analysis applied to microarray data. *Proc Natl Acad Sci U S A* 2001;**98**:10781–10786.

Fernholz LT, Morgenthaler S, Stahel W, editors. *Statistics in Genetics and in the Environmental Sciences*. Basel, Switzerland: Birkhauser-Verlag; 2001.

Fisher RA. The use of multiple measurements in taxonomic problems. *Ann Eugen* 1936;**7**:179–188.

Fisher RA. On the interpretation of χ^2 from contingency tables and the calculation of p. *J R Stat Soc Ser B* 1922;**85**:87–94.

Fisher RA. *Statistical Methods for Research Workers*. Oliver and Boyd; 1925.

Fisher RA. *The Design of Experiments*. 6th ed. London: Oliver and Boyd; 1951.

Fix E, Hodges J. Discriminatory analysis. nonparametric discrimination: consistency properties. Technical Report of the USAF School of Aviation Medicine, Randolph Field (TX); 1951.

Fraley C, Raftery AE. How many clusters? Which clustering method? Answers via model-based cluster analysis. *Comput J* 1998;**41**:578–588.

Freund Y, Schapire RE. A decision-theoretic generalization of on-line learning and an application to boosting. *J Comput Syst Sci* 1997;**55**:119–139.

Friedman JH. Exploratory projection pursuit. *J Am Stat Assoc* 1987;**82**:249–266.

Friedman JH. Regularized discriminant analysis. *J Am Stat Assoc* 1989;**84**:165–175.

Friedman JH. Flexible metric nearest neighbor classification. Technical Report of the Stanford University Statistics Department; 1994.

Friedman JH, Meulman JJ. Clustering objects on subsets of attributes. *J R Stat Soc Ser B* 2004;**66**:815–849.

Friedman JH, Stuetzle W. Projection pursuit regression. *J Am Stat Assoc* 1981;**76**:817–823.

Friedman JH, Tukey JW. A projection pursuit algorithm for exploratory data analysis. *IEEE Trans Comput* 1974;**C-23**:881–890.

Gabriel KR. The biplot graphical display of matrices with applications to principal component analysis. *Biometrika* 1971;**58**:453–467.

Gabriel KR, Odoroff CL. Biplots in biomedical research. *Stat Med* 1990;**9**:469–485.

Getz G, Levine E, Domany E. Coupled two-way clustering analysis of gene microarray data. *Proc Natl Acad Sci U S A* 2000;**97**:12079–12084.

Gentleman R, Carey V, Huber W, Irizarry R, Dudoit S. *Bioinformatics and Computational Biology Solutions using R and Bioconductor*. Springer; 2005.

Gibson G. Microarrays in ecology and evolution: a preview. *Ecology* 2002;**11**:17–24.

Glasbey CA, Ghazal P. Combinatorial image analysis of DNA microarray features. *Bioinformatics* 2003;**19**:194–203.

Gnanadesikan R. *Statistical Data Analysis of Multivariate Observations*. 2nd ed. New York: John Wiley & Sons; 1997.

Gnanadesikan R, Kettenring JR. Discriminant analysis and clustering. *Stat Sci* 1989;**4**:34–69.

Gohlmann H, Talloen W. *Gene Expression Studies Using Affymetrix Microarrays*. Taylor & Francis; 2009.

Golub TR, Slonim DK, Tamayo P, Huard C, Gaasenbeek M, Mesirov JP, Coller H, Loh ML, Downing JR, Caligiuri MA, Bloomfield CD, Lander ES. Molecular classification of cancer: class discovery and class prediction by gene expression monitoring. *Science* 1999;**286**:531–537.

Gonick L, Wheelis M. *A Cartoon Guide to Genetics*. New York: Harper Collins; 1991.

Gordon AD. *Classification*. Boca Raton (FL): Chapman and Hall/CRC; 1999.

Haab B, Dunham M, Brown P. Protein microarrays for highly parallel detection and quantitation of specific proteins and antibodies in complex solutions. *Genome Biol* 2001;**2**:Research 00004.1-Research 00004.13.

Hall P. Polynomial projection pursuit. *Ann Stat* 1989;**17**:589–605.

Hand DJ. *Construction and Assessment of Classification Rules*. New York: John Wiley & Sons; 1997.

Hartigan JA. Direct clustering of a data matrix. *J Am Stat Assoc* 1972;**67**:123–129.

Hartigan JA. *Clustering Algorithms*. New York: John Wiley & Sons; 1975.

Hastie T, Tibshirani R, Buja A. Flexible discriminant analysis. *J Am Stat Assoc* 1994;**89**:1255–1270.

Hastie T, Tibshirani R, Eisen MB, Alizadeh A, Levy R, Staudt L, Chan WC, Botstein D, Brown P. "Gene shaving" as a method for identifying distinct sets of genes with similar expression patterns. *Genome Biol* 2000;**1**: Research 0003.1-0003.21.

Hastie T, Tibshirani R, Friedman J. *Elements of Statistical Learning: Data Mining, Inference and Prediction, Second Edition*, Heidelberg: Springer-Verlag; 2009.

Hawkins DM, Kass GV. Automatic interaction detection. In: Hawkins DM, editors. Topics in Multivariate Analysis. Cambridge: Cambridge University Press; 1982.

Hearst M. SVM - trends and controversies. *IEEE Intell Syst* 1998;**13**:18.

Hedenfalk I, Duggan D, Chen Y, Radmacher M, Bittner M, Simon R, Meltzer P, Gusterson B, Esteller M, Kallioniemi OP, Wilfond B, Borg A, Trent J. Gene-expression profiles in hereditary breast cancer. *N Engl J Med* 2001;**344**:539–548.

Hoaglin DC. Exploratory data analysis. In: Kotz S, Johnson NL, Read CB, editors. *Encyclopedia of Statistical Sciences*. **Volume 2**. New York: John Wiley & Sons; 1982. p 579–583.

Hoaglin DC, Mosteller F, Tukey JW. *Understanding Robust and Exploratory Data Analysis*. New York: John Wiley & Sons; 1983.

Hochberg Y. A sharper Bonferroni procedure for multiple tests of significance. *Biometrika* 1988;**75**:800–803.

Hochreiter S, Bodenhofer U, Heusel M, Mayr A, Mitterecker A, Kasim A, Khamiakova T, Van Sanden S, Lin D, Talloen W, Bijnens L, Göhlmann HWH, Shkedy Z, Clevert D-A. FABIA: factor analysis for bicluster acquisition. *Bioinformatics* 2010;**26**(12):1520–1527.

Hoffmann R, Seidl T, Dugas M. Profound effect of normalization on detection of differentially expressed genes in oligonucleotide microarray data analysis. *Genome Biol* 2002;**3**:research 0033-1-0033-11.

Hollander M, Wolfe DA. *Nonparametric Statistical Methods*. 2nd ed. New York: John Wiley & Sons; 1999.

Holloway AJ, Van Laar RK, Tothill RW, Bowtell DD. Options available - from start to finish - for obtaining data from DNA microarrays II. *Nat Genet* 2002;**32**:481–489.

Holm S. A simple sequentially rejective multiple test procedure. *Scand J Stat* 1979;**6**:65–70.

Holmes I, Bruno WJ. Finding regulatory elements using joint likelihoods for sequence and expression profile data. In: Altman R, et al., editors. *Proceedings of the Eighth Annual International Conference on Intelligent Systems for Molecular Biology*. La Jolla (CA): AAAI Press; 2000. p 202–210.

Hosack DA, Dennis G Jr, Sherman BT, Lane HC, Lempicki RA. Identifying biological themes within lists of genes with EASE. *Genome Biol* 2003;**4**:R70.

Huber W, Heydebreck AV, Silvermaan H, Poustka A, Vingron M. Variance stabilization applied to microarray data calibration and to the quantification of differential expression. *Bioinformatics* 2002;**18**:1–9.

Iglewicz B and Hoaglin D. Volume 16: How to Detect and Handle Outliers, The ASQC Basic References in Quality Control: Statistical Techniques, Edward F. Mykytka, Editor, 1993.

Ihaka R, Gentleman R. R: a language for data analysis and graphics. *J Comput Graph Stat* 1996;**5**:299–314.

Irizarry RA, Bolstad BM, Collin F, Cope LM, Hobbs B, Speed TP. Summaries of Affymetrix GeneChip probe level data. *Nucleic Acids Res* 2003;**31**(4):1–8.

Irizarry RA, Hobbs B, Collin F, Beazer-Barclay YD, Antonellis KJ, Scherf U, Speed TP. Exploration, normalization, and summaries of high density oligonucleotide array probe level data. *Biostatistics* 2003;**4**(2):249–264.

Jin W, Riley R, Wolfinger RD, White KP, Passador-Gurgel G, Gibson G. Contributions of sex, genotype and age to transcriptional variance in Drosophila melanogaster. *Nat Genet* 2001;**29**:389–395.

Kanehisa M, Goto S. KEGG: Kyoto Encyclopedia of Genes and Genomes. *Nucl Acids Res* 2000;**28**:27–30.

Kasim A, Lin D, Van Sanden S, Clevert DA, Bijnens L, Göhhlmann H, Amaratunga D, Hochreiter S, Shkedy Z, Talloen W. Informative or noninformative calls for gene expression: a latent variable approach. *Stat Appl Genet Mol Biol* 2010;**9**(1):Article 4. doi: 10.2202/1544–6115.1460. Epub 2010 Jan 6.

Kaufman L, Rousseeuw PJ. *Finding Groups in Data: An Introduction to Cluster Analysis*. New York: John Wiley & Sons; 1990.

Kerr K, Afshari CA, Lee B, Bushel P, Martinez J, Walker NJ, Churchill GA. Statistical analysis of a gene expression microarray experiment with replication. *Stat Sin* 2002;**12**:203–218.

Kerr MK, Churchill GA. Bootstrapping cluster analysis: assessing the reliability of conclusions from microarray experiments. *Proc Natl Acad Sci U S A* 2000;**98**:8961–8965.

Kerr MK, Churchill GA. Statistical design and the analysis of gene expression microarray data. *Genet Res Camb* 2001a;**77**:123–128.

Kerr MK, Churchill GA. Experimental design for gene expression microarrays. *Biostatistics* 2001b;**2**:183–202.

Kerr MK, Martin M, Churchill GA. Analysis of variance for gene expression microarray data. *J Comput Biol* 2000;**7**:819–837.

Khan J, Wei JS, Ringner M, Saal LH, Ladanyi M, Westermann F, Berthold F, Schwab M, Antonescu CR, Peterson C, Meltzer PS. Classification and diagnostic prediction of cancers using gene expression profiling and artificial neural networks. *Nat Med* 2001;**7**:673–679.

Knezevic V, Leethanakul C, Bichsel VE, Worth JM, Prabhu VV, Gutkind JS, Liotta LA, Munson PJ, Petricoin EF, Krizman DB. Proteomic profiling of the cancer microenvironment by antibody arrays. *Proteomics* 2001;**1**:1271–1278.

Kodadek T. Protein microarrays: prospects and problems. *Chem Biol* 2001;**8**:105–115.

Kohonen T. *Self-organizing Maps*. Berlin, Heidelberg, New York: Springer-Verlag; 1995.

Kothapalli R, Yoder SJ, Mane S, Loughran TP Jr. Microarray results: how accurate are they? *BMC Bioinformatics* 2002;**3**:22.

Krzanowski WJ. Ranking principal components to reflect group structure. *J Chemom* 1992;**6**:97–102.

Krzanowski WJ. *Principles of Multivariate Analysis: A User's Perspective*. 2nd ed. New York: Oxford University Press; 2000.

Krzanowski WJ, Lai YT. A criterion for determining the number of groups in a data set using sum of squares clustering. *Biometrics* 1985;**44**:23–34.

Kuklin A, Petrov A, Shams S. Quality control in microarray image analysis. *GIT Imaging Microsc* 2001;**1**:2–3.

Lander ES. Array of hope. *Nat Genet Suppl* 1999;**21**:3–4.

Landgrebe J, Wurst W, Welzl G. Permutation validated principal components analysis of microarray data. *Genome Biol* 2002;**3**:1–11.

Lazzeroni L, Owen AB. Plaid models for gene expression data. *Stat Sin* 2002;**12**:61–86.

Lee MLT, Lu W, Whitmore GA, Beier D. Models for microarray gene expression data. *J Biopharm Stat* 2002;**12**:1–19.

Lee MLT, Kuo FC, Whitmore GA, Sklar J. Importance of replication in microarray gene expression studies: statistical methods and evidence from repetitive cDNA hybridizations. *Proc Natl Acad Sci U S A* 2000;**97**:9834–9839.

Lee YS, Buja A. Data mining criteria for tree-based regression and classification. Unpublished; 1999.

Lennon GG. High-throughput gene expression analysis for drug discovery. *Drug Discov Today* 2000;**5**:59–66.

Lewi PJ. Spectral mapping, a technique for classifying biological activity profiles of chemical compounds. *Arzneimttel Forschung (Drug Research)* 1976;**26**:1295–1300.

Li C, Wong WH. Model-based analysis of oligonucleotide arrays: model validation, design issues and standard error application. *Genome Biol* 2001a;**2**(8):research 0032–1–0032–11.

Li C, Wong WH. Model-based analysis of oligonucleotide arrays: expression index computation and outlier detection. *Proc Natl Acad Sci U S A* 2001b;**98**:31–36.

Lin LI-K. A concordance correlation coefficient to evaluate reproducibility. *Biometrics* 1989;**45**:255–268.

Lin SM, Johnson KF, editors. *Methods of Microarray Data Analysis: Papers from CAMDA 2000*. Kluwer Academic Publishers; 2002.

Lin D, Shkedy Z, Yekutieli D, Amaratunga D, Bijnens L, editors. *Modeling Dose-response Microarray Data in Early Drug Development Experiments Using R*. Springer-Verlag; 2012.

Lipshutz RJ, Fodor SPA, Gingeras TR, Lockhart DJ. High density synthetic oligonucleotide arrays. *Nat Genet Suppl* 1999;**21**:20–24.

Lo AY, Brunner LJ, Chan AT. Weighted Chinese restaurant processes and Bayesian mixture models. Unpublished; 2000.

Lockhart D, Dong H, Byrne M, Follettie M, Gallo M, Chee M, Mittmann M, Wang C, Kobayashi M, Horton H, Brown E. Expression monitoring by hybridization to high-density oligonucleotide arrays. *Nat Biotechnol* 1996;**14**:1675–1680.

Lonnstedt I, Speed TP. Replicated microarray data. *Stat Sin* 2002;**12**:31–46.

Lubomirski M, D'Andrea MR, Belkowski SM, Cabrera J, Dixon JM, and Amaratunga D. A consolidated approach to analyzing data from high throughput protein microarrays with an application to immune response profiling in humans. *Journal of Computational Biology* 2007;**14**:350–359.

MacBeath G. Protein microarrays and proteomics. *Nat Genet* 2002;**32**:526–532.

MacQueen JB. Some methods for classification and analysis of multivariate observations. *Proceedings of the 5th Berkeley Symposium on E Mathematical Statistics and Probability*. Volume 1. Berkeley: University of California Press; 1967. p 281–297.

Madeira SC, Oliveira AL. Biclustering algorithms for biological data analysis: a survey, *IEEE Trans Comput Biol Bioinform* 2004;**1**(1).

Manly BFJ. *Randomization and Monte Carlo Methods in Biology*. New York: Chapman and Hall; 1992.

Marcus R. The powers of some tests of the quality of normal means against an ordered alternative. *Biometrika* 1976;**63**:177–83.

Mardia KV, Kent JT, Bibby JM. *Multivariate Analysis*. London: Academic Press; 1979.

McCulloch CE, Searle SR. *Generalized, Linear and Mixed Models*. New York: John Wiley & Sons; 2001.

McLachlan GJ. *Discriminant Analysis and Statistical Pattern Recognition*. New York: John Wiley & Sons; 1992.

McLachlan GJ, Bean RW, Peel D. A mixture model-based approach to clustering of microarray expression data. *Bioinformatics* 2002;**18**:413–422.

Miller R. *Beyond ANOVA, Basics of Applied Statistics*. New York: John Wiley & Sons; 1986.

Moechars D, Vanacker N, Cryns K, Andries L, Mancini G, and Verheijen F. Sialin-deficient mice: a novel animal model for infantile free sialic acid storage disease. 2005. ISSD: Society for Neuroscience 35th Annual Meeting. Washington, USA.

Mootha VK, Lindgren CM, Eriksson KF, Subramanian A, Sihag S, Lehar J, Puigserver P, Carlsson E, Ridderstrale M, Laurila E, Houstis N, Daly MJ, Patterson N, Mesirov JP, Golub TR, Tamayo P, Spiegelman B, Lander ES, Hirschhorn JN, Altshuler D, Groop LC. PGC-1alpha-responsive genes involved in oxidative phosphorylation are coordinately downregulated in human diabetes. *Nat Genet* 2003;**34**:267–273.

Morgan JN, Sonquist JA. Problems in the analysis of survey data and a proposal. *J Am Stat Assoc* 1963;**58**:415–434.

Mosteller F, Tukey JW. *Data Analysis and Regression*. Reading (MA): Addison-Wesley; 1977.

Nadon R, Shoemaker J. Statistical issues with microarrays: processing and analysis. *Trends Genet* 2002;**18**:265–271.

Naef F, Lim DA, Patil N, Magnasco M. From features to expression: high-density oligonucleotide arrays analysis revisited. *Proceedings of the DIMACS Workshop on Analysis of Gene Expression Data*; 2001.

Newton MA, Kendziorski CM, Richmond CS, Blattner FR, Tsui KW. On differential variability of expression ratios: improving statistical inference about gene expression changes from microarray data. *J Comput Biol* 2001;**8**:37–52.

Newton MA, Quintana FA, den Boon JA, Sengupta S, Ahlquist P. Random-set methods identify distinct aspects of the enrichment signal in gene-set analysis. *Ann Appl Stat* 2007;**1**:85–106.

Nguyen DV, Arpat AB, Wang N, Carroll RJ. DNA microarray experiments: biological and technological aspects. *Biometrics* 2002;**58**:701–717.

Nguyen DV, Rocke DM. Tumor classification by partial least squares using microarray gene expression data. *Bioinformatics* 2002;**18**:39–50.

Oliver S. Guilt-by-association goes global. *Nature* 2000;**403**:601–603.

Pan W, Lin J, Le C. Model-based cluster analysis of microarray gene-expression data. *Genome Biol* 2002;**3**(2):research 0009.1–0009.8.

Pavlidis P, Qin J, Arango V, Mann JJ, Sibille E. Using the gene ontology for microarray data mining: a comparison of methods and application to age effects in human prefrontal cortex. *Neurochem Res* 2004;**29**:1213–1222.

Peddada S, Lobenhofer EK, Li L, Afshari CA, Weinberg CR, Umbach DM. Gene selection and clustering for time-course and dose-response microarray experiments using order-restricted inference. *Bioinformatics* 2003;**19**(7):834–841.

Peddada S, Harris S Harvey E. ORIOGEN: order restricted inference for ordered gene expression data. *Bioinformatics* 2005;**21**(20):3933–3934.

Peddada S, Harris S, Davidov O. Analysis of correlated gene expression data on ordered Categories. *J Indian Soc Agric Stat* 2010;**64**(1):45–60.

Peddada S, Umbrach DM, Harris S. Statistical analysis of gene expression studies with ordered experimental conditions. *Handbook Stat* 2012;**28**:39–65.

Pomeroy SL, Tamayo P, Gaasenbeek M, Sturla LM, Angelo M, McLaughlin ME, Kim JY, Goumnerova LC, Black PM, Lau C, Allen JC, Zagzag D, Olson JM, Curran T, Wetmore C, Biegel JA, Poggio T, Mukherjee S, Rifkin R, Califano A, Stolovitzky G, Louis DN, Mesirov JP, Lander ES, Golub TR. Prediction of central nervous system embryonal tumour outcome based on gene expression. *Nature* 2002;**415**:436–442.

Quackenbush J. Microarray data normalization and transformation. *Nat Genet* 2002;**32**:496–501.

Quinlan JR. *C4.5: Programs for Machine Learning*. San Mateo (CA): Morgan Kaufmann; 1993.

Raghavan N, Amaratunga D, Cabrera J, Nie A, Jie Q, McMillian M. On methods for gene function scoring as a means of facilitating the interpretation of microarray results. *J Comput Biol* 2006;**13**:798–809.

Raghavan N, De Bondt A, Talloen W, Moechars D, Gohhlmann H, Amaratunga D. The high-level similarity of some disparate gene expression measures, *Bioinformatics* 2007;**23**:3032–3038.

Raghavan N, Nie A, McMillian M, Amaratunga D. Fuzzy class prediction in toxicogenomics and other microarray applications. Unpublished; 2013.

Raghavan N, Nie A, McMillian M, Amaratunga D. A linear prediction rule based on ensemble classifiers for non-genotoxic carcinogenicity. *Stat Biopharm Res* 2011;**4**:185–193.

Rao CR. The utilization of multiple measurements in problems of biological classifications. *J R Stat Assoc [Ser B]* 1948;**10**:159–203.

Raychaudhuri S, Stuart JM, Altman RB. Principal components analysis to summarize microarray experiments: application to sporulation time series. *Pac Symp Biocomput* 2000;**5**:452–463.

Ripley BD. *Pattern Recognition and Neural Networks*. Cambridge: Cambridge University Press; 1996.

Robinson J. An asymptotic expansion for samples from a finite population. *Ann Stat* 1978;**6**(5):1005–1011.

Robertson T, Wright FT, Dykstra RL. *Order Restricted Statistical Inference*. New York: John Wiley & Sons; 1988.

Rocke DM, Durbin B. A model for measurement error for gene expression arrays. *J Comput Biol* 2001;**8**:557–569.

Rocke DM, Durbin B. Approximate variance-stabilizing transformations for gene expression microarrays. *J Comput Biol* 2002;**8**:557–569.

Rosset S, Zhu J. Piecewise linear regularized solution paths. *Ann Stat* 2007;**35**:1012–1030.

Sapir M, Churchill GA. Estimating the posterior probability of differential gene expression from microarray data. Unpublished; 2000.

Schadt EE, Li C, Ellis B, Wong WH. Feature extraction and normalization algorithms for high-density oligonucleotide gene expression array data. *J Cell Biochem* 2001;**84**(37):120–125.

Schadt EE, Li C, Su C, Wong WH. Analyzing high-density oligonucleotide gene expression array data. *J Cell Biochem* 2000;**80**:192–202.

Schena M. *DNA Microarrays: A Practical Approach*. Oxford: Oxford University Press; 1999.

Schena M, Shalon D, Davis RW, Brown PO. Quantitative monitoring of gene expression patterns with a complementary DNA microarray. *Science* 1995;**270**:467–470.

Schuchhardt J, Beule D, Malik A, Wolski E, Eickhoff H, Lehrach H, Herzel H. Normalization strategies for cDNA microarrays. *Nucl Acids Res* 2000;**28**:e47.

Seaman MA, Levin KR, Serlin RC. New developments in pairwise multiple comparisons: Some powerful and practicable procedures. *Psychol Bull* 1991;**110**:577–586.

Seber GAF. *Multivariate Observations*. New York: John Wiley & Sons; 1984.

Sidak Z. Rectangular confidence regions for the means of multivariate normal distributions. *J Am Stat Assoc* 1967;**62**:626–633.

Slonim DK. From patterns to pathways: gene expression data analysis comes of age. *Nat Genet* 2002;**32**:502–508.

Slonim DK, Tamayo P, Mesirov JP, Golub TR, Lander ES. Class prediction and discovery using gene expression data. Proceedings of RECOMB IV; 2000. p 263–271.

Smyth GK. Linear models and empirical Bayes methods for assessing differential expression in microarray experiments. *Stat Appl Genet Mol Biol* 2004;**3**(1):Article 3.

Smyth GK. Limma: linear models for microarray data. In: Gentleman R, Carey V, Dudoit S, Irizarry R, Huber W, editors. *Bioinformatics and Computational Biology Solutions using R and Bioconductor*. New York: Springer-Verlag; 2005. p 397–420.

Sokal RR, Michener CD. A statistical method for evaluating systematic relationships. *Univ Kansas Sci Bull* 1958;**38**:1409–1438.

Sonquist JA, Morgan JN. The Detection of Interaction Effects, Survey Research Center, Monograph No. 35, Ann Arbor: Institute for Social Research, University of Michigan; 1964.

Sorlie T, Perou CM, Tibshirani R, Aas T, Geisler S, Johnsen H, Hastie T, Eisen MB, van De Rijn M, Jeffrey SS, Thorsen T, Quist H, Matese JC, Brown PO, Botstein D, Lonning PE, Borresen-Dale AL. Gene expression patterns of breast carcinomas distinguish tumor subclasses with clinical implications. *Proc Natl Acad Sci U S A* 2001;**98**:10869–10874.

Spellman PT, Sherlock G, Zhang MQ, Iyer VR, Anders K, Eisen MB, Brown PO, Botstein D, Futcher B. Comprehensive identification of cell cycle-regulated genes of the yeast Saccharomyces cerevisiae by microarray hybridization. *Mol Biol Cell* 1998;**9**:3273–3297.

Storey JD. The positive False Discovery Rate: a Bayesian interpretation and the q-value. Technical Report of the Stanford University Department of Statistics; 2001.

Storey JD. A direct approach to false discovery rates. *J R Stat Soc [Ser B]* 2002;**64**:479–498.

Storey JD, Tibshirani R. Estimating false discovery rates under dependence, with applications to DNA microarrays. Technical Report of the Stanford University Department of Statistics; 2001.

Strachan T, Read AP. *Human Molecular Genetics*. 2nd ed. New York: John Wiley & Sons; 1999.

Subramanian A, Tamayo P, Mootha VK, Mukherjee S, Ebert BL, Gillette MA, Paulovich A, Pomeroy SL, Golub TR, Lander ES, Mesirov JP. Gene set enrichment analysis: a knowledge-based approach for interpreting genome-wide expression profiles. *Proc Natl Acad Sci U S A* 2005;**102**:15545–15550.

Sugden RA, Smith TMF. Edgeworth approximation to the distribution of the sample mean under simple random sampling. *Stat Probab Lett* 1997;**34**:293–299–; *Correct Stat Probab Lett* 1998;**37**:317.

Slawski M, Daumer M, Boulesteix AL. CMA: a comprehensive Bioconductor package for supervised classification with high dimensional data. *BMC Bioinformatics* 2008.

Talloen W, Clevert D, Hochreiter S, Amaratunga D, Bijnens L, Kass S, and Göhlmann H. Gene selection: filtering microarray probesets based on probe level consistency. *Bioinformatics* 2007;**23**:2897–2902.

Talloen W, Hochreiter S, Bijnens L, Kasim A, Shkedy Z, Amaratunga D, Gahlmann H. Filtering data from high-throughput experiments based on measurement reliability. *Proc Natl Acad Sci U S A* 2010;**107**(46):E173–E174.

Tamayo P, Slonim D, Mesirov J, Zhu Q, Kitareewan S, Dmitrovsky E, Lander ES, Golub TR. Interpreting patterns of gene expression with self-organizing maps: methods and application to hematopoietic differentiation. *Proc Natl Acad Sci U S A* 1999;**96**:2907–2912.

Tavazoie S, Hughes JD, Campbell MJ, Cho RJ, Church GM. Systematic determination of genetic network architecture. *Nat Genet* 1999;**22**:281–285.

The Gene Ontology Consortium. Gene ontology: tool for the unification of biology. *Nat Genet* 2000;**25**:25–29.

Therneau T, Tschumper RC, Jelinek D. Sharpening spots: correcting for bleedover in cDNA array images. *Math Biosci* 2002;**176**:1–15.

Tibshirani R. Regression shrinkage and selection via the lasso. *J R Stat Soc [Ser B]* 1996;**58**(1):267–288.

Tibshirani R, Hastie T, Narasiman B, Chu G. Diagnosis of multiple cancer types by shrunken centroids of gene expression. *Proc Natl Acad Sci U S A* 2002;**99**:6567–6572.

Tibshirani R, Hastie T, Narasimhan B, Eisen M, Sherlock G, Brown P, Botstein D. Exploratory screening of genes and clusters from microarray experiments. *Stat Sin* 2002;**12**:47–60.

Tibshirani R, Walther G, Botstein D, Brown P. Cluster validation by prediction strength. Technical Report of the Stanford University Department of Statistics; 2001.

Tibshirani R, Walther G, Hastie T. Estimating the number of clusters in a dataset via the gap statistic. *J R Stat Soc [Ser B]* 2001;**64**:411–423.

Toronen P, Kolehmainen M, Wong G, Castren E. Analysis of gene expression data using self-organizing maps. *FEBS Lett* 1999;**451**:142–146.

Triola MF. *Elementary Statistics Using Excel*. Reading (MA): Addison Wesley; 2001.

Triola MF. *Elementary Statistics*. 8th ed. Reading (MA): Addison Wesley; 2002.

Tseng GC, Oh MK, Rohlin L, Liao JC, Wong WH. Issues in cDNA microarray analysis: quality filtering, channel normalization, models of variations and assessment of gene effects. *Nucl Acids Res* 2001;**29**:2549–2557.

Tukey JW. The future of data analysis. *Ann Math Stat* 1962;**33**:1–67.

Tukey JW. *Exploratory Data Analysis*. Reading (MA): Addison-Wesley; 1977.

Tukey JW. We need both exploratory and confirmatory. *Am Stat* 1980;**34**:23–25.

Tukey JW. The Collected Works of John W. In: Jones LV, editor. *Tukey: Philosophy and Principles of Data Analysis 1949–1964*. **Volume 3**. Pacific Grove (CA): Wadsworth and Brooks/Cole; 1986.

Tusher VG, Tibshirani R, Chu G. Significance analysis of microarrays applied to the ionizing radiation response. *Proc Natl Acad Sci U S A* 2001;**98**:5116–5121.

Van Der Laan MJ, Bryan J. Gene expression analysis with the parametric bootstrap. *Biostatistics* 2001;**2**:445–461.

Velleman PF, Hoaglin DC. *Applications, Basics and Computing of Exploratory Data Analysis*. Boston (MA): Duxbury Press; 1981.

Vingron M. Bioinformatics needs to adopt statistical thinking. *Bioinformatics* 2001;**17**:389–390.

Walker MG, Volkmuth W, Sprinzak E, Hodgson D, Klingler T. Prediction of gene function by genome-scale expression analysis: prostate cancer-associated genes. *Genome Res* 1999;**9**:1198–1203.

Ward JH. Hierarchical grouping to optimize an objective function. *J Am Stat Assoc* 1963;**58**:236–244.

Wang X, Ghosh S, Guo SW. Quantitative quality control in microarray image processing and data acquisition. *Nucl Acids Res* 2001;**29**:e75.

Westfall PH, Young SS. *Resampling-Based Multiple Testing: Examples and Methods for P-Value Adjustment*. New York: John Wiley & Sons; 1993.

Wijesinha M, Amaratunga D. A comparison of methods for identifying differentially expressed genes in microarray experiments. *Proceedings of the Joint Statistical Meetings Biopharmaceutical Section*. Miami, FL; 2011.

Wilson EB, Hilferty MM. The distribution of chi-square. *Proc Natl Acad Sci U S A* 1931;**17**:694.

Williams DA. A test for differences between treatment means when several dose levels are compared with a zero dose control. *Biometrics* 1971;**27**:103–117.

Williams DA. The comparison of several dose levels with a zero dose control. *Biometrics* 1972;**28**:519–531.

Wolfinger RD, Gibson G, Wolfinger ED, Bennett L, Hamadeh H, Bushel P, Afshari C, Paules RS. Assessing gene significance from cDNA microarray expression data via mixed models. *J Comput Biol* 2001;**8**:625–637.

Wouters L, Gohlmann HW, Bijnens L, Molenberghs G, Lewi PJ. Graphical exploration of gene expression data: a comparative study of three multivariate methods. *Biometrics* 2003;**59**:1131–1139.

Yang YH, Buckley MJ, Dudoit S, Speed TP. Comparison of methods for image analysis on cDNA microarray data. Technical Report of the Department of Statistics, University of California at Berkeley; 2000.

Yang YH, Buckley MJ, Speed TP. Analysis of microarray images. *Brief Bioinform* 2001;**2**:341–349.

Yang YH, Dudoit S, Lu P, Speed TP. *Normalization for cDNA microarray data*. In:Bittner ML, Chen Y, Dorsel AN, Dougherty ER, editors. *Microarrays: Optical Technologies and Informatics*. **Volume 466**. Proceedings of SPIE; 2001.

Yang YH, Dudoit S, Lu P, Lin DM, Peng V, Ngai J, Speed TP. Normalization for cDNA microarray data: a robust composite method addressing single and multiple slide systematic variation. *Nucl Acids Res* 2002;**30**(4):e15.

Yang YH, Speed T. Design issues for cDNA microarray experiments. *Nat Rev Genet* 2002;**3**:579–588.

Yeang CH, Ramaswamy S, Tamayo P, Mukherjee S, Rifkin RM, Angelo M, Reich M, Lander ES, Mesirov J, Golub T. Molecular classification of multiple tumor types. *Bioinformatics* 2001;**17**:S316-S322.

Yeung KY, Fraley C, Murua A, Raftery AE, Ruzzo WL. Model-based clustering and data transformations for gene expression data. *Bioinformatics* 2001;**17**:977–987.

Yeung KY, Haynor DR, Ruzzo WL. Validating clustering for gene expression data. *Bioinformatics* 2001;**17**:309–318.

Yeung KY, Ruzzo WL. Principal component analysis for clustering gene expression data. *Bioinformatics* 2001;**17**:763–774.

Yuketieli D, Benjamini Y. Resampling based false discovery rate controlling multiple test procedures for correlated test statistics. *J Stat Plann Inference* 1999;**82**:171–196.

Zhang H, Yu CY, Singer B, Xiong M. Recursive partitioning for tumor classification with gene expression microarray data. *Proc Natl Acad Sci U S A* 2001;**98**:6730–6735.

Zhang X, Amaratunga D, Roeder K. Identifying differentially expressed genes for class prediction using classification error and gene clustering. Unpublished; 2002.

Zou H, Hastie T. Regularization and variable selection via the elastic net. *J R Stat Soc [Ser B]* 2005;**67**(2):301–320.

Index

Exploration and Analysis of DNA Microarray and Other High-Dimensional Data, Second Edition.
Dhammika Amaratunga, Javier Cabrera, Ziv Shkedy.

WILEY SERIES IN PROBABILITY AND STATISTICS

ESTABLISHED BY WALTER A. SHEWHART AND SAMUEL S. WILKS

The ***Wiley Series in Probability and Statistics*** is well established and authoritative. It covers many topics of current research interest in both pure and applied statistics and probability theory. Written by leading statisticians and institutions, the titles span both state-of-the-art developments in the field and classical methods.

Reflecting the wide range of current research in statistics, the series encompasses applied, methodological and theoretical statistics, ranging from applications and new techniques made possible by advances in computerized practice to rigorous treatment of theoretical approaches.

This series provides essential and invaluable reading for all statisticians, whether in academia, industry, government, or research.

† ABRAHAM and LEDOLTER · Statistical Methods for Forecasting
AGRESTI · Analysis of Ordinal Categorical Data, *Second Edition*
AGRESTI · An Introduction to Categorical Data Analysis, *Second Edition*
AGRESTI · Categorical Data Analysis, *Second Edition*
ALTMAN, GILL, and McDONALD · Numerical Issues in Statistical Computing for the Social Scientist
AMARATUNGA and CABRERA · Exploration and Analysis of DNA Microarray and Protein Array Data
AMARATUNGA, CABRERA, and SHKEDY . Exploration and Analysis of DNA Microarray and Other High-Dimensional Data, *Second Edition*
ANDĚL · Mathematics of Chance
ANDERSON · An Introduction to Multivariate Statistical Analysis, *Third Edition*
* ANDERSON · The Statistical Analysis of Time Series
ANDERSON, AUQUIER, HAUCK, OAKES, VANDAELE, and WEISBERG · Statistical Methods for Comparative Studies
ANDERSON and LOYNES · The Teaching of Practical Statistics
ARMITAGE and DAVID (editors) · Advances in Biometry
ARNOLD, BALAKRISHNAN, and NAGARAJA · Records
* ARTHANARI and DODGE · Mathematical Programming in Statistics
* BAILEY · The Elements of Stochastic Processes with Applications to the Natural Sciences
BAJORSKI · Statistics for Imaging, Optics, and Photonics
BALAKRISHNAN and KOUTRAS · Runs and Scans with Applications
BALAKRISHNAN and NG · Precedence-Type Tests and Applications
BARNETT · Comparative Statistical Inference, *Third Edition*
BARNETT · Environmental Statistics
BARNETT and LEWIS · Outliers in Statistical Data, *Third Edition*
BARTHOLOMEW, KNOTT, and MOUSTAKI · Latent Variable Models and Factor Analysis: A Unified Approach, *Third Edition*
BARTOSZYNSKI and NIEWIADOMSKA-BUGAJ · Probability and Statistical Inference, *Second Edition*
BASILEVSKY · Statistical Factor Analysis and Related Methods: Theory and Applications

*Now available in a lower priced paperback edition in the Wiley Classics Library.
†Now available in a lower priced paperback edition in the Wiley–Interscience Paperback Series.

BATES and WATTS · Nonlinear Regression Analysis and Its Applications
BECHHOFER, SANTNER, and GOLDSMAN · Design and Analysis of Experiments for Statistical Selection, Screening, and Multiple Comparisons
BEIRLANT, GOEGEBEUR, SEGERS, TEUGELS, and DE WAAL · Statistics of Extremes: Theory and Applications
BELSLEY · Conditioning Diagnostics: Collinearity and Weak Data in Regression
† BELSLEY, KUH, and WELSCH · Regression Diagnostics: Identifying Influential Data and Sources of Collinearity
BENDAT and PIERSOL · Random Data: Analysis and Measurement Procedures, *Fourth Edition*
BERNARDO and SMITH · Bayesian Theory
BHAT and MILLER · Elements of Applied Stochastic Processes, *Third Edition*
BHATTACHARYA and WAYMIRE · Stochastic Processes with Applications
BIEMER, GROVES, LYBERG, MATHIOWETZ, and SUDMAN · Measurement Errors in Surveys
BILLINGSLEY · Convergence of Probability Measures, *Second Edition*
BILLINGSLEY · Probability and Measure, *Anniversary Edition*
BIRKES and DODGE · Alternative Methods of Regression
BISGAARD and KULAHCI · Time Series Analysis and Forecasting by Example
BISWAS, DATTA, FINE, and SEGAL · Statistical Advances in the Biomedical Sciences: Clinical Trials, Epidemiology, Survival Analysis, and Bioinformatics
BLISCHKE and MURTHY (editors) · Case Studies in Reliability and Maintenance
BLISCHKE and MURTHY · Reliability: Modeling, Prediction, and Optimization
BLOOMFIELD · Fourier Analysis of Time Series: An Introduction, *Second Edition*
BOLLEN · Structural Equations with Latent Variables
BOLLEN and CURRAN · Latent Curve Models: A Structural Equation Perspective
BOROVKOV · Ergodicity and Stability of Stochastic Processes
BOSQ and BLANKE · Inference and Prediction in Large Dimensions
BOULEAU · Numerical Methods for Stochastic Processes
* BOX and TIAO · Bayesian Inference in Statistical Analysis
BOX · Improving Almost Anything, *Revised Edition*
* BOX and DRAPER · Evolutionary Operation: A Statistical Method for Process Improvement
BOX and DRAPER · Response Surfaces, Mixtures, and Ridge Analyses, *Second Edition*
BOX, HUNTER, and HUNTER · Statistics for Experimenters: Design, Innovation, and Discovery, *Second Editon*
BOX, JENKINS, and REINSEL · Time Series Analysis: Forcasting and Control, *Fourth Edition*
BOX, LUCEÑO, and PANIAGUA-QUIÑONES · Statistical Control by Monitoring and Adjustment, *Second Edition*
* BROWN and HOLLANDER · Statistics: A Biomedical Introduction
CAIROLI and DALANG · Sequential Stochastic Optimization
CASTILLO, HADI, BALAKRISHNAN, and SARABIA · Extreme Value and Related Models with Applications in Engineering and Science
CHAN · Time Series: Applications to Finance with R and S-Plus®, *Second Edition*
CHARALAMBIDES · Combinatorial Methods in Discrete Distributions
CHATTERJEE and HADI · Regression Analysis by Example, *Fourth Edition*
CHATTERJEE and HADI · Sensitivity Analysis in Linear Regression
CHERNICK · Bootstrap Methods: A Guide for Practitioners and Researchers, *Second Edition*
CHERNICK and FRIIS · Introductory Biostatistics for the Health Sciences
CHILÈS and DELFINER · Geostatistics: Modeling Spatial Uncertainty, *Second Edition*
CHOW and LIU · Design and Analysis of Clinical Trials: Concepts and Methodologies, *Second Edition*

*Now available in a lower priced paperback edition in the Wiley Classics Library.
†Now available in a lower priced paperback edition in the Wiley–Interscience Paperback Series.

CLARKE · Linear Models: The Theory and Application of Analysis of Variance
CLARKE and DISNEY · Probability and Random Processes: A First Course with Applications, *Second Edition*
* COCHRAN and COX · Experimental Designs, *Second Edition*
COLLINS and LANZA · Latent Class and Latent Transition Analysis: With Applications in the Social, Behavioral, and Health Sciences
CONGDON · Applied Bayesian Modelling
CONGDON · Bayesian Models for Categorical Data
CONGDON · Bayesian Statistical Modelling, *Second Edition*
CONOVER · Practical Nonparametric Statistics, *Third Edition*
COOK · Regression Graphics
COOK and WEISBERG · An Introduction to Regression Graphics
COOK and WEISBERG · Applied Regression Including Computing and Graphics
CORNELL · A Primer on Experiments with Mixtures
CORNELL · Experiments with Mixtures, Designs, Models, and the Analysis of Mixture Data, *Third Edition*
COX · A Handbook of Introductory Statistical Methods
CRESSIE · Statistics for Spatial Data, *Revised Edition*
CRESSIE and WIKLE · Statistics for Spatio-Temporal Data
CSÖRGŐ and HORVÁTH · Limit Theorems in Change Point Analysis
DAGPUNAR · Simulation and Monte Carlo: With Applications in Finance and MCMC
DANIEL · Applications of Statistics to Industrial Experimentation
DANIEL · Biostatistics: A Foundation for Analysis in the Health Sciences, *Eighth Edition*
* DANIEL · Fitting Equations to Data: Computer Analysis of Multifactor Data, *Second Edition*
DASU and JOHNSON · Exploratory Data Mining and Data Cleaning
DAVID and NAGARAJA · Order Statistics, *Third Edition*
* DEGROOT, FIENBERG, and KADANE · Statistics and the Law
DEL CASTILLO · Statistical Process Adjustment for Quality Control
DEMARIS · Regression with Social Data: Modeling Continuous and Limited Response Variables
DEMIDENKO · Mixed Models: Theory and Applications with R, *Second Edition*
DENISON, HOLMES, MALLICK and SMITH · Bayesian Methods for Nonlinear Classification and Regression
DETTE and STUDDEN · The Theory of Canonical Moments with Applications in Statistics, Probability, and Analysis
DEY and MUKERJEE · Fractional Factorial Plans
DILLON and GOLDSTEIN · Multivariate Analysis: Methods and Applications
* DODGE and ROMIG · Sampling Inspection Tables, *Second Edition*
* DOOB · Stochastic Processes
DOWDY, WEARDEN, and CHILKO · Statistics for Research, *Third Edition*
DRAPER and SMITH · Applied Regression Analysis, *Third Edition*
DRYDEN and MARDIA · Statistical Shape Analysis
DUDEWICZ and MISHRA · Modern Mathematical Statistics
DUNN and CLARK · Basic Statistics: A Primer for the Biomedical Sciences, *Fourth Edition*
DUPUIS and ELLIS · A Weak Convergence Approach to the Theory of Large Deviations
EDLER and KITSOS · Recent Advances in Quantitative Methods in Cancer and Human Health Risk Assessment
* ELANDT-JOHNSON and JOHNSON · Survival Models and Data Analysis
ENDERS · Applied Econometric Time Series, *Third Edition*
† ETHIER and KURTZ · Markov Processes: Characterization and Convergence

*Now available in a lower priced paperback edition in the Wiley Classics Library.
†Now available in a lower priced paperback edition in the Wiley–Interscience Paperback Series.

EVANS, HASTINGS, and PEACOCK · Statistical Distributions, *Third Edition*
EVERITT, LANDAU, LEESE, and STAHL · Cluster Analysis, *Fifth Edition*
FEDERER and KING · Variations on Split Plot and Split Block Experiment Designs
FELLER · An Introduction to Probability Theory and Its Applications, Volume I, *Third Edition*, Revised; Volume II, *Second Edition*
FITZMAURICE, LAIRD, and WARE · Applied Longitudinal Analysis, *Second Edition*
* FLEISS · The Design and Analysis of Clinical Experiments
FLEISS · Statistical Methods for Rates and Proportions, *Third Edition*
† FLEMING and HARRINGTON · Counting Processes and Survival Analysis
FUJIKOSHI, ULYANOV, and SHIMIZU · Multivariate Statistics: High-Dimensional and Large-Sample Approximations
FULLER · Introduction to Statistical Time Series, *Second Edition*
† FULLER · Measurement Error Models
GALLANT · Nonlinear Statistical Models
GEISSER · Modes of Parametric Statistical Inference
GELMAN and MENG · Applied Bayesian Modeling and Causal Inference from ncomplete-Data Perspectives
GEWEKE · Contemporary Bayesian Econometrics and Statistics
GHOSH, MUKHOPADHYAY, and SEN · Sequential Estimation
GIESBRECHT and GUMPERTZ · Planning, Construction, and Statistical Analysis of Comparative Experiments
GIFI · Nonlinear Multivariate Analysis
GIVENS and HOETING · Computational Statistics
GLASSERMAN and YAO · Monotone Structure in Discrete-Event Systems
GNANADESIKAN · Methods for Statistical Data Analysis of Multivariate Observations, *Second Edition*
GOLDSTEIN · Multilevel Statistical Models, *Fourth Edition*
GOLDSTEIN and LEWIS · Assessment: Problems, Development, and Statistical Issues
GOLDSTEIN and WOOFF · Bayes Linear Statistics
GREENWOOD and NIKULIN · A Guide to Chi-Squared Testing
GROSS, SHORTLE, THOMPSON, and HARRIS · Fundamentals of Queueing Theory, *Fourth Edition*
GROSS, SHORTLE, THOMPSON, and HARRIS · Solutions Manual to Accompany Fundamentals of Queueing Theory, *Fourth Edition*
* HAHN and SHAPIRO · Statistical Models in Engineering
HAHN and MEEKER · Statistical Intervals: A Guide for Practitioners
HALD · A History of Probability and Statistics and their Applications Before 1750
† HAMPEL · Robust Statistics: The Approach Based on Influence Functions
HARTUNG, KNAPP, and SINHA · Statistical Meta-Analysis with Applications
HEIBERGER · Computation for the Analysis of Designed Experiments
HEDAYAT and SINHA · Design and Inference in Finite Population Sampling
HEDEKER and GIBBONS · Longitudinal Data Analysis
HELLER · MACSYMA for Statisticians
HERITIER, CANTONI, COPT, and VICTORIA-FESER · Robust Methods in Biostatistics
HINKELMANN and KEMPTHORNE · Design and Analysis of Experiments, Volume 1: Introduction to Experimental Design, *Second Edition*
HINKELMANN and KEMPTHORNE · Design and Analysis of Experiments, Volume 2: Advanced Experimental Design
HINKELMANN (editor) · Design and Analysis of Experiments, Volume 3: Special Designs and Applications
HOAGLIN, MOSTELLER, and TUKEY · Fundamentals of Exploratory Analysis of Variance

*Now available in a lower priced paperback edition in the Wiley Classics Library.
†Now available in a lower priced paperback edition in the Wiley–Interscience Paperback Series.

* HOAGLIN, MOSTELLER, and TUKEY · Exploring Data Tables, Trends and Shapes
* HOAGLIN, MOSTELLER, and TUKEY · Understanding Robust and Exploratory Data Analysis

HOCHBERG and TAMHANE · Multiple Comparison Procedures
HOCKING · Methods and Applications of Linear Models: Regression and the Analysis of Variance, *Third Edition*
HOEL · Introduction to Mathematical Statistics, *Fifth Edition*
HOGG and KLUGMAN · Loss Distributions
HOLLANDER, WOLFE, and CHICKEN · Nonparametric Statistical Methods, *Third Edition*
HOSMER and LEMESHOW · Applied Logistic Regression, *Second Edition*
HOSMER, LEMESHOW, and MAY · Applied Survival Analysis: Regression Modeling of Time-to-Event Data, *Second Edition*
HUBER · Data Analysis: What Can Be Learned From the Past 50 Years
HUBER · Robust Statistics
† HUBER and RONCHETTI · Robust Statistics, *Second Edition*
HUBERTY · Applied Discriminant Analysis, *Second Edition*
HUBERTY and OLEJNIK · Applied MANOVA and Discriminant Analysis, *Second Edition*
HUITEMA · The Analysis of Covariance and Alternatives: Statistical Methods for Experiments, Quasi-Experiments, and Single-Case Studies, *Second Edition*
HUNT and KENNEDY · Financial Derivatives in Theory and Practice, *Revised Edition*
HURD and MIAMEE · Periodically Correlated Random Sequences: Spectral Theory and Practice
HUSKOVA, BERAN, and DUPAC · Collected Works of Jaroslav Hajek— with Commentary
HUZURBAZAR · Flowgraph Models for Multistate Time-to-Event Data
JACKMAN · Bayesian Analysis for the Social Sciences
† JACKSON · A User's Guide to Principle Components
JOHN · Statistical Methods in Engineering and Quality Assurance
JOHNSON · Multivariate Statistical Simulation
JOHNSON and BALAKRISHNAN · Advances in the Theory and Practice of Statistics: A Volume in Honor of Samuel Kotz
JOHNSON, KEMP, and KOTZ · Univariate Discrete Distributions, *Third Edition*
JOHNSON and KOTZ (editors) · Leading Personalities in Statistical Sciences: From the Seventeenth Century to the Present
JOHNSON, KOTZ, and BALAKRISHNAN · Continuous Univariate Distributions, Volume 1, *Second Edition*
JOHNSON, KOTZ, and BALAKRISHNAN · Continuous Univariate Distributions, Volume 2, *Second Edition*
JOHNSON, KOTZ, and BALAKRISHNAN · Discrete Multivariate Distributions
JUDGE, GRIFFITHS, HILL, LÜTKEPOHL, and LEE · The Theory and Practice of Econometrics, *Second Edition*
JUREK and MASON · Operator-Limit Distributions in Probability Theory
KADANE · Bayesian Methods and Ethics in a Clinical Trial Design
KADANE AND SCHUM · A Probabilistic Analysis of the Sacco and Vanzetti Evidence
KALBFLEISCH and PRENTICE · The Statistical Analysis of Failure Time Data, *Second Edition*
KARIYA and KURATA · Generalized Least Squares
KASS and VOS · Geometrical Foundations of Asymptotic Inference
† KAUFMAN and ROUSSEEUW · Finding Groups in Data: An Introduction to Cluster Analysis
KEDEM and FOKIANOS · Regression Models for Time Series Analysis
KENDALL, BARDEN, CARNE, and LE · Shape and Shape Theory

*Now available in a lower priced paperback edition in the Wiley Classics Library.
†Now available in a lower priced paperback edition in the Wiley–Interscience Paperback Series.

KHURI · Advanced Calculus with Applications in Statistics, *Second Edition*
KHURI, MATHEW, and SINHA · Statistical Tests for Mixed Linear Models
* KISH · Statistical Design for Research
KLEIBER and KOTZ · Statistical Size Distributions in Economics and Actuarial Sciences
KLEMELÄ · Smoothing of Multivariate Data: Density Estimation and Visualization
KLUGMAN, PANJER, and WILLMOT · Loss Models: From Data to Decisions, *Third Edition*
KLUGMAN, PANJER, and WILLMOT · Loss Models: Further Topics
KLUGMAN, PANJER, and WILLMOT · Solutions Manual to Accompany Loss Models: From Data to Decisions, *Third Edition*
KOSKI and NOBLE · Bayesian Networks: An Introduction
KOTZ, BALAKRISHNAN, and JOHNSON · Continuous Multivariate Distributions, Volume 1, *Second Edition*
KOTZ and JOHNSON (editors) · Encyclopedia of Statistical Sciences: Volumes 1 to 9 with Index
KOTZ and JOHNSON (editors) · Encyclopedia of Statistical Sciences: Supplement Volume
KOTZ, READ, and BANKS (editors) · Encyclopedia of Statistical Sciences: Update Volume 1
KOTZ, READ, and BANKS (editors) · Encyclopedia of Statistical Sciences: Update Volume 2
KOWALSKI and TU · Modern Applied U-Statistics
KRISHNAMOORTHY and MATHEW · Statistical Tolerance Regions: Theory, Applications, and Computation
KROESE, TAIMRE, and BOTEV · Handbook of Monte Carlo Methods
KROONENBERG · Applied Multiway Data Analysis
KULINSKAYA, MORGENTHALER, and STAUDTE · Meta Analysis: A Guide to Calibrating and Combining Statistical Evidence
KULKARNI and HARMAN · An Elementary Introduction to Statistical Learning Theory
KUROWICKA and COOKE · Uncertainty Analysis with High Dimensional Dependence Modelling
KVAM and VIDAKOVIC · Nonparametric Statistics with Applications to Science and Engineering
LACHIN · Biostatistical Methods: The Assessment of Relative Risks, *Second Edition*
LAD · Operational Subjective Statistical Methods: A Mathematical, Philosophical, and Historical Introduction
LAMPERTI · Probability: A Survey of the Mathematical Theory, *Second Edition*
LAWLESS · Statistical Models and Methods for Lifetime Data, *Second Edition*
LAWSON · Statistical Methods in Spatial Epidemiology, *Second Edition*
LE · Applied Categorical Data Analysis, *Second Edition*
LE · Applied Survival Analysis
LEE · Structural Equation Modeling: A Bayesian Approach
LEE and WANG · Statistical Methods for Survival Data Analysis, *Fourth Edition*
LEPAGE and BILLARD · Exploring the Limits of Bootstrap
LESSLER and KALSBEEK · Nonsampling Errors in Surveys
LEYLAND and GOLDSTEIN (editors) · Multilevel Modelling of Health Statistics
LIAO · Statistical Group Comparison
LIN · Introductory Stochastic Analysis for Finance and Insurance
LITTLE and RUBIN · Statistical Analysis with Missing Data, *Second Edition*
LLOYD · The Statistical Analysis of Categorical Data
LOWEN and TEICH · Fractal-Based Point Processes
MAGNUS and NEUDECKER · Matrix Differential Calculus with Applications in Statistics and Econometrics, *Revised Edition*

*Now available in a lower priced paperback edition in the Wiley Classics Library.
†Now available in a lower priced paperback edition in the Wiley–Interscience Paperback Series.

MALLER and ZHOU · Survival Analysis with Long Term Survivors
MARCHETTE · Random Graphs for Statistical Pattern Recognition
MARDIA and JUPP · Directional Statistics
MARKOVICH · Nonparametric Analysis of Univariate Heavy-Tailed Data: Research and Practice
MARONNA, MARTIN and YOHAI · Robust Statistics: Theory and Methods
MASON, GUNST, and HESS · Statistical Design and Analysis of Experiments with Applications to Engineering and Science, *Second Edition*
McCULLOCH, SEARLE, and NEUHAUS · Generalized, Linear, and Mixed Models, *Second Edition*
McFADDEN · Management of Data in Clinical Trials, *Second Edition*
* McLACHLAN · Discriminant Analysis and Statistical Pattern Recognition
McLACHLAN, DO, and AMBROISE · Analyzing Microarray Gene Expression Data
McLACHLAN and KRISHNAN · The EM Algorithm and Extensions, *Second Edition*
McLACHLAN and PEEL · Finite Mixture Models
McNEIL · Epidemiological Research Methods
MEEKER and ESCOBAR · Statistical Methods for Reliability Data
MEERSCHAERT and SCHEFFLER · Limit Distributions for Sums of Independent Random Vectors: Heavy Tails in Theory and Practice
MENGERSEN, ROBERT, and TITTERINGTON · Mixtures: Estimation and Applications
MICKEY, DUNN, and CLARK · Applied Statistics: Analysis of Variance and Regression, *Third Edition*
* MILLER · Survival Analysis, *Second Edition*
MONTGOMERY, JENNINGS, and KULAHCI · Introduction to Time Series Analysis and Forecasting
MONTGOMERY, PECK, and VINING · Introduction to Linear Regression Analysis, *Fifth Edition*
MORGENTHALER and TUKEY · Configural Polysampling: A Route to Practical Robustness
MUIRHEAD · Aspects of Multivariate Statistical Theory
MULLER and STOYAN · Comparison Methods for Stochastic Models and Risks
MURTHY, XIE, and JIANG · Weibull Models
MYERS, MONTGOMERY, and ANDERSON-COOK · Response Surface Methodology: Process and Product Optimization Using Designed Experiments, *Third Edition*
MYERS, MONTGOMERY, VINING, and ROBINSON · Generalized Linear Models. With Applications in Engineering and the Sciences, *Second Edition*
NATVIG · Multistate Systems Reliability Theory With Applications
† NELSON · Accelerated Testing, Statistical Models, Test Plans, and Data Analyses
† NELSON · Applied Life Data Analysis
NEWMAN · Biostatistical Methods in Epidemiology
NG, TAIN, and TANG · Dirichlet Theory: Theory, Methods and Applications
OKABE, BOOTS, SUGIHARA, and CHIU · Spatial Tesselations: Concepts and Applications of Voronoi Diagrams, *Second Edition*
OLIVER and SMITH · Influence Diagrams, Belief Nets and Decision Analysis
PALTA · Quantitative Methods in Population Health: Extensions of Ordinary Regressions
PANJER · Operational Risk: Modeling and Analytics
PANKRATZ · Forecasting with Dynamic Regression Models
PANKRATZ · Forecasting with Univariate Box-Jenkins Models: Concepts and Cases
PARDOUX · Markov Processes and Applications: Algorithms, Networks, Genome and Finance
PARMIGIANI and INOUE · Decision Theory: Principles and Approaches
* PARZEN · Modern Probability Theory and Its Applications
PEÑA, TIAO, and TSAY · A Course in Time Series Analysis

*Now available in a lower priced paperback edition in the Wiley Classics Library.
†Now available in a lower priced paperback edition in the Wiley–Interscience Paperback Series.

PESARIN and SALMASO · Permutation Tests for Complex Data: Applications and Software
PIANTADOSI · Clinical Trials: A Methodologic Perspective, *Second Edition*
POURAHMADI · Foundations of Time Series Analysis and Prediction Theory
POURAHMADI · High-Dimensional Covariance Estimation
POWELL · Approximate Dynamic Programming: Solving the Curses of Dimensionality, *Second Edition*
POWELL and RYZHOV · Optimal Learning
PRESS · Subjective and Objective Bayesian Statistics, *Second Edition*
PRESS and TANUR · The Subjectivity of Scientists and the Bayesian Approach
PURI, VILAPLANA, and WERTZ · New Perspectives in Theoretical and Applied Statistics
† PUTERMAN · Markov Decision Processes: Discrete Stochastic Dynamic Programming
QIU · Image Processing and Jump Regression Analysis
* RAO · Linear Statistical Inference and Its Applications, *Second Edition*
RAO · Statistical Inference for Fractional Diffusion Processes
RAUSAND and HØYLAND · System Reliability Theory: Models, Statistical Methods, and Applications, *Second Edition*
RAYNER, THAS, and BEST · Smooth Tests of Goodnes of Fit: Using R, *Second Edition*
RENCHER and SCHAALJE · Linear Models in Statistics, *Second Edition*
RENCHER and CHRISTENSEN · Methods of Multivariate Analysis, *Third Edition*
RENCHER · Multivariate Statistical Inference with Applications
RIGDON and BASU · Statistical Methods for the Reliability of Repairable Systems
* RIPLEY · Spatial Statistics
* RIPLEY · Stochastic Simulation
ROHATGI and SALEH · An Introduction to Probability and Statistics, *Second Edition*
ROLSKI, SCHMIDLI, SCHMIDT, and TEUGELS · Stochastic Processes for Insurance and Finance
ROSENBERGER and LACHIN · Randomization in Clinical Trials: Theory and Practice
ROSSI, ALLENBY, and McCULLOCH · Bayesian Statistics and Marketing
† ROUSSEEUW and LEROY · Robust Regression and Outlier Detection
ROYSTON and SAUERBREI · Multivariate Model Building: A Pragmatic Approach to Regression Analysis Based on Fractional Polynomials for Modeling Continuous Variables
* RUBIN · Multiple Imputation for Nonresponse in Surveys
RUBINSTEIN and KROESE · Simulation and the Monte Carlo Method, *Second Edition*
RUBINSTEIN and MELAMED · Modern Simulation and Modeling
RUBINSTEIN, RIDDER, and VAISMAN · Fast Sequential Monte Carlo Methods for Counting and Optimization
RYAN · Modern Engineering Statistics
RYAN · Modern Experimental Design
RYAN · Modern Regression Methods, *Second Edition*
RYAN · Sample Size Determination and Power
RYAN · Statistical Methods for Quality Improvement, *Third Edition*
SALEH · Theory of Preliminary Test and Stein-Type Estimation with Applications
SALTELLI, CHAN, and SCOTT (editors) · Sensitivity Analysis
SCHERER · Batch Effects and Noise in Microarray Experiments: Sources and Solutions
* SCHEFFE · The Analysis of Variance
SCHIMEK · Smoothing and Regression: Approaches, Computation, and Application
SCHOTT · Matrix Analysis for Statistics, *Second Edition*
SCHOUTENS · Levy Processes in Finance: Pricing Financial Derivatives
SCOTT · Multivariate Density Estimation: Theory, Practice, and Visualization
* SEARLE · Linear Models
† SEARLE · Linear Models for Unbalanced Data

*Now available in a lower priced paperback edition in the Wiley Classics Library.
†Now available in a lower priced paperback edition in the Wiley–Interscience Paperback Series.

† SEARLE · Matrix Algebra Useful for Statistics
† SEARLE, CASELLA, and McCULLOCH · Variance Components
SEARLE and WILLETT · Matrix Algebra for Applied Economics
SEBER · A Matrix Handbook For Statisticians
† SEBER · Multivariate Observations
SEBER and LEE · Linear Regression Analysis, *Second Edition*
† SEBER and WILD · Nonlinear Regression
SENNOTT · Stochastic Dynamic Programming and the Control of Queueing Systems
* SERFLING · Approximation Theorems of Mathematical Statistics
SHAFER and VOVK · Probability and Finance: It's Only a Game!
SHERMAN · Spatial Statistics and Spatio-Temporal Data: Covariance Functions and Directional Properties
SILVAPULLE and SEN · Constrained Statistical Inference: Inequality, Order, and Shape Restrictions
SINGPURWALLA · Reliability and Risk: A Bayesian Perspective
SMALL and McLEISH · Hilbert Space Methods in Probability and Statistical Inference
SRIVASTAVA · Methods of Multivariate Statistics
STAPLETON · Linear Statistical Models, *Second Edition*
STAPLETON · Models for Probability and Statistical Inference: Theory and Applications
STAUDTE and SHEATHER · Robust Estimation and Testing
STOYAN · Counterexamples in Probability, *Second Edition*
STOYAN, KENDALL, and MECKE · Stochastic Geometry and Its Applications, *Second Edition*
STOYAN and STOYAN · Fractals, Random Shapes and Point Fields: Methods of Geometrical Statistics
STREET and BURGESS · The Construction of Optimal Stated Choice Experiments: Theory and Methods
STYAN · The Collected Papers of T. W. Anderson: 1943–1985
SUTTON, ABRAMS, JONES, SHELDON, and SONG · Methods for Meta-Analysis in Medical Research
TAKEZAWA · Introduction to Nonparametric Regression
TAMHANE · Statistical Analysis of Designed Experiments: Theory and Applications
TANAKA · Time Series Analysis: Nonstationary and Noninvertible Distribution Theory
THOMPSON · Empirical Model Building: Data, Models, and Reality, *Second Edition*
THOMPSON · Sampling, *Third Edition*
THOMPSON · Simulation: A Modeler's Approach
THOMPSON and SEBER · Adaptive Sampling
THOMPSON, WILLIAMS, and FINDLAY · Models for Investors in Real World Markets
TIERNEY · LISP-STAT: An Object-Oriented Environment for Statistical Computing and Dynamic Graphics
TSAY · Analysis of Financial Time Series, *Third Edition*
TSAY · An Introduction to Analysis of Financial Data with R
UPTON and FINGLETON · Spatial Data Analysis by Example, Volume II: Categorical and Directional Data
† VAN BELLE · Statistical Rules of Thumb, *Second Edition*
VAN BELLE, FISHER, HEAGERTY, and LUMLEY · Biostatistics: A Methodology for the Health Sciences, *Second Edition*
VESTRUP · The Theory of Measures and Integration
VIDAKOVIC · Statistical Modeling by Wavelets
VIERTL · Statistical Methods for Fuzzy Data
VINOD and REAGLE · Preparing for the Worst: Incorporating Downside Risk in Stock Market Investments

*Now available in a lower priced paperback edition in the Wiley Classics Library.
†Now available in a lower priced paperback edition in the Wiley–Interscience Paperback Series.

WALLER and GOTWAY · Applied Spatial Statistics for Public Health Data
WEISBERG · Applied Linear Regression, *Third Edition*
WEISBERG · Bias and Causation: Models and Judgment for Valid Comparisons
WELSH · Aspects of Statistical Inference
WESTFALL and YOUNG · Resampling-Based Multiple Testing: Examples and Methods for *p*-Value Adjustment
* WHITTAKER · Graphical Models in Applied Multivariate Statistics
WINKER · Optimization Heuristics in Economics: Applications of Threshold Accepting
WOODWORTH · Biostatistics: A Bayesian Introduction
WOOLSON and CLARKE · Statistical Methods for the Analysis of Biomedical Data, *Second Edition*
WU and HAMADA · Experiments: Planning, Analysis, and Parameter Design Optimization, *Second Edition*
WU and ZHANG · Nonparametric Regression Methods for Longitudinal Data Analysis
YIN · Clinical Trial Design: Bayesian and Frequentist Adaptive Methods
YOUNG, VALERO-MORA, and FRIENDLY · Visual Statistics: Seeing Data with Dynamic Interactive Graphics
ZACKS · Stage-Wise Adaptive Designs
* ZELLNER · An Introduction to Bayesian Inference in Econometrics
ZELTERMAN · Discrete Distributions—Applications in the Health Sciences
ZHOU, OBUCHOWSKI, and McCLISH · Statistical Methods in Diagnostic Medicine, *Second Edition*

*Now available in a lower priced paperback edition in the Wiley Classics Library.
†Now available in a lower priced paperback edition in the Wiley–Interscience Paperback Series.